HIGH G FLIGHT

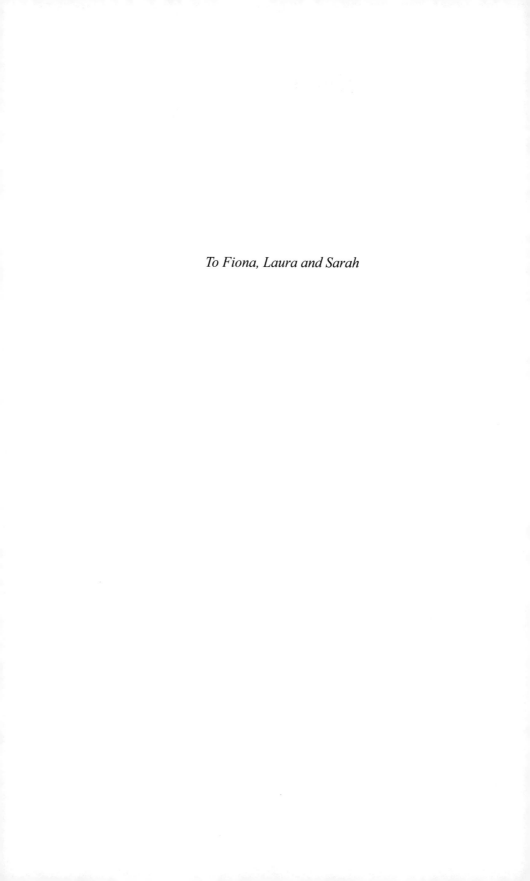

To Fiona, Laura and Sarah

High G Flight
Physiological Effects and Countermeasures

DAVID G. NEWMAN
MB, BS, DAvMed, MBA, PhD, FRAeS, FAsMA, FACAsM, FAICD, FAIM
Monash University, Australia

ASHGATE

Published by
Ashgate Publishing Limited
Wey Court East
Union Road
Farnham
Surrey, GU9 7PT
England

Ashgate Publishing Company
110 Cherry Street
Suite 3-1
Burlington, VT 05401-3818
USA

www.ashgate.com

British Library Cataloguing in Publication Data
A catalogue record for this book is available from the British Library

The Library of Congress has cataloged the printed edition as follows:
Newman, David G. (David Glen), 1965- author.
  High G flight : physiological effects and countermeasures / by David G. Newman.
     pages cm
  Includes bibliographical references and index.
  ISBN 978-1-4724-1457-1 (hardback) -- ISBN 978-1-4724-1458-8 (ebook) -- ISBN 978-1-4724-1459-5 (epub) 1. Gravity--Physiological effect. 2. Gravity--Physiological effect--Protection. 3. Acceleration (Physiology)--Protection. 4. Air pilots--Health and hygiene. 5. Flight--Physiological aspects. I. Title.
  QP82.2.G7N48 2015
  571.4'35--dc23

2014044652

ISBN 9781472414571 (hbk)
ISBN 9781472414588 (ebk – PDF)
ISBN 9781472414595 (ebk – ePUB)

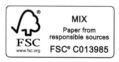

Printed in the United Kingdom by Henry Ling Limited, at the Dorset Press, Dorchester, DT1 1HD

Contents

List of Figures	*xi*
Foreword by Lieutenant General (Dr) Thomas W. Travis	*xiii*
Preface	*xv*
Acknowledgements	*xvii*
List of Abbreviations	*xix*

PART I: MECHANICS OF G

1	**The Physics of Gravity**	**3**
	Mechanics	3
	Gravity	4
	What is Gravity?	4
	Newton's Universal Law of Gravitation	5
	Newton's Laws of Motion	7
	Acceleration Due to Motion	8
	The Mechanics of Circular Motion	9
	Acceleration Due to Gravity	12
	Gravity and Weight	13
	Einstein's Contribution	14
	Kepler and Newton	15
	Conclusion	17
2	**High G Flight**	**19**
	Acceleration Nomenclature	19
	Magnitude	19
	Direction	20
	Acceleration in the Flight Environment	21
	Generating G in Flight	22
	Physiological Consequences of High G Exposure	23
	+Gx Acceleration	24
	+Gy Acceleration	24
	+Gz Acceleration	24

Flight Operations Involving High G   26
  Military Flight Operations   26
  Civilian Aerobatic Flight   30
  Commercial Spaceflight Operations   33
Conclusion   35

PART II: PHYSIOLOGY OF G

3   The Cardiovascular System at +1 Gz   **39**
Haemodynamic Relationships   39
Hydrostatic Pressure (HP)   40
  Hydrostatic Indifference Point   41
Upright Posture   42
  Hydrostatic Pressure and the Giraffe   43
Countermeasures to Orthostasis   45
  Venous Valves   45
  Venous Volume-Pressure Relationship   45
  Microcirculatory Changes   45
  The Muscle Pump   46
  The Respiratory Pump   46
The Baroreflexes   46
  Anatomical Structure of the Baroreflexes   47
  Function of the Baroreflexes   49
  Heart Rate Effects   52
  Blood Pressure Effects   52
  Regulation of Blood Pressure   53
The Role of the Vestibular System   54
Conclusion   55

4   The Cardiovascular System at High Gz   **57**
Effects of Acceleration on the Circulation   57
Effect of Acceleration on Vision   60
  Grey-out   60
  Black-out   60
Almost Loss of Consciousness (A-LOC)   61
  Prevalence of A-LOC   63
G-Induced Loss of Consciousness (G-LOC)   63
  Historical Aspects of G-LOC   63
  Characteristics of a G-LOC Episode   65
  Prevalence of G-LOC   68

The Effect of Rate of Change of +Gz   68
A Word on Negative Gz   70
Conclusion   72

5   Respiratory Effects of G   **73**
The Respiratory System at +1 Gz   73
Respiratory Effects of High Gz Exposure   76
Acceleration Atelectasis   78
Respiratory Effects of High Gx Exposure   79
Respiratory Effects of High Gy Exposure   81
Conclusion   81

6   Musculoskeletal Effects of G   **83**
+Gz-Induced Neck Injuries   83
Prevalence   83
Risk Factors   84
Types of Injury   88
Operational Impact   89
Preventive Measures   90
Spine Injuries   94
Prevalence   94
Risk Factors   95
Types of Injury   95
Preventive Measures   96
Conclusion   96

7   Miscellaneous Clinical Effects of G   **97**
Cardiac Effects   97
Arrhythmias   97
Morphologic Changes   98
Cognitive Changes   100
Vestibular Effects   101
Auditory Function   103
Visual Function   104
Endocrine and Biochemical Changes   105
Trauma   106
Vascular Effects   106
Respiratory System   107
Abdominal Trauma   107
Orthopaedic Issues   108
Skin Effects   108
Conclusion   109

PART III: TOLERANCE AND ADAPTATION

8   Tolerance to High G   **113**
      Defining and Measuring G Tolerance   113
      G-Time Tolerance Curve   115
      Individual Factors Affecting G Tolerance   118
        Individual Variation   118
        Anthropometry and Gender   118
        Blood Volume Changes   119
        Hypoxia   119
        Caffeine   119
        Fatigue   120
        Physical Conditioning   120
        Miscellaneous Factors   124
      Flight-Related Factors Affecting G Tolerance   125
        Seat-Back Angle   125
        The Flight Manoeuvre   126
        Frequency of Exposure   126
        The Push–Pull Effect   127
        Centrifuge Training   128
      Conclusion   129

9   Cardiovascular Adaptation to Acceleration   **131**
      Is Adaptation an Advantage?   131
      Adaptation to Microgravity   133
      Investigative Techniques   135
        Head-Up Tilt (HUT)   136
        Lower-Body Negative Pressure   137
        Standing   137
        The Squat–Stand Test   138
      Adaptation of the Baroreflexes   138
        The Influence of Exercise on Baroreflex Function   140
      Cardiovascular Adaptation to G   141
        Animal Studies   141
        +Gz Training Studies in Humans   142
      Future Research Directions   148
      Conclusion   149

PART IV: COUNTERMEASURES

10   The Anti-G Straining Manoeuvre   **153**
      The Physiological Basis of the Anti-G Straining
      Manoeuvre (AGSM)   153

	Muscle Tensing	154
	Expiratory Strain	154
	Timing of the Breathing Cycle	155
	Types of AGSM	157
	Advantages	159
	Disadvantages	160
	Conclusion	161
11	**The G-Suit**	**163**
	History of the G-Suit	163
	Mode of Operation	164
	Advantages	167
	Disadvantages	169
	Advanced G-Suit Designs	169
	Anti-G Valve (AGV) Developments	172
	Conclusion	172
12	**Positive Pressure Breathing for G Protection**	**173**
	Physiology of Positive Pressure Breathing for G Protection (PBG)	173
	Pressure Schedule	175
	The Role of the G-Suit	176
	Pressure Syncope	176
	Efficient Pressure Transmission	176
	PBG and AGSM in Combination	177
	The Role of Chest Counterpressure	178
	Is Counterpressure Necessary?	179
	The Pressure Regulator	180
	Pressure Variations	181
	Advantages of Positive Pressure Breathing for G Protection (PBG)	182
	Increased +Gz Tolerance	183
	Reported Problems with Positive Pressure Breathing for G Protection (PBG)	183
	Adverse Pressure Problems	184
	Mask Leakage	184
	Arm Pain	184
	Acceleration Atelectasis	186
	Increased Thermal Burden	187
	Conclusion	187
References		*189*
Index		*233*

List of Figures

1.1	A spacecraft in orbit	9
1.2	The geometry of circular motion	10
1.3	The geometry of an ellipse	16

2.1	Inertial vectors used to describe the direction of G	21
2.2	An aircraft in turning flight	23
2.3	A typical air combat manoeuvre – rolling scissors	27
2.4	Gz-time plot in an F/A-18 during air combat manoeuvring (ACM)	28
2.5	Gz-time plot in an F/A-18 for a single 1 v 1 air combat manoeuvring (ACM) engagement	28
2.6	Aresti diagrams for aerobatic flight manoeuvres	32

3.1	Upright posture and blood pressure (BP) changes	41
3.2	Arterial blood pressure (BP) response to upright postural change	49
3.3	The baroreflex in operation – blood pressure (BP) decrease	50
3.4	The baroreflex in operation – blood pressure (BP) increase	51

4.1	Blood pressure (BP) changes with high +Gz exposure	58
4.2	Rushmer's human–giraffe comparison	59
4.3	The outside loop as an example of a –Gz flight manoeuvre	71

| 5.1 | Lung volumes and capacities under normal resting conditions | 74 |
| 5.2 | Lung volumes and capacities under +5 Gz conditions | 77 |

| 6.1 | The 'Check 6' head position during air combat manoeuvring (ACM) | 86 |

8.1	The simulated air combat manoeuvring (SACM) centrifuge profile	114
8.2	The Stoll G-time tolerance curve	116
8.3	The effect of G onset rates on G tolerance	116
8.4	A manoeuvre resulting in the push–pull effect (PPE)	128

9.1	The effect of cardiovascular adaptation on the G-time tolerance curve	132
9.2	Cardiovascular responses to head-up tilt (HUT), G-adapted pilots vs non-pilots	145
9.3	Longitudinal training effect of +Gz exposure on cardiovascular responses to head-up tilt (HUT)	146

10.1 Anti-G straining manoeuvre (AGSM) effect on
      arterial blood pressure (BP)   156

11.1 Standard G-suit   165

12.1 Positive pressure breathing for G protection (PBG)
      pressure schedule   175
12.2 Chest counterpressure garment (CCPG)   179
12.3 Typical positive pressure breathing for G protection (PBG)
      ensemble as worn by a fast jet pilot   182

Foreword

When Dr Newman asked me to pen the Foreword to this book I jumped at the chance. The topic is one I have personally addressed for more than two decades, doing both bench-level design work on aircrew G-protective equipment, and sweating as a centrifuge subject to man-rate resulting prototypes. I know G well, having been mission qualified in the F-4, the F-15, the F-16, and, as an RAF exchange officer, the RAF Hawk, doing high-G test work on prototype aircrew equipment, gear which later evolved into pilot flight equipment for the F-22, legacy USAF fighters (to include the F-15 and F-16), and now the Typhoon and the F-35.

This background has brought a professional association with many international leaders in aviation medicine, physiology and human performance. One of many notable examples is the late Dr John Ernsting, whom I knew from my time at Brooks AFB, and then as an exchange officer with the RAF at Farnborough. Of course, these professional relationships were enriched and enhanced by groups such as the NATO Aeromedical Working Group, which I was privileged to chair for several years, and through the five-nation Air Standardization Coordinating Committee (ASCC), now the Air and Space Interoperability Council (ASIC). In fact, it was at an annual meeting of this body that I first met Dr Newman. In the years that ensued we have followed each other's careers and work, David staying very much involved academically and in research, while my military duties drew me into command and executive responsibilities. That is why being asked to review and write a Foreword for this important book is a real pleasure! And this opportunity allows me to share some perspectives I have learned through my own work, as well as the work of others, as an experienced high-performance pilot who happens to also be board-certified as an aerospace medicine physician.

In the early days of agile high-G flight, many nations lost aircraft and crew to G-induced loss of consciousness, or G-LOC. As a fighter pilot and physician, I was frequently tapped to investigate or consult on fatal G-LOC mishaps, and I personally felt the impact of these tragedies. Searching for cures as well as causes, I soon became aware of the protective potential of pressure-breathing for G (PBG) and the beneficial effects of a full-coverage anti-G suit. These new garments provided more complete coverage and better circulatory support than the 1940s vintage five-bladder suit. In 1988, compelled by a particularly bad year of GLOC losses, the USAF opted to field these technologies sequentially rather than develop an integrated system. PBG went operational before the full-coverage anti-G suit, and many questioned its effectiveness in that it was only a partial solution. This was particularly true in upright seats, such as the F-15.

In a reclined seat with more elevated lower limbs, such as the F-16, return of blood flow was better and PBG seemed to work better because the pump (the heart) remained well primed to push blood to the eyes and brain under high-acceleration forces. The F-22 later brought a full-coverage suit and PBG together for the first time and demonstrated a synergy so effective that full-coverage G-suits have since been mandated for all PBG-equipped aircraft.

So effective is the combination of these measures that many pilots can reach +9 Gz in an almost relaxed state (yours truly included). And while this certainly does support safety of flight and reduce the chances of a GLOC, many of us became more and more convinced that the true value of this technology was performance enhancement. A fully occupied pilot (mentally and physically) shouldn't have to worry about the timing or effectiveness of an anti-G straining manoeuvre. The aircrew should worry about achieving mission objectives and defeating the adversary, or at least surviving to fight another day. The physiologic support provided by the complete anti-G ensemble (PBG and full-coverage trousers) enhances performance and decreases the need to pay attention to something unrelated to the task at hand. And that is why many of us for so many years have laboured to understand the physiology involved, develop the technology and then obtain warfighter support for the funding and fielding of such technology. By the way, the same garments can support pressure breathing for altitude (PBA), as high as 60–65,000 feet, heights readily and routinely attainable by our newest generation of fighter aircraft – but that is another story.

Clearly this Foreword is from the perspective of a military Airman regarding the application of the physiology explained in Dr Newman's book, and others before it. It is also worth stating that the work must continue, because every time the operational community decides it knows all it needs to know to crack a problem such as countering acceleration forces, new challenges arise. If this is the first text you have ever read on the topic, you will find it very enlightening. If you have been in the field for some or many years, I think you will agree this is a very useful updated treatment of a persistent physiological issue for those who fly. I hope you find this topic as interesting and professionally fulfilling as I have for the last 25 years.

Lieutenant General (Dr) Thomas W. Travis,
USAF, MC, CFS

Preface

In writing this book, my aim was to bring together into a single volume the considerable body of scientific literature dealing with human exposure to the high +Gz environment. Somewhat surprisingly, perhaps, this has never been done before. Humans exist in a gravity-dependent environment. In the world of high-performance military fast jets and civilian competition aerobatic aircraft, humans are now exposed to an increasingly complicated acceleration environment. Much is known about the human performance and physiological limitations that such exposure creates in humans. The intent of this book is to illustrate this depth of knowledge, but also to highlight what remains to be discovered.

The purpose of this book is not to give an exhaustive treatment of human physiology. There are other books that do this very well. Much of that knowledge is assumed in this book, with the emphasis here being on how the normal physiological systems are affected by and respond to exposure to the high G environment, and what can be done to protect the human from the adverse consequences of this exposure.

My professional interest in the high G environment spans several decades. As an aviation medicine specialist and flight surgeon in the Royal Australian Air Force (RAAF), my experience involved support of tactical fighter operations, as well as conducting aviation medicine training for aircrew, particularly in terms of high G physiology. I undertook a PhD while in the RAAF, based on my personal flying experiences where G seemed to be easier to deal with as a result of regular exposure. As a result, my research interests were centred on cardiovascular adaptation to repetitive high +Gz exposure, but I was also interested in G tolerance as well as G-induced neck injuries (after personally sustaining one!).

My RAAF service allowed me to fly regularly in high-performance aircraft such as the Macchi MB326H, the Hawk, and the F/A-18Hornet, as well as a Harrier T10 while on exchange in the UK with the RAF. As a pilot, I have flown aerobatics and high G manoeuvres in a wide variety of aircraft, from light trainers right through to fast jets, from -3 Gz to +9 Gz. I have also been involved in research, development, testing and man-rating of human centrifuges. This wide range of exposure to G has allowed me to personally experience many of the issues covered in this book, from visual symptoms to cardiac arrhythmias, from vestibular disturbance to loss of consciousness, among others.

This book is in four parts. The first part deals with the mechanics, physics and mathematics of G, as well as how G is generated in flight, how it is calculated and given direction. This part also deals with the different environments where high G in aviation is applicable: military operations, civilian aerobatics and spaceflight operations. Part II explores the physiological and clinical implications of high G exposure. Part III deals with the various factors that determine an individual's G tolerance, as well as the emerging body of scientific knowledge concerning cardiovascular adaptation to the high G environment. Finally, Part IV considers the various countermeasures that have been developed, mainly for military applications, to increase a person's ability to tolerate exposure to the high G environment.

I have tried to produce a book as comprehensive as possible, while at the same time being as readable as possible. That was no easy task, and some compromise was inevitable. As a result, some readers may find certain topics not covered as thoroughly as they might like, or not included at all. I have specifically limited the book to the manoeuvring environment of aviation. Any errors or omissions, if there are any, are entirely mine.

I was very conscious during the writing of this book that a significant number of talented, dedicated and brilliant people had spent a lot of time and effort seeking to understand the consequences of human exposure to high G force. Their combined work has helped make the high G environment safer for all those who operate within it. It is my hope that my efforts in consolidating this century of research work into this book will help your understanding of the complexities of the high G environment and the physiological challenges associated with it. If that is the case, then I will be very satisfied.

Dr David G. Newman,
Melbourne, Australia

Acknowledgements

I would like to thank the many people who have helped make this book possible. Firstly, I am extremely grateful to all the fast jet pilots that participated in many of the experiments I conducted into the cardiovascular effects of high G exposure on human physiology. I also would like to thank them for all the many hours of flight time in fast jets that they spent with me, exploring the consequences of high G force on a first-hand basis.

I would like to particularly thank Lieutenant General Thomas W. Travis, United States Air Force, for writing the Foreword to this book. I have known Tom for many years, and his experience as a military flight surgeon, fast jet pilot and G researcher made him an ideal and obvious choice for writing the Foreword. He knows the challenges of the high +Gz world very well. His generosity in so readily agreeing to write the Foreword, given his extremely busy schedule, is something I am very grateful for. Tom, you are a true gentleman. A special thank you to Professor Robin Callister for being a great supervisor during my PhD research into the effects on cardiovascular physiology of high +Gz exposure. Robin remains a good friend, academic mentor and professional colleague, and I owe her a great debt of thanks.

Finally, I would like to thank my wonderful family. Their love, support, understanding and encouragement over many years have made my work in high G research and this book possible. Saying thank you here does not really seem enough! My amazing wife Fiona has listened to me talk about G for over 25 years. Her understanding, patience and support know no bounds, and for that I am truly thankful. She is a very special woman. Thanks also to my two talented daughters, Laura (who did many of the figures in the book) and Sarah. I am truly lucky to have such a fantastic family. They are my greatest source of inspiration, and this book is dedicated to them.

List of Abbreviations

ACM	Air Combat Manoeuvring
ACTH	Adrenocorticotropic Hormone
ADH	Anti-Diuretic Hormone
AEA	Aircrew Equipment Assembly
AGS	Anti-gravity Suit
AGSM	Anti-G Straining Manoeuvre
AGV	Anti-G Valve
A-LOC	Almost Loss of Consciousness
AOA	Angle of Attack
ASCC	Air Standardization Coordinating Committee
ASIC	Air and Space Interoperability Council
ATAGS	Advanced Technology Anti-G Suit
ATSB	Australian Transport Safety Bureau
BFM	Basic Fighter Manoeuvres
BP	Blood Pressure
BPPV	Benign Paroxysmal Positional Vertigo
CCPG	Chest Counterpressure Garment
CD	Cardiovascular Deconditioning
CF	Canadian Forces
CID	Cardiovascular Index of Deconditioning
CLL	Central Light Loss
CO	Cardiac Output
COMBAT EDGE	Combined Advanced Technology Enhanced Design Anti-G Ensemble
DFS	Dynamic Flight Simulation
DP	Diastolic Pressure
ECGS	Extended Coverage G-Suit
EDV	End-Diastolic Volume
EMG	Electromyography
ERV	Expiratory Reserve Volume
FAI	Federation Aeronautique International
FCAGT	Full Coverage Anti-G Trouser
FRC	Functional Residual Capacity
FVP	Forearm Venous Pressure
FVR	Forearm Vascular Resistance
g	Acceleration due to Earth's Gravity
G	Multiples of g; Gravitational constant

GIVD	G-Induced Vestibular Dysfunction
G-LOC	G-induced Loss of Consciousness
GOR	Gradual Onset Run
HDNF	Head-Down Neck Flexion
HIP	Hydrostatic Indifference Point
HMD	Helmet-Mounted Display
HOTAS	Hands On Throttle And Stick
HP	Hydrostatic Pressure
HR	Heart Rate
HUT	Head-Up Tilt
IC	Inspiratory Capacity
IRV	Inspiratory Reserve Volume
JHMCS	Joint Helmet Mounted Cueing System
LBNP	Lower Body Negative Pressure
LVEDV	Left Ventricular End Diastolic Volume
MAP	Mean Arterial Pressure
MAST	Military Anti Shock Trousers
MFD	Multi-Function Display
mmHg	Millimetres of mercury
MRI	Magnetic Resonance Imaging
MSA	Multiple System Atrophy
MSDRS	Maintenance Status Display and Recording System
NATO	North Atlantic Treaty Organisation
NIRS	Near-Infrared Spectroscopy
NTS	Nucleus of the Tractus Solitarius
NVG	Night Vision Goggles
PASG	Pneumatic Anti Shock Garment
PBG	Positive Pressure Breathing for G Protection
PFD	Primary Flight Display
PLL	Peripheral Light Loss
PP	Pulse Pressure
PPE	Push-Pull Effect
PVC	Premature Ventricular Contraction
RAAF	Royal Australian Air Force
RAF	Royal Air Force
ROR	Rapid Onset Run
RSAGV	Rate Sensitive Anti-G Valve
RV	Residual Volume
SA	Situational Awareness
SACM	Simulated Air Combat Manoeuvring profile.
SHR	Spontaneously Hypertensive Rat
SP	Systolic Pressure
SPECT	Single Photon Emission Computed Tomography
SST	Squat–Stand Test

STANAG	NATO Standardisation Agreement
SV	Stroke Volume
SVPB	Supraventricular Premature Beats
TACM	Tactical Air Combat Manoeuvring profile
TLC	Total Lung Capacity
TPR	Total Peripheral Resistance
TV	Tidal Volume
TVC	Thrust Vectoring Control
USAF	United States Air Force
USN	United States Navy
VC	Vital Capacity
VR	Venous Return
VSR	Vestibulosympathetic Reflex

PART I
Mechanics of G

Chapter 1
The Physics of Gravity

Humans exist in a gravity-dependent environment. In order to fully appreciate the physiological consequences of human exposure to high-gravitational forces, it is useful first to have a thorough understanding of what is meant by the terms gravity and acceleration, since they will be used frequently throughout this book. This chapter will examine the mathematics and physics underlying these important terms.

Mechanics

Initially, it is helpful to define some important terms in mechanics that will be used repeatedly throughout this book. Speed is the term used to denote a change in distance with respect to time. It is a scalar quantity, reflecting magnitude only. When both the magnitude and direction of change in distance with time are considered, the term velocity is used rather than speed. Velocity is a vector quantity. When velocity experiences a rate of change with respect to time, acceleration is said to have occurred. It can also be thought of as the second derivative of distance with respect to time. Acceleration is of course also a vector quantity, having both magnitude and direction. The magnitude of acceleration, and the direction in which it is applied, will be examined in more detail in Chapter 2.

The terms speed, velocity, acceleration and force (to be discussed later with Newton's Laws of Motion) are straightforward terms. Unfortunately, in many cases they are used interchangeably and in the wrong technical sense. This is worth briefly discussing, for the sake of clarity. Speed and velocity are often used to represent the same thing, which as has been seen above, is not technically correct. One is a scalar quantity, the other is a vector. In many cases, speed is used when velocity might be the more correct term. In the lexicon of acceleration physiology, the terms force and acceleration are also very often used interchangeably. This can create some confusion on the part of readers, particularly those new to the field. The situation is made worse when the terms G force and G acceleration are used on an interchangeable basis. Ultimately, it does not matter which term is used, as long as there is some consistency. As readers will see in later sections of this chapter, the interchangeable use of force and acceleration is a by-product of one of Newton's Laws of Motion – force and acceleration are proportional to each other. In this book, the term G force will be used to represent the force applied to a body undergoing an acceleration. This will become clearer as this chapter develops.

Gravity

While acceleration is a relatively straightforward notion, gravity is a rather more nebulous concept. While gravity is understood on an intuitive level, little is known of its actual nature. The question of just what exactly gravity is has puzzled physicists for many years (Freedman and van Nieuwenhuizen, 1978; Narlikar, 1996; Will, 1974), and remains the subject of much ongoing work (a detailed analysis of which is well beyond the scope of this book).

What is Gravity?

Current thinking, based initially on the work of the theoretical physicist Albert Einstein (1879–1955), is that gravity is a wave-form. Einstein's General Relativity Theory predicts the existence of gravitational waves, which are considered to be ripples in (or warping of) the space–time continuum produced by violent events such as exploding stars (Wald, 1984). The Theory describes the observed gravitational attraction between such masses as being a result of warping of space and time by those very masses. As an example, Einstein's General Relativity Theory underpins the modern understanding of black holes, an astronomic phenomenon where gravitational attraction is so strong that nothing can escape from them, not even light (Gallo and Marolf, 2009; Narlikar, 1996; Wald, 1984).

Gravitational waves have so far never been detected, but several experiments are currently underway around the world, involving the use of ground-based and space-based interferometers, as well as pulsar timing arrays (based at radiotelescope facilities such as that in Parkes, New South Wales, Australia). One of the earliest detection devices was the so-called Weber bar, developed by Joseph Weber (1919–2000). This bar, made of solid aluminium, was isolated from external vibrations. While Weber claimed to have detected gravitational waves with his device in the 1960s, repeat experiments by other researchers have failed to confirm his findings, and his claim has largely been discredited (Bartusiak, 2000). Modern forms of the Weber bar are in use for the purposes of detecting gravitational waves. These include large pieces of pure metals such as niobium which are supercooled to near absolute zero. The passage of gravitational waves through this metal sets up a series of detectable vibrations within the metal's atoms. These efforts at detecting gravitational waves are extraordinarily difficult and complex, and have to date produced no peer-reviewed, generally accepted, concrete and empirical evidence.

The difficulty with such experiments is that gravitational waves are inherently difficult to detect. They are thought to be rare, occurring anywhere from once a decade to once a century. In addition, their physical properties make them particularly problematic. Their wavelength is thought to be very long (about 300 km), their amplitude is very small (millions of times smaller than the diameter of an atom) and their speed of travel is on an astronomical scale (they could pass through the Earth in 0.04 seconds).

According to the latest thinking in Quantum Field Theory, it is speculated that the gravitational force is mediated by the hypothetical elementary particle the 'graviton', similar to the role of the photon in electromagnetism (Dyson, 2013; Trippe, 2013; Vayenas and Souentie, 2012; Will, 1998). Work to detect both gravitational waves and the existence of gravitons remains ongoing.

Newton's Universal Law of Gravitation

What is clear, however, is that gravity influences all aspects of life on Earth, as all biological, mechanical and physical processes occur within a gravitational environment. Gravity is one of the four fundamental forces in nature, and is the weakest of them all. The others are electromagnetic force, the strong nuclear force holding the nuclei of atoms together, and the weak force responsible for radioactive decay (all of which are beyond the scope of this book). Gravity influences the motion of tides, due to the intermittent influence of the gravitational pull of the Moon while in orbit around the Earth, and is responsible for the sensation of weight that humans experience on Earth.

Gravity was first comprehensively described in a scientific sense by Sir Isaac Newton (1642–1727). His classic work, *Philosophiae Naturalis Principia Mathematica* (*The Mathematical Principles of Natural Philosophy*), was published in Latin in July, 1687. This treatise expounded the three Laws of Motion and the Universal Law of Gravitation, and made Newton internationally famous (Feynman, 1965, 1985, 1996; Goodstein and Goodstein, 1997; Kane and Sternheim, 1984; Narlikar, 1996; Westfall, 1993; White, 1997). These Laws now demand some attention, for they form the theoretical foundation for subsequent chapters of this book.

The Universal Law of Gravitation was developed by Newton as a consequence of his work on planetary motion (Feynman, 1996; Goodstein and Goodstein, 1997; Howard, 1965; Kane and Sternheim, 1984; Narlikar, 1996). This Law is a fundamentally important principle of nature, and defines gravity in mechanical terms as the force of attraction that exists between two bodies separated by a particular distance. It has as its central premise the idea that all objects in the universe attract each other in a mathematically predictable way. This attractive or gravitational force is dependent on the relative masses of the objects and the distance separating them. If two objects, of mass m and m', are separated by a distance r, then the attractive or gravitational force between them is expressed in the following formula;

$$F = G.\frac{m.m'}{r^2}$$

where: F = gravitational force,

               G = the gravitational constant, which has been shown to have a
               measured value of $6.67 \times 10^{-11} N.m^2.kg^{-2}$.

where: m = metre

               N = Newton unit of force, where 1 Newton is defined as the force
               required to accelerate a 1 kilogram mass at 9.8 metres per
               second^{-2}

               kg = kilogram.

The value of the gravitational constant, G, was first experimentally measured by the English physicist Henry Cavendish (1731–1810). Credited with the discovery of hydrogen, Cavendish was also famous for what became known as the 'Cavendish experiment', where a torsion balance was used in a laboratory to measure the gravitational attraction between two objects. This experiment allowed Cavendish to determine the mass and density of the Earth, and in so doing was able to derive a value for the gravitational constant, G.

The gravitational force is directed along a line joining the centres of both objects. The magnitude of the gravitational force generated by an object is therefore a direct function of the mass of the object and an inverse function of the square of the separating distance. The greater the mass, and the closer the objects, the stronger the attractive force. A human being on the Earth's surface is subjected to the gravitational attraction of the Earth's mass, and the Earth in turn experiences a gravitational attraction to the human on its surface. Due to the large difference in relative mass (about 70 kg for the human, and 5.98×10^{24} kg for the Earth), the gravitational attraction of the human is negligible compared with that of the Earth (Kane and Sternheim, 1984).

From a planetary motion perspective, Newton's Universal Law of Gravitation represented the culmination of centuries of thought. The early views on planetary motion were geocentric, in that it was thought that the planets orbited the Earth. This view was championed by Aristotle and Ptolemy. The work of the Polish astronomer and mathematician Nicholas Copernicus (1473–1543) formulated a heliocentric view of the solar system, with planets orbiting around the Sun rather than the Earth. Johannes Kepler (1571–1630) was then able to show that planetary orbits were elliptical rather than circular, and Galileo was able to provide supporting evidence from direct astronomical observations. Newton's Universal Law of Gravitation and the three Laws of Motion were able to confirm Kepler's Laws of Planetary Motion and effectively confirm the helicocentric nature of the solar system.

Newton's theories were subsequently confirmed experimentally by several others, notably the French mathematician Pierre Simon Laplace (1749–1827),

Urbain Jean Joseph Le Verrier (1811–77) and John Couch Adams (1819–92). Laplace's mathematical work showed strong agreement between predicted and observed planetary motion, confirming the validity of Newton's Law of Universal Gravitation. The Frenchman Le Verrier and the Englishman Adams are credited with the discovery of the planet Neptune, as a result of their independent work on the orbit of Uranus. This orbit did not appear to conform to Newton's Law of Gravitation. The lack of agreement between the observed orbit of Uranus and that predicted by Newton's Law led them to deduce the existence of another nearby planet, which was exerting a gravitational pull on Uranus. The new planet, Neptune, was duly discovered.

Newton's Laws of Motion

Newton's three Laws of Motion are integral to an accurate and comprehensive understanding of acceleration and its physiological consequences. Much of Newton's work represented an evolution of thought from predecessors such as the Greek philosopher Aristotle (384–322 BC) and the Italian physicist and astronomer Galileo (1564–1642). Aristotle understood motion in a qualitative sense. His idea was that objects tended to move towards an ideal (or potential) position from their current (actual) position, and that this motion was the result of a force acting on the objects. He opined that a constant force is required on an object to produce a constant velocity. Galileo took these ideas a step further and developed the theory that a force acting on an object resulted in an acceleration of the object. In contrast to Aristotle, he believed that an object in a state of constant velocity has *no* force acting on it. He also considered the effects of friction in terms of opposing the applied force on an object. Newton's significant contribution was to define the relationship between force and acceleration in a quantitative sense.

Newton's First Law of Motion states that an object will remain in a state of rest or of uniform motion in a straight line unless acted on by a force. This force, if applied to the object, can produce a change in speed and/or direction. The object will thus experience an acceleration. For example, if an object is travelling at a certain speed and is acted on by a force that changes only its direction of travel, it is said to have been accelerated in its new direction.

Newton's Second Law states that the force acting on a body is the product of that body's mass and the acceleration it undergoes as a result. The equation describing this is thus;

$$F = m.a$$

where: F = force

                 m = mass of the body

                 a = acceleration

It is worth mentioning the concept of inertia at this point. The force applied to the object must overcome the object's inherent inertia in order to achieve an acceleration. Inertia is a function of mass, which is the quantity of matter in a given object. The greater the mass, the greater is the inertia of the object. To accelerate an object of large mass by a certain amount, a larger force must be applied. Thus, an important aspect of Newton's Second Law is that force is proportional to acceleration.

Newton's Third Law is perhaps the most significant in practical and physiological terms. This Third Law states that for every action, there is an equal and opposite reaction. When the action involved is acceleration, the equal and opposite reaction is inertia. This is clear from Newton's Second Law: acceleration must be applied to an object to overcome its inertia (which is effectively resisting movement of the object). Thus, inertia (which as has been seen is a function of its inherent mass) opposes acceleration directionally, but is equal to it in terms of magnitude. Newton's Third Law is fundamentally important to the subject of this book, as it encapsulates the basic physiological responses to applied acceleration. This will be elaborated on in subsequent chapters.

Acceleration Due to Motion

As an example of these important Laws of Motion, consider an object attached to a piece of string rotating in a circle at constant speed. The rotating object has several forces acting upon it. The first is a tangential force that will cause the object to travel in a straight line if the string should break. This is the natural tendency of the object. From Newton's First Law, a force must therefore be acting upon the object to keep it travelling in a circle. The object is travelling at a particular angular velocity, but the direction of its travel changes constantly. There is therefore by definition an acceleration acting upon the object, which is directed towards the centre of rotation.

In accordance with Newton's Second Law, this angular acceleration is proportional to the force applied to the object, given that it's mass is constant. This force, which is also directed towards the centre of the circle, is known as centripetal force.

In accordance with Newton's Third Law, there must be an equal yet opposite force balancing the centripetal force. This is known as the centrifugal force, and is directed away from the centre of the circle. Centripetal force is active, whereas centrifugal force is reactive and inertial.

In the example given, the object on the end of the string is essentially the same as an aircraft in a circular turn, a planet in orbit around another, or a satellite or spacecraft in orbit around the Earth. The physics is fundamentally the same. In the case of an orbiting spacecraft, the gravitational attraction of the Earth is

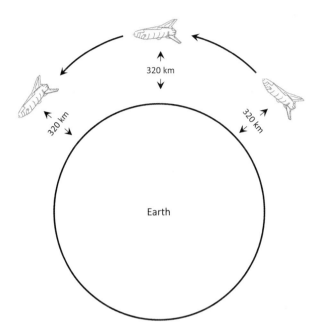

Figure 1.1   A spacecraft in orbit

exactly counterbalanced by the centrifugal force generated by the spacecraft's orbit at that altitude. In this situation, the spacecraft is effectively falling towards the surface of the Earth at the same rate that the surface of the rotating Earth 'falls away' from the spacecraft. This is shown in Figure 1.1. The spacecraft and its occupants are effectively weightless, as the gravitational force is not resisted by the Earth's surface. For such orbital flight conditions to be maintained at a certain constant height above the Earth's surface, the spacecraft must travel at a constant, extremely high speed. For example, to maintain its low-Earth orbit (at a height of approximately 300 km above the surface of the Earth), the Space Shuttle had to maintain an orbit speed of approximately 28,000 km per hour (a speed equivalent to Mach 25, or 25 times the speed of sound).

The Mechanics of Circular Motion

It is now important to mathematically consider the nature of the circular motion of an object. The magnitude of the centripetal acceleration, and therefore the centripetal force, of an object undergoing circular motion at constant speed (as shown in Figure 1.2) can be mathematically determined in the following way.

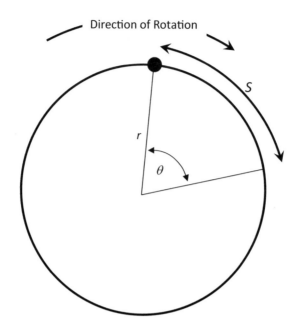

Figure 1.2   The geometry of circular motion

If the object in Figure 1.2 moves along an arc of circumference S, with the circle having a radius of r, the angle subtended by this motion, θ, is given by:

$$\theta = \frac{S}{r}$$

where: θ = angular position (in radians).

In accordance with Newton's First Law, the object would have a natural tendency to move in a tangent to any point on the arc of travel, and it would do so with a certain velocity. This is known as its tangential velocity. However, there is a centripetal force acting on that object to keep it describing a circle of radius r. This force, directed towards the centre of the circle, can be calculated following the logical steps below, where simple mechanics are applied to the object describing a circular path.

The tangential velocity is a function of the change in subtended angle (distance travelled) per unit change in time. This expression is given by the following expression:

$$dv = v.\tan d\theta$$

where: v = tangential velocity
dv = change in velocity
$d\theta$ = change in angular position.

Since at small angles the size of the tangent is correspondingly very small, the equation can be simplified to:

$$dv = v.d\theta$$

Since the change in angular position will occur relative to a time interval, adding the time interval to the equation converts the expression to one involving angular acceleration:

$$\frac{dv}{dt} = v.\frac{d\theta}{dt}$$

where: $\frac{dv}{dt}$ = angular acceleration, a

v = tangential velocity

$\frac{d\theta}{dt}$ = the instantaneous rate of change of direction, or angular velocity, ω.

By making angular acceleration the subject of the equation, and substituting ω. for the angular velocity expression, the equation then becomes:

$$a = v.\omega$$

If the object makes one full revolution about the centre of rotation in time t, it will have travelled a distance equal to the circumference of the circle of radius r that it has described. The object's tangential velocity v is thus a function of circumference and time, and is given by the expression:

$$v = \frac{2\pi r}{t}$$

When the object makes a complete rotation of the circle, it has travelled a distance equal to the circumference, and the expression becomes:

$$\theta = \frac{S}{r} = \frac{2\pi r}{r} = 2\pi$$

In terms of angular velocity, one full revolution in time t is equal to the circumference of the circle, or 2π. Angular velocity is therefore:

$$\omega = \frac{d\theta}{dt} = \frac{2\pi}{t}$$

Substituting the equation above for angular velocity into the previous one for tangential velocity, the resultant equation becomes:

$$v = \frac{2\pi}{t} r = \omega.r$$

Rearranging this equation to make angular velocity the subject gives:

$$\omega = \frac{v}{r}$$

Substituting this equation for angular velocity into the equation for angular acceleration results in the following expression:

$$a = v . \omega = v . \frac{v}{r} = \frac{v^2}{r}$$

This equation allows the magnitude of angular (centripetal) acceleration to be determined. With this, centripetal force F_C can then be simply determined using Newton's Second Law:

$$F_C = m.a = m \frac{v^2}{r}$$

From this equation it becomes apparent that centripetal force is directly proportional to velocity and indirectly proportional to radius of rotation. In practical terms, therefore, an object undergoing a tight turn (small r) at high speed (large v) will experience a large centripetal force. In accordance with Newton's Third Law, this also holds true for centrifugal acceleration and force, albeit the direction of application of both of these will be opposite to that of centripetal acceleration and force, respectively.

Acceleration Due to Gravity

Armed now with an understanding of gravitational force, angular velocities and centripetal/centrifugal accelerations, it is now possible for the important relationship between the concepts of gravity and weight to be carefully considered. It is not as straightforward as might first be presumed.

A person standing on the Earth's surface will experience two significant forces. One is the force generated by the mass of the Earth itself, which is a function of its inherent overall mass. This force is given by Newton's Universal Law of Gravitation, as discussed earlier. The person on the Earth's surface is also subjected to the centrifugal force developed by virtue of the fact that the Earth is a rotating object. By finding the difference between these two forces, the weight of the person can be defined. This can be resolved in simple terms to a gravitational force, F_g, which attracts the person to the Earth's centre, a relationship given by a special form of Newton's Second Law:

$$F_g = m.g$$

where m = mass of the person

           g = acceleration due to the Earth's gravity, 9.8 ms^{-2}.

The term g above is thus a resultant of the gravitational force (based on the Universal Law of Gravitation) and the centrifugal force (based on the metrics of the rotating Earth).

Gravity and Weight

The expression above introduces the important concept of weight. Weight can be defined as the force exerted by the mass of an accelerating body (Green, 2006a). An object's weight will vary according to its mass and the acceleration to which it is subjected. As seen earlier, an object's mass is a function of how much matter it contains. As such, mass is an inherent property of the object and is independent of its physical or chemical state. Since mass tends to be constant, weight is therefore proportional to acceleration. On the surface of the Earth, therefore, weight is thus equal to F_g:

$$W = m.g = F_g$$

Importantly, it is not the active component of this force that is experienced subjectively as weight, but rather the reactive or inertial component, in accordance with Newton's Third Law of Motion.

An object on the surface of the Earth will experience a centripetal acceleration due to gravity, g, of 9.8 m/s^2. This value of g is dependent on the mass of the Earth and also on the distance between the object and the centre of the Earth. The value of g can vary from 9.832 m/s^2 at the North Pole to 9.796 m/s^2 in Denver, Colorado which is at an altitude of 1,638 metres. Thus, the value of g varies in accordance with Newton's Inverse-Square Law of Gravitation.

As we have already seen, the magnitude of the Earth's gravitational force varies, in accordance with the Inverse-Square Law, with distance from the surface. The further one travels from the Earth's surface, the lower the gravitational pull back towards Earth. At a sufficient distance from the surface, objects are able to remain in orbit at a particular height above Earth by maintaining a constant high speed. This concept is exploited by modern satellite technology and by spacecraft such as the Space Shuttle, Soyuz rockets and the International Space Station. Satellites and spacecraft carrying humans enter orbits at varying heights above the surface of the Earth (depending on many factors). The force of gravity at these heights is quite low, and is generally only enough to prevent the object from escaping further away into true space. In this situation, the centrifugal force generated by the object's orbit is exactly counterbalanced by the gravitational attraction of the Earth.

As an example, when it was in operation the Space Shuttle typically entered orbit with a gravitational force of only 0.07 times the force of Earth's gravity acting on it. This is known as microgravity and, while not true zero gravity (as occurs in true space), it is nevertheless a close approximation, especially in a physiological sense.

The variation of the terrestrial gravitational force with distance from the surface results in Earth's atmosphere having a specific vertical profile in terms of density and pressure. Both of these variables reduce with distance from the Earth's surface. At a distance of around 700 km from the Earth's surface, collisions between air molecules are extremely infrequent. This level represents the upper level of the atmosphere, beyond which molecules tend to escape into true space.

Weight and mass are often used interchangeably, but it is important to have a thorough understanding of these two terms in view of subsequent sections of this book. An object's mass is a function of how much matter it contains. Weight, as we have seen above, is an expression of the gravitational force acting on an object. Weight will vary from place to place for any given object, whereas mass will remain constant.

An object of a certain mass on the surface of the Earth will have a certain weight due to the force of gravity acting on the mass and accelerating it towards the centre of the Earth at a rate equal to g. All objects on the surface of the Earth will accelerate towards the centre of the Earth at the same rate, their weight varying in proportion with their mass. On the surface of the Moon, the gravity field is only 1/6th that of Earth's, (that is, 0.17 times the Earth's gravity, or 1.63 m.s^{-2}), because the Moon is a much smaller planet and thus has much less mass. That explains the relative ease with which the Apollo astronauts were able to move around the Moon's surface despite all their heavy and cumbersome life support systems. On the Moon, these astronauts effectively weighed 1/6th of their normal (or Earth-referenced) weight, while their mass obviously remained constant. Conversely, if an astronaut was to stand on the surface of Jupiter, their effective weight would be approximately 2.5 times greater than their Earth-referenced weight, due to the much greater mass of Jupiter (some 300 times greater than that of the Earth) generating a higher level of gravity (24.9 ms^{-2}).

Einstein's Contribution

Newtonian mechanics essentially hold true for ordinary objects at ordinary velocities within the known universe. Newton's Laws, however, do not hold true at the atomic scale and at speeds approaching the speed of light (3 x 10^8 ms^{-2}). While an exhaustive analysis of why this is the case is well and truly beyond the scope of this book, it is worth making some brief comments by way of explanation. Einstein's Special Relativity Theory gave the speed of light the role of being the upper limit for the speed of all interactions. This is in contrast to

Newton's Universal Law of Gravitation, which implied an instantaneous effect over any possible distance. The General Relativity Theory was an attempt to resolve this mutual conflict, and when it was published in 1915 it significantly altered the traditional understanding of gravity. Einstein's General Relativity Theory (as mentioned earlier) holds that gravity is a manifestation of the curvature or distortion of the space–time continuum. In other words, the geometry of space–time has become non-Euclidean in nature (Narlikar, 1996). In practical terms, this means that light is bent by the force of gravity. This has been scientifically established by astronomical experiments which revealed that starlight curves as it passes the sun.

Similarly, time itself is influenced by the force of gravity. Absolute time and absolute space are thus terms made somewhat redundant by Einstein's Special Relativity Theory. Time therefore is a relative term, and according to the Theory, time runs faster the higher above the Earth one travels (and the less the force of gravity becomes as a result). For the purposes of everyday activity however, Newton's Laws of Motion provide a satisfactory explanation for the behaviour of masses relative to each other. The reader may be heartened to know that this particularly applies to the consequences of exposure to acceleration on human physiology, as will be seen in later chapters.

Kepler and Newton

To illustrate just how important and encompassing Newton's Laws are, it is worth a brief and final digression to consider Kepler's contribution to planetary motion, and how an integration of Newton's and Kepler's work produces the Inverse-Square Law of Gravitation. Kepler developed the next big breakthrough in the understanding of planetary motion after the earlier work of Copernicus. Through direct observation of the planets, Kepler discovered that planetary orbits are generally in the form of an ellipse, rather than a pure circle. Based on this work, he elaborated what have become known as Kepler's three Laws of Planetary Motion:

1. A planet orbits in an ellipse, with the Sun as one of the ellipse's foci.
2. The radial line from the Sun to the planet sweeps out equal areas in equal time intervals.
3. The square of the time (T) taken by the planet to complete one orbit is proportional to the cube of the semi-major axis (r) of the orbit.

The semi-major axis is an important geometric component of an ellipse. The major axis of an ellipse is where the longest diameter occurs, and is the distance between the widest parts of the ellipse (passing through the centre and both elliptical foci). The semi-major axis is one half of the major axis. It runs from the centre of the ellipse, through one of the two foci, and then to the edge of the ellipse. In the case of a circle, the semi-major axis is equal to the radius.

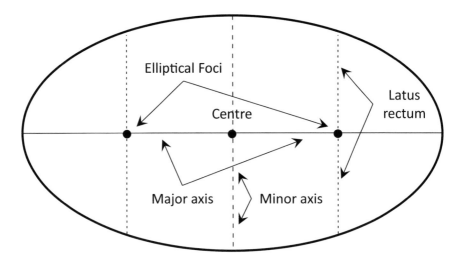

Figure 1.3   The geometry of an ellipse

Kepler's Third Law can be expressed mathematically as:

$$\frac{T^2}{r^3} = k$$

Where: T = time to complete one orbit

r = major axis of the orbit

k = constant

Kepler's Third Law thus states that the relationship between T and r (as shown in the equation above) is the same for all planets.

For the sake of completing the circle, as it were, it is possible to consider the motion of an object in a circle using Kepler's Third Law. A planet of mass m completes a circular orbit of another planet in time T. The circumference of the circle is given by $2\pi r$. With this in mind, the velocity of the planet is given by:

$$v = \frac{2\pi r}{t}$$

The force acting on this planet is given by Newton's Second Law:

$$F = m.a = m\frac{v^2}{r}$$

Putting the expression for v into the expression for force, the resultant expression is:

$$F = m. \frac{(\frac{2\pi r}{T})^2}{r} = \frac{m4\pi^2 r}{T^2}$$

Kepler's Third Law can be rewritten to make T the subject of the equation:

$$T^2 = k.r^3$$

Substituting this equation for T into the equation for force (above) results in:

$$F = \frac{m4\pi^2 r}{kr^3} = \frac{m4\pi^2}{kr^2}$$

Since this particular planet has a known mass, the equation can be simplified as shown, taking into account the known constant values which act now as a proportionality factor:

$$F \propto \frac{1}{r^2}$$

The end result of this manipulation is that the force acting on the object is inversely proportional to the square of the distance from the centre of the planet it is orbiting. This is the same inverse-square relationship captured in Newton's Universal Law of Gravitation. Integrating Newton's Laws of Motion with Kepler's work confirms the inverse-square nature of gravitation. Sir Isaac Newton's elegant and pioneering work was thus fundamental in developing classical mechanics, and his contribution to modern scientific thinking is rightly seen as monumental.

Conclusion

Human beings are constantly exposed to a gravitational environment by virtue of their existence on the surface of the Earth. However, it is possible to alter the gravitational force on an object within the Earth's gravitational field by accelerating the object. The applied acceleration can be greater or less than the normal level of gravitational force. Modern aircraft, whether military fighters or civilian aerobatic aircraft, can generate significant levels of angular acceleration, and in so doing expose the pilot to a raft of potentially adverse physiological consequences. Similarly, spaceflight can subject humans to a wide range of gravitational forces, ranging from microgravity in the case of low-Earth orbit, or relatively high levels of gravitational force during launch and re-entry procedures.

This chapter has hopefully armed the reader with an understanding of the general concepts of gravity and angular acceleration. These concepts are important, as they form the foundation on which the physiological consequences of exposure to a high G force environment are considered in subsequent chapters of this book. These physiological consequences and indeed the countermeasures developed to combat them are more easily understood if the basic mechanics of circular motion are remembered. In the next chapter, a brief analysis of the manner in which accelerations and gravitational forces are generated in flight will be presented.

Chapter 2
High G Flight

The previous chapter considered the general concept of gravity, angular acceleration and the Laws of Motion. The purpose of this chapter is to relate these Laws of Motion specifically to the flight environment. This is important, as it will form the foundation for the remainder of this book in its discussion of the physiological consequences of human exposure to this environment and the various countermeasures developed to increase human tolerance.

Acceleration Nomenclature

Investigation of the physiological effects of exposure to high G acceleration requires that the position of the subject relative to the G vector is clearly identified, in order to prevent confusion. To this end, a standardised nomenclature has been developed and widely adopted to describe the direction of application of G in relation to the three major spatial axes of the human body (Blomqvist and Stone, 1983; Burton and Whinnery, 1996; Green, 2006a). Before discussing this directional coordinate system, it is first critically important to discuss what is meant by the term 'G' and how this variable is calculated.

Magnitude

G is a dimensionless ratio which expresses the applied acceleration that an object undergoes as a multiple of the normal acceleration due to Earth's gravity. This relationship is expressed thus:

$G = a.g^{-1}$
where a = applied acceleration
                    g = acceleration due to gravity (9.8 ms^{-2}).

The applied acceleration that an object experiences when it is undergoing circular motion was discussed in detail in Chapter 1. Applied acceleration in circular motion is a function of the velocity of the object and the radius of the circle described in the manoeuvre. The end result of this relationship (see Chapter 1) might be a number such as 19.6 ms^{-2}. This figure makes little intuitive sense, particularly in terms of the likely physiological consequences.

Use of the term G allows the description of acceleration to be simplified. It takes into account the fact that acceleration can be achieved in several ways, but the effect (either physiological or mechanical) is the same. In practical terms, it does not matter how the acceleration is produced. In that sense, G is an extremely useful and simple tool for expressing the magnitude of an acceleration, by using the acceleration due to the force of gravity as a reference value. In so doing, it gives a more intuitive context for developing an understanding of the likely physiological consequences of exposure to an acceleration environment. In the example above, the 19.6 ms^{-2} turn is 2 multiples of the Earth's gravity, 9.8 ms^{-2}. The manoeuvre can thus be described as a 2 G turn. This is intuitive, as the effects of a 2 G turn are therefore twice what would usually be experienced at 1 G.

The term 'G force' has entered common usage. Strictly speaking, G is not a ratio of force but of acceleration. However, given that mass is a constant, force is therefore proportional to acceleration in accordance with Newton's Second Law of Motion. As such, the related terms G force and G acceleration are frequently used interchangeably. For the purpose of this book, as mentioned in Chapter 1, the term G force will be used.

Direction

While magnitude of G is easily calculated, the other key aspect is the direction in which the G is applied. In order to standardise the description of acceleration, a three-axis coordinate system has been adopted, which is used by international convention to describe the direction of an applied acceleration. This system is illustrated in Figure 2.1. Acceleration can be applied in the longitudinal axis (z), the transverse axis (x) or the lateral axis (y). The acceleration is also expressed as either positive (+) or negative (−). For example, a transverse centripetal acceleration acting from chest-to-back is denoted as −Gx, whereas the same acceleration acting in the opposite direction (that is, back-to-chest) is +Gx. This system can be used to describe either an applied acceleration (centripetal) or its inertial (centrifugal) component. From a physiological point of view, the inertial vectors are the most important, as it is these that drive the various physiological consequences of high G exposure to be discussed throughout this book.

In describing inertial vectors, the positive and negative signs are reversed, such that a chest-to-back inertial vector is denoted as +Gx. This reflects the fact that centripetal and centrifugal accelerations are equal in magnitude but act in diametrically opposed directions. It is important to clearly identify which form of acceleration is being described to avoid confusion. For the purposes of this book, inertial vectors will be used throughout, unless otherwise stated.

Based on these conventions, an object on the Earth's surface (such as a human being) will undergo an applied acceleration of 9.8 ms^{-2} in the z axis. The terrestrial level of gravitational force is thus arbitrarily defined as +1 Gz. With increasing distance from the Earth, the strength of the gravitational field diminishes.

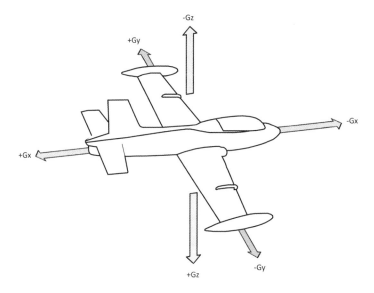

Figure 2.1   Inertial vectors used to describe the direction of G

In Earth orbit, the gravitational force is generally only able to prevent the orbiting object from escaping further away into true space. Astronauts in the Space Shuttle or the International Space Station experience very low levels of gravity (known as microgravity, μG), during orbital spaceflight, typically in the region of 10^{-4} to 10^{-5}Gz.

Acceleration in the Flight Environment

Armed now with an understanding of how G is calculated and how direction is assigned, the next step is to consider how G force can be developed during flight. Accelerations in the flight environment are typically classified in the following way;

- Short duration (< 1 second): ground impact, mid-air collisions.
- Medium duration (0.5–2 seconds): catapult launches, carrier deck landings, ejections.
- Long duration (>2 seconds): normal aviation activities, especially air combat manouevring (ACM), basic fighter manoeuvres (BFM), and aerobatic flight.

Short- and medium-duration accelerations produce characteristic physiological problems. Short-duration accelerations obviously result in significant trauma to the human occupant of the aircraft commensurate with the size of the impact forces, which may well be non-survivable. Medium duration accelerations in carrier operations are in the Gx plane and are generally well tolerated. Ejecting from an aircraft produces a large +Gz force over a short time period which is generally well tolerated but does tend to produce typical and well documented injury patterns (Newman, 2014). Both short- and medium-duration accelerations are beyond the intended scope of this book. Long-duration accelerations in the ±Gz axis are by far the most physiologically significant for a pilot, and thus these will form the basis for the rest of this book.

Generating G in Flight

The wings of an aircraft are designed to generate lift. This lift supports the weight of the aircraft and allows it to fly. In straight and level flight, the lift generated by the wings (the lift vector) is equal in magnitude but opposite in direction to the weight of the aircraft (that is, the gravitational force developed by the product of the aircraft's mass and the acceleration due to gravity, g). The lift generated thus tends to oppose the natural tendency of the aircraft to return to the Earth's surface due to the effect of gravity. The occupants of the aircraft when it is in this mode of flight are subjected to the normal gravitational field of the Earth, that is, +1 Gz.

Flight occurs in a three-dimensional medium and is a dynamic activity. In the flight environment, acceleration is a particularly important variable. There are basically two types of acceleration available to an aircraft – linear and radial. Most aircraft have insufficient thrust to produce physiologically important linear acceleration quantities (although as will be seen later, spacecraft can often generate high levels of linear acceleration during the launch phase). However, radial accelerations are very common, and occur whenever the aircraft changes direction.

Manipulation of the lift vector allows the aircraft to change direction in flight and manoeuvre as required. During a manoeuvre, such as a banked turn or a loop, the aircraft will describe part of a circle (with the pilot's head generally directed towards the centre) and thereby generate a degree of radial, or angular, acceleration. The aircraft acts in a very similar way to the object at the end of a string discussed in Chapter 1 (and shown in Figure 1.1), with the same forces described by Newton's Laws of Motion acting upon the aircraft and the pilot, that is, centripetal force and centrifugal force. If the aircraft executes a tight turn (small *r*) at high speed (large *v*) it will generate a large centripetal acceleration and a large opposing centrifugal acceleration. An example of such a flight manoeuvre is shown in Figure 2.2.

During manoeuvring flight, the pilot's head is generally directed towards the centre of the circle described by the aircraft. The resultant acceleration is in the head-to-foot or +Gz axis (and is known as 'positive G') and is the most common acceleration generated by flight. Thus, an aircraft undergoing an angular acceleration of 19.6 ms^{-2} (2 x 9.8ms^{-2}) is said to be 'pulling +2 Gz' (twice the normal acceleration due to gravity). Similarly, the inertial force experienced by the pilot of an F/A-18 fighter aircraft in a 7.5 G turn is therefore described as +7.5 Gz.

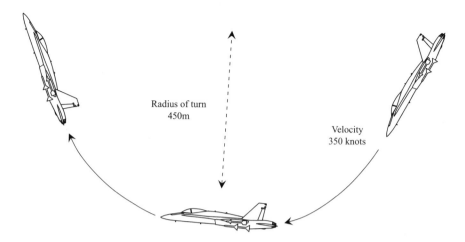

Figure 2.2   An aircraft in turning flight

Most aircraft are capable of +2 Gz. An aircraft maintaining altitude in a 60° banked turn will generate +2 Gz. Modern jet fighter aircraft such as the F-16 and the JAS-39 Gripen are capable of up to +9 Gz, while civilian competition aerobatic aircraft can generate more than +10 Gz. The value of +Gz in the manoeuvre shown in Figure 2.2 is +7.35 Gz.

If the aircraft in Figure 2.2 was inverted, the pilot's head would be directed away from the centre of the circle during the manoeuvre. The magnitude of the resultant Gz force would be the same (7.35 Gz) but the direction of acceleration would be opposite (negative rather than positive). According to the convention shown in Figure 2.1, this is known as –Gz or 'negative G'. The Gz limits of a particular aircraft are largely determined by aerodynamic and engine performance factors inherent in the aircraft's design. Most military fast jet and training aircraft can generate –3 Gz, but civilian competition aerobatic aircraft can easily generate up to –4 Gz.

Physiological Consequences of High G Exposure

Given that G exposure can occur in three different axes of direction, it is worth briefly summarising the physiological consequences of such exposure. While Gx and Gy accelerations can have an impact on physiological function, it is Gz acceleration that has the predominant effect on the human during long-duration flight-based manoeuvring. Indeed, this aspect will form the major scope of this book, as the physiological consequences of exposure to military flight operations, spaceflight and aerobatic flight are considered. This section provides a general summary of the key issues involved in long-duration accelerations in the three main axes.

+Gx Acceleration

Transverse accelerations, at right angles to the long axis of the body, are generally well tolerated. In the conventional flight environment, they are due to linear accelerations such as a catapult launch from or an arrested landing back onto an aircraft carrier, or a rocket-assisted take-off. However, the magnitude of these accelerations tends to be small relative to the tolerance of the human body, and as such physiological consequences are rare. As will be seen later in this chapter, spaceflight imposes considerable Gx loads during the launch phase.

When transverse accelerations do cause physiological consequences, the respiratory system is the most affected (Green, 2006a). At levels in the order of +2 Gx, arm weight and abdominal pressure increase. At +3 Gx, breathing becomes difficult, while at +5 Gx, chest and abdominal pain becomes increasingly more severe and is aggravated by inspiration. As +Gx increases, the breathing difficulties become more pronounced. At approximately +12 Gx the weight of the chest wall is increased to the point where breathing is extremely difficult.

Exposure to even higher levels of +Gx depends very much on the willingness of the individual participant to continue with the exposure (Green, 2006a). It is the respiratory effects of +Gx exposure and its consequent fatigue penalty that ultimately tend to limit human tolerance. –Gx accelerations are tolerated a little better, due to the inertial forces lifting the abdominal contents away from the infero-posterior part of the thoracic cavity. The same fundamental respiratory effects take place, but tolerance tends to be higher. These respiratory effects of ±Gx exposure are considered in more detail in Chapter 5.

+Gy Acceleration

Lateral accelerations do not tend to have significant physiological effects, and indeed are quite rare in the conventional flight environment. The unsupported neck of a pilot may be at risk during exposure to ±Gy acceleration (Newman and Ostler, 2011), and at levels in the order of ±3 to ±4 Gy the respiratory system may be affected. It has been suggested by some authors that the increased mediastinal weight at such Gy levels may lead to sequential inflation and deflation of the left and right lungs relative to each other (Green, 2006a). This may have considerable implications for respiratory function which would probably be the end-point for human tolerance.

+Gz Acceleration

The human body is particularly sensitive to acceleration in the longitudinal or z axis. As has been seen previously, weight is altered by the level of applied +Gz. The soft tissues of the face will sag, and general mobility can be adversely affected. The arms and legs will weigh proportionally more under high levels of +Gz, but the muscles responsible for their movement will be no stronger. At approximately +8 Gz movement of the upper limbs above the head becomes impossible (Green, 2006a). To enable the pilot to activate key switches and controls during high +Gz flight, most modern fast jet aircraft employ a Hands on Throttle and Stick (HOTAS) system, whereby these key switches and controls are located on the throttle and control column, effectively within finger reach (Newman, 2014).

If a pilot wearing a protective helmet allows their head to flex forward under approximately +4 Gz, the head cannot then be raised until the +Gz load has been reduced. Neck injuries are thus common sequelae of frequent and chronic exposure to the high +Gz environment (Andersen, 1988; Green, 2003; Knudson et al., 1988; Newman, 1997a, 1997b; Vanderbeek, 1988), and are considered in detail in Chapter 6.

The cardiovascular system is especially susceptible to adverse effects from Gz exposure, and can ultimately be unable to sustain adequate cerebral perfusion at a +Gz level of +4.5 to 5.5 Gz. This results in G-Induced Loss of Consciousness (G-LOC), discussed in more detail in Chapter 4. With the use of anti-G countermeasures to be discussed in later chapters, pilots can tolerate up to +9 Gz. With the increasing agility of modern fast jet aircraft, some research effort and consideration has been given to extending this tolerance limit, out to potentially +12 Gz (Burns et al., 2001).

The respiratory system is progressively affected by higher levels of +Gz acceleration (Burton and Whinnery, 1996; Green, 2006a; Lombard et al., 1948). This is examined in detail in Chapter 5. Other body systems are affected by exposure to the +Gz environment. There is an endocrinological response, with rises documented in anti-diuretic hormone (ADH), catecholamines and cortisol in response to the stress of the acceleration (Burton and Whinnery, 1996; Green, 2006a), proteinuria in subjects exposed to high +Gz has been observed (Noddeland et al., 1986), as have non-pathological, transient cardiac arrhythmias (Blomqvist and Stone, 1983; Burton and Whinnery, 1996; Comens et al., 1987; Green, 2006a; Whinnery et al., 1990; Zuidema, 1956). All of these effects are discussed in greater detail in Part II of this book.

Negative Gz (–Gz) essentially causes the same fundamental problems but in a different direction from +Gz acceleration. –Gz is poorly tolerated due to the unpleasant subjective sensations that it generates. Feelings of head fullness, facial puffiness, eye distension and neck pressure tend to limit deliberate exposure, with these symptoms becoming particularly unpleasant at –3 Gz. In general, –Gz tends to be a feature of civilian aerobatic flight rather than military fast jet operations.

Flight Operations Involving High G

Having considered the physics of the high +Gz environment, it is now appropriate to explore the different flight environments in which significant levels of +Gz might be generated. There are three broad categories of long-duration G exposure that will be considered throughout this book. They are:

- military flight operations;
- civilian aerobatic flight;
- commercial spaceflight operations.

Military Flight Operations

Almost all military pilots, as part of their flight training, will undergo some exposure to the high +Gz environment. Basic aerobatics are often conducted as part of military flight training, in order to create confidence in the pilot, teach them aircraft handling techniques and recovery from unusual attitudes. Fast jet operations, however, are where the vast majority of high +Gz exposure occurs. The nature of military fast jet operations and the high level of risk involved have been extensively described elsewhere (Knapp and Johnson, 1996; Newman, 2014). A modern high-performance military fast jet aircraft operates in an extremely fluid three-dimensional environment, and as such the G environment it operates in is extremely complex (Newman, 2014). In fast jet operations, high +Gz loads are produced during ACM (otherwise known colloquially as 'dog-fighting'), air-to-surface weapons delivery profiles, evasive manoeuvres and general aerobatic flight. An example of an ACM flight manoeuvre is shown in Figure 2.3. The centrifugal forces generated during such manoeuvring flight are important, as these are the forces that the pilot experiences physiologically and the aircraft must withstand structurally.

ACM imposes the most frequent and stressful series of accelerative changes on both the airframe and the pilot. ACM is an extremely demanding, fluid and highly dangerous form of flying. It usually involves frequent and repetitive excursions to high +Gz levels, and peak +Gz levels in the order of +11 Gz have been recorded during ACM engagements. Sustained operations at levels of above +1 Gz are not unusual, but are certainly of significance when one takes into account the fact that the average mission duration is generally around one hour. Both the aircraft and the fighter pilot are subjected to a tremendous amount of high-speed, repetitive manoeuvring under significant loads during a typical mission.

The RAAF uses the Boeing F/A-18 Hornet in the advanced tactical fighter role. This modern and highly sophisticated twin-engined jet fighter is an all-weather, night and day aircraft, capable of fulfilling both the fighter (air-to-air) role and the attack (air-to-ground) role. It has a service ceiling of about 50,000 feet and is capable of supersonic speeds up to Mach 1.8 (approximately 1,900 kph). The F/A-18's G limits are +7.5 Gz to –3 Gz.

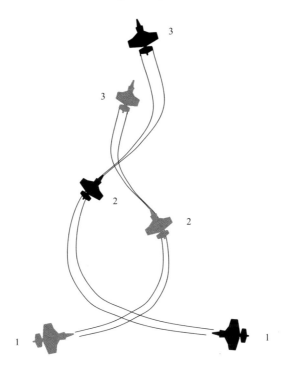

Figure 2.3   A typical air combat manoeuvre – rolling scissors

There are other jet fighters in service around the world that have similar or better G load factors. The United States Air Force's (USAF) air superiority fighter, the F-15 Eagle, is also capable of +7.5 Gz. By contrast, the Lockheed F-16 Fighting Falcon fighter is capable of sustained load factors of up to +9 Gz (Holland and Freeman, 1995), as is the JAS-39 Gripen and the Eurofighter Typhoon.

The pilot of the military fast jet operates in a physiologically hostile environment. During ACM, significant acceleration forces are repetitively applied to the fighter pilot, and the potential adverse physiological consequences, for example, G-LOC, will be extensively described in Part II of this book. During the course of an ACM training sortie, the fighter pilot may often experience G loads of +6 Gz or more, sometimes up to a maximum peak of +7.5 or +9 Gz.

Figure 2.4 shows the Gz levels experienced by a fast jet pilot as a function of time during a typical ACM sortie.

Figure 2.5 shows a specific 1 vs 1 manoeuvring engagement, which demonstrates the significant and repetitive +Gz loads experienced by a fast jet pilot over a relatively short period of time.

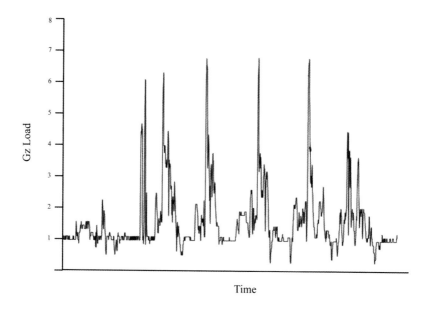

Figure 2.4 **Gz-time plot in an F/A-18 during air combat manoeuvring (ACM)**

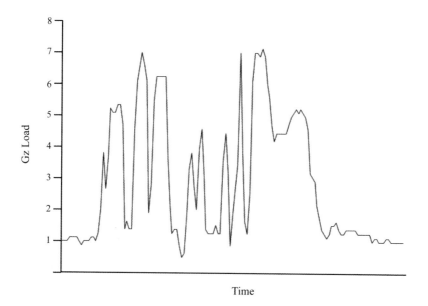

Figure 2.5 **Gz-time plot in an F/A-18 for a single 1 v 1 air combat manoeuvring (ACM) engagement**

The nature and characteristics of the Gz environment during ACM in the F/A-18 fighter aircraft have been extensively investigated (Newman and Callister, 1999). Both offensive and defensive manoeuvres in this aircraft involve a frequently changing force environment, with multiple high G excursions and high peak +Gz levels being recorded. Using data downloaded from the aircraft's Maintenance Status Display and Recording System (MSDRS), it was found that around 9 per cent of a typical 1 v 1 ACM sortie is spent at moderate-to-high +Gz levels, and the average +Gz level for such a sortie is around +1.5 Gz (Newman and Callister, 1999). This is effectively the baseline level, against which the pilot is subjected to frequent peaks to +7 Gz and beyond. Around 20 per cent of the flight is spent at +2 Gz and beyond, with some flights showing 61 excursions beyond a +2 Gz threshold (Newman and Callister, 1999). The high intensity and frequency of these force environment changes confirm the physiologically challenging nature of ACM in high-performance fighter aircraft such as the F/A-18. When the repetitive high +Gz excursions involved in ACM are taken into account, the challenge to the pilot's cardiovascular system can be readily appreciated. Not only must the pilot be able to tolerate a high-onset exposure to +7 Gz but they must also do so frequently throughout the sortie. The cardiovascular challenges of such exposure are considered in detail in Chapters 3 and 4.

Actual in-flight assessments of the ±Gz environments of particular fighter aircraft have been documented by several authors (Gillingham et al., 1985; Lau and Steinleitner, 1994; Newman and Callister, 1999; Oksa et al., 1996). Gillingham et al. (1985) examined several fighter aircraft including the F-15 and F-16. Their data for ACM in the F-15 (which has similar Gz limits to the F/A-18) in terms of time spent at or above certain Gz levels were roughly similar to those obtained for the ±Gz environment of the F/A-18 (Newman and Callister, 1999). Other studies have shown similar ±Gz-vs-time curves for different fighter aircraft types (Lau and Steinleitner, 1994; Oksa et al., 1996).

Future generations of fast jet aircraft are likely to have expanded performance and manoeuvring envelopes (Newman, 2014). Such sixth generation fighters will be characterised by their super-agile nature. This unprecedented level of aircraft manoeuvrability will involve full control authority at high angles of attack (AOA) in the post-stall region of the flight envelope (Alcorn et al., 1996; Boyum et al., 1995; Ericsson, 1995; Newman, 1998; Newman and Ostler, 2011). These aircraft will be designed with extremely relaxed stability criteria and will make use of various advanced aerodynamic features such as thrust vectoring control (TVC), canard foreplanes, and advanced digital flight control systems. The end result of this will be to give the aircraft a significantly enlarged operating envelope, with improvements in turn radius, rate of turn, directional change, rate of deceleration, AOA, low-speed flight, pitch rate and nose authority. They will also be more fuel efficient, have greater top-end speed (multi-Mach number), and be highly stealthy, with sophisticated sensor systems and digital information processing capabilities.

From a human factors and performance limitations perspective, these aircraft put the pilot in a more demanding environment by virtue of the super-agile characteristics of the aircraft (Newman, 2014). While conventional fighter aircraft have a +Gz environment predominantly in the Gz axis (Newman and Callister, 1999), super-agile aircraft are capable of performing manoeuvres with rapid, complex multi-axis motion, with excursions in the Gz, Gx and Gy axes (Newman and Ostler, 2011). This type of manoeuvring environment will have significant implications for human tolerance, particularly in terms of the need to withstand such sudden multi-axis G applications. Indeed, it is likely that G forces in the Gx and Gy axes will become more significant in these highly agile aircraft of the future.

It should be remembered that the high +Gz environment is no longer restricted to fast jet operations. Helicopters fulfilling the attack mission are becoming increasingly agile, with +Gz levels up to +4.5 Gz (Shender, 2001). The +Gz environment of these helicopters (including the AH-64 Apache and the Eurocopter Tiger) is such that the aircrew in these aircraft are exposed to the same adverse physiological consequences of G exposure as their fast jet colleagues.

The specifics of the helicopter G environment are somewhat different from the fast jet equivalent. Helicopter operations tend to be conducted at lower speed and at lower altitudes, but the risks of a G-LOC episode at 150 knots during low-level nap-of-the-earth tactical operations are just as serious as the higher altitude G-LOC event in an F-16. In both cases, the time remaining to ground impact may exceed the pilot's recovery time, leading to a fatal outcome. Given the increasing use of helicopters in the modern battlefield, and the greater sophistication and agility of the latest generation of these aircraft, it is important to recognise the risks of G exposure in aircrew operating these aircraft. The interaction of this G environment with known G tolerance reducing factors (fatigue, dehydration and so on) makes this even more important. This is discussed in more detail in Chapter 8.

Civilian Aerobatic Flight

Civilian aerobatic flight operations are quite different from military fast jet operations. In the civilian setting, aerobatics are performed for enjoyment, as an end in themselves, or for varying levels of competition. The types of aircraft used are quite different as well, as are their G environments.

Most civilian competition aerobatic aircraft are relatively small, single- or dual-seat aircraft with a single piston engine. The wing often employs a symmetrical aerofoil design, with a zero angle of incidence. This gives the aircraft a similar level of performance when inverted as when it is up the right way. The aircraft tend to be relatively light in comparison to their engine performance, thus giving a high power-to-weight ratio. They often have extremely high peak +Gz levels (to +10 Gz and beyond) and high rates of roll (sometimes greater than 400° per second). These parameters result in a particularly agile aircraft, but one which cannot sustain such high G loads for very long. The manoeuvres thus tend to be very abrupt and sometimes quite violent (Adler et al., 2013).

The G envelope of aerobatic aircraft has been reported on by several authors (Adler et al., 2013; Beyer and Daily, 2004). In a case report of a pilot presenting with abdominal pain (see Chapter 7), the G environment of the Extra 300 aerobatic aircraft was found to range from +8 Gz to –6 Gz (Beyer and Daily, 2004). Adler et al. (2013) found a similar level of G performance in the Sukhoi Su-31 aerobatic aircraft. In contrast with military fast jet aircraft, civilian aerobatic aircraft tend to explore the –Gz component of the manoeuvring envelope much more, especially in unlimited competition.

While a comprehensive review of aerobatics is beyond the scope of this book, some general observations can be made to help put the physiological consequences of high +Gz exposure into context. Aerobatic manoeuvres involve operating the aircraft around its longitudinal or lateral axes, sometimes in combination. A rolling manoeuvre is performed around the longitudinal axis, while a pitch-up or pitch-down manoeuvre is performed around the aircraft's lateral axis. In general, aerobatics involves various rolling manoeuvres and looping or turning manoeuvres, and sudden transitions between them. A spin is a complex manoeuvre, in which the aircraft is first stalled then flicked into a corkscrew descending spiral around the yaw axis.

Other manoeuvres include a stall turn, where the aircraft climbs vertically until zero airspeed, then is turned via sudden application of rudder through 180° before descending vertically. More advanced manoeuvres include the tail-slide (similar to a stall turn, but the aircraft slides vertically downward tail-first) and the Lomcovak. This latter manoeuvre is an advanced form of freestyle aerobatic exercise, and involves combinations of movement in all three axes. It is a particularly disorienting manoeuvre for the pilot, given the high degree of roll rate involved and the multi-axial nature of the flight path. It can also involve –Gz applications as well as +Gz.

A sequence of aerobatic manoeuvres is described via the Aresti system. This system, developed originally by the Spanish pilot Colonel Don Jose Luis Aresti Aguirre (1919–2003) as the Aresti Aerocriptographic System, was officially adopted by the Federation Aeronautique International (FAI) in the 1960s. The FAI is the official world body responsible for governing air sports (including aerobatic competitions), as well as aviation-related world records.

The Aresti system of aerobatic notation gives a standardised way of graphically representing each type of aerobatic manoeuvre. The FAI currently uses this notation in the Aresti Catalogue, which is the FAI standards document that describes the permitted aerobatic manoeuvres for competition use, and how these manoeuvres should be flown. The Catalogue groups possible manoeuvres into nine groups, known as families.

In Aresti notation, +Gz manoeuvres (upright flight) are represented by solid lines, whereas –Gz manoeuvres (inverted flight) are represented by dashed lines. Triangles represent manoeuvres such as stalls, and arrows represent rolling manoeuvres (with numbers showing the number of any roll segments to be flown). Examples of such manoeuvres are shown in Figure 2.6.

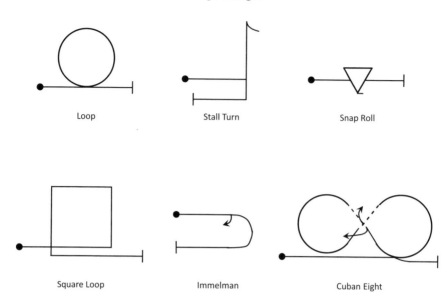

Figure 2.6   Aresti diagrams for aerobatic flight manoeuvres

The main aim with competition aerobatics is to demonstrate a high level of accuracy and precision when executing the various manoeuvres. The aerobatic sequence is flown inside an area of airspace known as the 'aerobatic box'. This is generally a cube of airspace, with side dimensions of 1,000 metres. This box can vary in height above the ground, depending on the level of competition. The box tends to be closer to the ground for higher levels of competition.

Judging is based on the accuracy and precision of the manoeuvres, as well as whether the pilot remained within the aerobatic box. Points are scored from 0 to 10 (a perfect score), with points deducted for flight outside the box.

Aerobatic flight is not without is dangers. It involves high levels of manoeuvring often in close proximity to the ground. The high level of +Gz involved in these manoeuvres (especially at unlimited competition level) increases the risk of adverse physiological consequences. In an Australian analysis of aerobatic aircraft accidents, a total of 51 accidents involving some 70 occupants in the period 1980–2010 were identified in the Australian Transport Safety Bureau (ATSB) accident and incident database (Newman, 2012). Of these, there were 27 fatal accidents (a rate of 53 per cent) resulting in 36 fatalities. The major cause of these fatal accidents was loss of control by the pilot in 44 per cent of cases. While very difficult to establish with any degree of certainty, it is likely that a proportion of these pilot loss of control events are related to G-LOC, which is discussed in detail in Chapter 4. Similarly, the 26 per cent of fatal accidents attributed to terrain impact may also have included a subset of G-LOC events.

In a similar study in the United States, 494 accidents involving aerobatic aircraft were studied (DeVoogt and van Doorn, 2009). More than 80 per cent of these accidents were fatal, the main cause of which was failure to maintain altitude. These findings are consistent with other studies that show that the biggest risk for accident-related fatality is aerobatic manoeuvring (O'Hare et al., 2003). The weight of evidence in the scientific literature thus demonstrates that aerobatic operations have a higher inherent level of risk than non-aerobatic operations. This level of risk requires an appreciation by the aerobatic pilot of the various adverse physiological effects of +Gz exposure.

Commercial Spaceflight Operations

With the advent of commercial spaceflight ventures, there is more opportunity now for the average person to travel into space than ever before (Aerospace Medical Association, 2011; Blue et al., 2012; Campbell and Garbino, 2011; Carminati et al., 2011; Jennings et al., 2010; Rayman et al., 2002; Wu et al., 2012). Over 250 people from some 30 different countries have paid a fee to fly into space with Virgin Galactic alone (Campbell and Garbino, 2011). Spaceflight per se involves long-duration exposure to microgravity (when in Earth orbit) or zero gravity (during interplanetary travel). As such, a discussion of the physiological consequences of human exposure to long-term extremely low G levels is beyond the intended scope of this book. There are two aspects of spaceflight, however, that do warrant a brief consideration here. The launch phase and the return to Earth phase of spaceflight expose the astronaut to high G levels, on a relative basis.

Astronauts being launched into space, whether on a Soyuz rocket, onboard the Space Shuttle, or onboard a commercial launch vehicle, all tend to adopt the same orientation with respect to the launch forces involved. Typically an astronaut will occupy their seat with the frontal aspect of their body facing the intended direction of travel. With the firing of the rocket, the forces involved in the launch are thus in the Gx direction. Typical Gx values during conventional rocket launches (Mercury, Apollo Soyuz and so on) are in the region of +8 Gx, while the Space Shuttle subjected the crew to a maximum Gx on launch of only +3.4 Gx (Nicogossian and Nachtwey, 1989). The physiological consequences of this Gx exposure generally are manifest mostly in the respiratory system, and are discussed in further detail in Chapter 5.

In what can be called the conventional return to Earth mode, astronauts will parachute to the ground or water while sitting in their seats. The forces involved in re-entry and landing are thus effectively in the opposite direction to those of the launch phase, and can be up to a peak of -6 Gx during re-entry. In general, however, the average force is much less and is applied over a sufficiently large period of time that there are very few adverse physiological consequences.

However, for return to Earth in the Space Shuttle, the forces were quite different. These vehicles involve the seated occupants returning to Earth in the same orientation as passengers in a conventional aircraft. The forces involved, while relatively small, are applied in the +Gz axis and for a protected period of time. The Space Shuttle exposed returning astronauts to only +1.2 Gz, but for a period of up to 20 minutes (Nicogossian and Nachtwey, 1989). This is potentially significant, given that those astronauts had adapted to a Gz environment of effectively 0 Gz over a 10–14 day period. The physiological consequences of such +Gz exposure on return from space are similar to those seen in aerobatic flight operations (but on an arguably lesser scale), with potentially adverse cardiovascular consequences being the most significant (Blamick et al., 1988; Blomqvist and Stone, 1983; Bungo, 1989; Bungo et al., 1985; Bungo and Johnson, 1983; Convertino, 1990; Convertino et al., 1989; Eichler et al., 2004; Fritsch-Yelle et al., 1994; Ten Harkel et al., 1992; Tomaselli et al., 1990). These are discussed in detail in Chapters 3 and 4.

The flight profile for commercial suborbital spaceflight operations is likely to be different again (Aerospace Medical Association, 2011; Campbell and Garbino, 2011). There will be only a brief period of exposure to 0 Gz, giving no chance for adaptation as would occur with longer-duration spaceflight. Virgin Galactic's 'Spaceship Two' commercial suborbital operation will involve a conventional horizontal take-off underneath the carrier aircraft 'White Knight Two' and subsequent climb to approximately 50,000 ft. At that altitude, Spaceship Two is launched from the carrier aircraft. During this 70-second boost phase, the peak G will be 3.8 (mostly in the +Gx axis, with a short-term spike in the +Gz axis).

The participants will spend approximately 4 minutes in 0 G, before a 25-minute duration unpowered glide return to landing. The deceleration phase will have a maximum peak of 6 G. Interestingly, the six spaceflight participants will have reclining seats that will give the resultant G exposure in the Gx axis, whereas the two-man flight crew will have conventional seats and as such will experience their G load predominantly in the +Gz axis. As a result, there has been considerable interest in the health status of participants and in establishing medical guidelines for such commercial spaceflight operations (Aerospace Medical Association, 2011; Blue et al., 2012; Carminati et al., 2011; Jennings et al., 2010; Rayman et al., 2002; Wu et al., 2012). Given the rapid transition from 0 Gz to +Gz levels greater than +1Gz, suborbital commercial spaceflight can create a type of 'push–pull effect' (PPE) (discussed in Chapter 8). According to Campbell and Garbino (2011), the effect on landing and re-entry +Gz tolerance of such prior 0 Gz exposure remains to be understood. Centrifuge studies suggest that even people with well-controlled medical issues can tolerate the likely G environment well (Blue et al., 2012; Wu et al., 2012).

Conclusion

High levels of applied +Gz acceleration have tremendous physiological implications for the human occupants of high-performance military aircraft, civilian aerobatic aircraft and spacecraft. Flying high-performance fighter aircraft and competition aerobatic aircraft in the high +Gz environment represents a significant orthostatic challenge unmatched by any other human endeavour or activity, in terms of the magnitude of the applied G force. The next part of this book will consider the physiological implications of exposure to the high +Gz environment. Due to its orientation in the long axis of the body, the cardiovascular system is by far and away the system most affected by exposure to +Gz acceleration. The cardiovascular consequences of exposure to high +Gz are considered in extensive detail in the next two chapters.

PART II
Physiology of G

Chapter 3
The Cardiovascular System at +1 Gz

The human body is particularly sensitive to acceleration in the Gz axis. This is largely due to the behaviour of the cardiovascular system under the influence of head-to-foot or Gz accelerations. The cardiovascular system is effectively a closed-loop fluid-filled system, with blood flow being primarily driven by a dynamic pressure generated by the pumping action of the heart.

In this chapter, the function of the cardiovascular system in the normal environment of +1 Gz acceleration will be examined. In particular, the emphasis of this chapter will be on the dynamic regulation of blood pressure (BP) and HR when the system is exposed to postural change in a +1 Gz environment. This is important, since in order to understand the implications of cardiovascular exposure to high G force, it is particularly helpful to understand how the cardiovascular system functions under more normal +1 Gz conditions.

Haemodynamic Relationships

Firstly, it is helpful to briefly review some important haemodynamic relationships, as they will be frequently referred to throughout the next two chapters. BP is a fundamental issue. Mean arterial pressure (MAP) is the key regulated variable of the cardiovascular system, and is the variable most closely monitored by the baroreflexes, discussed later in this chapter (Rowell, 1986). MAP is effectively an average pressure, and is given by the following expression:

$$MAP = DP +$$
where: $\quad$ DP = diastolic pressure
$\qquad$ SP = systolic pressure

MAP is not simply the average between the minimum (diastolic) and the maximum (systolic) pressures. Rather, the MAP equation reflects the pressure distribution over time in the cardiac cycle, with diastole accounting for approximately two-thirds of the cycle.

The heart will pump out a certain volume of blood per beat. This is defined as stroke volume (SV). Cardiac output (CO) is the volume of blood pumped from the heart per minute, and is given by:

CO = SV x HR
where: SV = stroke volume
HR = heart rate.

Another important variable is the state of vascular tone in the circulatory system. This is known as total peripheral resistance (TPR) and is given by:

TPR = MAP/(HR x SV).

TPR is an indicator of how constricted the peripheral blood vessels are, which in turn reflects their state of compliance. A high level of vasoconstriction leads to increased resistance to blood flow, leading to a correspondingly high value for TPR.

Putting MAP as the subject of the equation above gives:

MAP = HR x SV x TPR.

This relationship shows that MAP (the key regulated cardiovascular variable) is the product of HR, SV and TPR. Any change in vascular tone, HR and SV will result in a change in arterial pressure.

Hydrostatic Pressure (HP)

In an upright human, the cardiovascular system can be considered as a simple vertical column of fluid, extending from head to foot. This column of fluid is subjected to a force known as HP. HP is defined as the pressure exerted by a column of fluid and is proportional to the magnitude of the applied acceleration. Under applied +Gz, the column of blood in the cardiovascular system weighs proportionally more than it did under the normal situation of +1 Gz. As a result of this hydrostatic effect, the vascular pressure above the heart is reduced, and the vascular pressure below the heart is increased. The relative change in pressure per Gz is a function of distance from the heart. The overall pressure gradient from head to foot under +1 Gz conditions is shown in Figure 3.1. This shows that arterial pressure at the level of the base of the brain in the upright posture is approximately 78 mmHg (millimetres of mercury), at the femoral artery it is around 145 mmHg, and at the ankle it is approximately 195 mmHg.

In mathematical terms, HP is a function of three variables, expressed in the following formula:

HP = $\rho.g.h$
where: HP = hydrostatic pressure
ρ = fluid density
g = acceleration due to gravity
h = height of the fluid column.

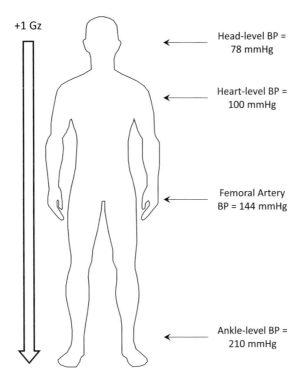

Figure 3.1 Upright posture and blood pressure (BP) changes

Under normal conditions, the cardiovascular system only has to deal with changes in the value of *h*. Assuming adequate hydration, a fit and well person will generally not experience significant changes in blood density, and during normal operations of daily life the G environment will not change from that due to the force of Earth's gravity. However, postural changes, as in assuming the upright position from a supine or prone position, will alter the direction that the G vector is applied in (remembering that in the upright position it is in the head-to-foot axis) and the value of *h* (while not physically changing) will now play a much more significant role in driving HP effects on the column of blood than it did while the person was prone or supine.

Hydrostatic Indifference Point

Since pressures above the heart decrease and those below the heart increase, there is a point in the cardiovascular system where the pressure remains constant irrespective of body position. This is known as the Hydrostatic Indifference Point (HIP), first described by Wagner in 1886, and is effectively the centre of gravity for the vascular system (Gauer and Thron, 1965). Investigators have determined that the HIP in humans is located close to the diaphragm, 5–6 cm below the upper end of the venous hydrostatic column (Rowell, 1986). This contrasts with the position of the HIP in animals such as the dog, whose HIP is located at right atrial level (Guyton and Hall, 1996; Rowell, 1986, 1993).

The position of the HIP is not anatomically fixed. It is a dynamic point within the vascular system, and its position is determined by several factors. Indeed, during tilting from supine to upright the HIP in humans varies continuously. The compliance of the vascular system, the degree of peripheral resistance and the magnitude of intravascular pressure all determine the position of the HIP. Any decrease in compliance, or increase in peripheral resistance, will shift the HIP headward. Conversely, a decrease in vascular filling pressure (that is, due to haemorrhage, heat stress or applied acceleration) will result in a footward shift in the location of the HIP.

Upright Posture

Postural changes that occur during activities of daily life alter the HP component acting upon the cardiovascular system. The average human spends about two-thirds of their day upright, which is a hydrostatically unfavourable state. The principle effect on the cardiovascular system of assuming an upright posture (an orthostatic challenge) is an immediate hydrostatically-induced redistribution of intravascular volume. The majority of this redistributed volume comes from the low-pressure venous side of the circulation. Researchers have shown that about 500 to 600 mls of blood moves into the lower limb veins and another 200 to 300 mls shifts into the buttock and pelvic veins (Rowell, 1986, 1993). This volume shift is significant, and it must be remembered that this redistribution occurs during quiet standing in a +1 Gz environment.

Sjostrand (1952) further established that about 78 per cent of this redistributed blood volume comes from intrathoracic vessels (which thus act as a blood volume reservoir). During postural changes (such as those occurring with normal daily activities) significant amounts of blood volume are shifted from one end of the circulation to the other, with the middle part of the circulation (that is, the abdominal or splanchnic region) remaining essentially unaffected (Rowell, 1986, 1993; Sjostrand, 1952). The state of the circulation during the orthostatic challenge of upright posture has been described as reflecting a 'functional haemorrhage into the dependent vascular bed' (Gauer and Thron, 1965).

Upright posture represents a significant challenge to the human circulation due to the latter's intrinsic properties. Approximately 75 per cent of the human blood volume is contained in the compliant low-pressure venous system, with only about 15–20 per cent within the high-pressure arterial side of the circulation (Rowell, 1986). When upright, about 70–75 per cent of the total blood volume is below the level of the heart. Indeed, approximately 65 per cent of venous return (VR) to the heart travels via the inferior vena caval system. Because of the distensible, elastic properties of the dependent vascular bed, the total blood volume is effectively too small to fill the circulatory system in upright posture. If the vascular container consisted of a series of rigid tubes rather than distensible ones this posture would be more tolerable for humans.

The redistribution of intravascular volume due to the HP gradient, therefore, is dependent on the position of the body, the characteristics of the blood vessels and the nature and strength of the gravitational field. The redistribution of blood volume to the capacitance vessels of the lower limbs results in an increased mean transit time for the larger volume of blood present. In this sense the term 'peripheral pooling' that is often used to describe the redistribution of blood volume to the lower limbs is actually a misnomer. Peripheral pooling implies that blood is stagnant in the peripheral venous system, which it is not. Rather, due to the increased blood volume and the capacitance of the blood vessels the transit time through the lower limbs is increased.

When upright, the human heart must generate a dynamic pressure that is able to overcome the hydrostatic challenge to cerebral perfusion. However, ventricular filling and therefore SV are secondarily affected by the hydrostatically-mediated volume redistribution. Ventricular filling pressure decreases as a result of decreased VR. This then results in a decrease in SV, in accordance with the Frank–Starling length–tension relationship. Changes in ventricular filling pressure due to intravascular volume redistribution thus have a significant effect on the pump performance of the heart. Heart volume decreases during upright posture, by up to 130 mls in men and 90 mls in women (Gauer and Thron, 1965). CO can only be maintained by either an increase in heart rate (HR) or an increase in cardiac contractility. This latter mechanism is limited, for even at rest under normal conditions the left ventricular ejection fraction is 70 per cent.

With a large decrease in ventricular filling pressure, SV will decrease and HR must therefore increase to at least maintain CO, if not increase it. SV falls to a level of 50–60 per cent of the recumbent level. HR increases by 10 to 20 beats per minute, but generally this increase is not enough to prevent a fall in CO to 60–80 per cent of the recumbent level. Systolic pressure tends to remain relatively constant, while DP rises. This then tends to reduce arterial pulse pressure (PP). However, TPR increases by 30–40 per cent, which accounts for the overall reduction in regional blood flow (to the splanchnic viscera, kidneys, skin and skeletal muscle). Autoregulation limits the fall in cerebral blood flow to 6 per cent (Rowell, 1986). Without autoregulation, of course, this reduction would obviously be greater. As a result, in the upright steady state, MAP tends to be maintained at the supine level, but in some cases may have increased slightly.

Hydrostatic Pressure and the Giraffe

To put the concept of HP and the attendant circulatory effects into perspective, it is worth digressing at this point to consider a unique example. In the animal world, the giraffe (*Giraffa Camelopardalis*) is perhaps the animal singularly most affected by the challenge of upright posture (Warren, 1974). As such, it represents a useful animal model for the cardiovascular consequences of exposure to a high +Gz environment.

The most striking and obvious feature of the giraffe is, of course, its long neck, quite apart from its overall size. A full-grown giraffe can be up to 6 metres tall, with a neck length of approximately 2 metres. The magnitude of this brain–heart hydrostatic barrier represents a tremendous orthostatic challenge to this particular animal. Several unique features of the giraffe's circulatory system, however, allow it to maintain an optimum cerebral perfusion despite the hydrostatic effect it experiences. Firstly, the arterial walls in the neck are extremely thick and muscular, in order to tolerate the high driving pressures generated by the heart. They possess abundant elastic connective tissue, and the lumina are small relative to overall vessel diameter. In a quietly standing giraffe, MAP at brain level is about 90 mmHg. Left ventricular systolic pressures have been measured in the range of 260–285 mmHg. This large driving pressure is essential in order to overcome the hydrostatic barrier in the neck, which represents a pressure differential of about 118 mmHg for a brain–heart distance of 160 cm. Contrast this with the brain–heart distance in man of about 30 cm for a pressure differential of some 22 mmHg.

Mean aortic pressure in the giraffe has been measured at 220 mmHg, while left ventricular end-DP is about 10–18 mmHg. Clearly the giraffe's heart empties forcefully with each heart beat, and the muscular arterial walls tend to result in a high peripheral resistance. These factors tend to sustain cerebral perfusion at the required level.

The effect of gravity will facilitate VR to the heart from the cerebral circulation in the upright position. However, a new and rather unique problem arises when drinking is considered. To drink, the giraffe must lower its head to ground level. In so doing, it places its cerebral circulation and the subsequent VR to the heart at a distinct hydrostatic disadvantage. VR must be made against a large hydrostatic barrier created by a height differential of about 4 metres. To ensure appropriate VR when its head is lowered, the giraffe has a unique feature in the venous system of the neck. The neck veins have a system of valves oriented in such a way as to prevent backflow of blood into the brain when the head is lowered below the level of the heart, as in drinking. In the upright position, these valves do not interfere with normal gravity-dependent flow back to the heart. In that respect they function much like the venous valves in the lower limbs of humans.

The legs of the giraffe are encased in a tightly adherent non-distensible hide. This confers some hydrostatic countermeasure to the animal, as it tends to maintain a high transmural pressure in the capacitance vessels. This then ensures that peripheral pooling is minimised, and also reduces the fluid filtration and translocation that could be expected to occur as a secondary effect of the large HP head.

The giraffe is thus well equipped to deal with the HP effects generated by its size and unique anatomical features. It is well adapted to upright posture. The human cardiovascular system also does not simply allow hydrostatic forces to redistribute intravascular volume to the point of circulatory compromise. If it did, humans would never have been able to adopt the upright position, as syncope would inevitably result every time. Instead, the cardiovascular system mounts a dynamic response to any postural change. It does so by utilising various compensatory mechanisms which deal with the effects of postural changes on the circulation. These are considered in the next section.

Countermeasures to Orthostasis

The cardiovascular system must be able to deal with orthostatic challenges to prevent circulatory embarrassment when assuming the upright position. If there are no compensatory mechanisms brought to bear, the sequestration of blood volume in the dependent vascular bed will eventually deny the heart an adequate VR with which to generate the required level of cerebral perfusion. The end result of this series of events is loss of consciousness. To prevent such circulatory compromise from occurring, the cardiovascular system has several mechanisms for dealing with the effects of postural changes on the circulation. These include certain structural elements within the cardiovascular system (the venous valves, the venous volume-pressure relationship and microcirculatory changes), and several dynamic mechanisms (the muscle pump, the respiratory pump and the various baroreceptor-mediated responses).

Venous Valves

The veins of the lower limbs contain a series of one-way valves that facilitate the return of blood to the heart against the HP gradient (Blomqvist and Stone, 1983; Rowell, 1986). These valves effectively break up the hydrostatic column of blood. On assumption of the upright posture, the increasing arterial pressure fills the veins and the valves open in a heartward progression. Eventually there is an uninterrupted hydrostatic column between the right atrium and the feet, with the valves tending to prevent retrograde flow.

Venous Volume-Pressure Relationship

The distensible nature of the veins gives them a capacitance role. As such, large changes in volume result in small changes in transmural pressure (Rowell, 1986). This is an important evolutionary feature, in that large volume changes (such as in haemorrhage) do not affect venous (and therefore arterial) pressure significantly. The compliant nature of the veins allows significant volume changes to be accommodated with little overall detriment. As volume increases, however, the veins become progressively less compliant (Rowell, 1993). This tends to limit the degree of peripheral pooling that can occur.

Microcirculatory Changes

Compliance of the low-pressure venous side of the circulation in the dependent parts of the body tends to vary during upright posture, due to the effects of HP. At the microvascular level, increased blood volume in the lower limb veins leads to increased capillary HP, and therefore to greater amounts of fluid filtration into the extravascular tissues (oedema formation). However, over time, the extravascular tissue pressure rises and tends to counterbalance the intravascular pressure, reducing filtration pressure and thus the rate of tissue filtration and the amount of fluid loss. This is the Starling–Landis principle (Rowell, 1993).

However, while the extravascular pressure effects tend to reduce venous capacitance, the viscoelastic properties of the veins themselves tend to offset this effect to an extent by allowing their volume to expand (increased capacitance) while maintaining a set transmural pressure. Nonetheless, oedema is thus a self-limiting phenomenon that restricts filtration and changes in venous transmural pressure (which tends to remain constant despite the hydrostatic effect of upright posture). As a consequence, lower limb vascular capacitance is also restricted.

The Muscle Pump

In addition to its primary roles of postural stabilisation and locomotion, the musculature of the lower limbs acts as an accessory pump or 'second heart' (Rowell, 1986). The importance of this muscle pump should not be overlooked. According to Rowell (1986), totally passive upright posture with no input from the muscle pump is a potentially lethal stress for humans. Hydrostatically-mediated peripheral sequestration of blood volume can eventually result in ventricular filling pressure being reduced to an inadequate level to maintain SV and CO. In the presence of competent venous valves, the muscle pump is able to generate driving forces of 90 mmHg. SV is returned to normal levels by even modest contractions of the lower limb anti-gravity muscles (Rowell, 1986). The action of the muscle pump is routinely exploited by soldiers standing on parade for considerable periods of time. These individuals rhythmically contract their lower limb muscles to maintain their SV and thus avoid syncope.

The Respiratory Pump

In a similar way, the respiratory cycle acts to augment VR. Inspiration accelerates the central discharge of vena caval blood through an increase in intra-abdominal pressure relative to intra-thoracic pressure. Expiration reduces intra-abdominal pressure and encourages cephalad blood flow from the thorax as the diaphragm relaxes and ascends (Rowell, 1986, 1993). In conjunction with these respiratory movements, the liver acts as a 'pre-right ventricular sump' (Rowell, 1986, 1993). Diaphragmatic movements during breathing affect hepatic venous outflow in a sequence out-of-phase with caval blood flow. Inspiration compresses hepatic veins, while raising of the diaphragm during expiration allows hepatic venous outflow. This tends to smooth out fluctuations in central venous pressure due to respiratory movements.

The Baroreflexes

Perhaps the most significant and well-studied of the cardiovascular compensatory mechanisms are the baroreflexes. These consist of the arterial baroreflexes on the high-pressure side of the circulation, and the cardiopulmonary baroreflexes on the low-pressure side.

The application of Engineering Control Theory to physiological research has led to the baroreflexes being considered as a closed-loop negative feedback control system, the sole purpose of which is to control arterial BP within a specific range (Dorf, 1989; Kalmus, 1966; Milhorn, 1966; Shinners, 1998). As a negative feedback loop, the human baroreflex system is designed to maintain BP at an optimum functional level. It does this by using any deviation from normal values as a mismatch or error signal with which to drive the control loop back towards restoration of the predetermined optimum level (Dorf, 1989; Guyton and Hall, 1996).

The error signal is proportional to the difference between the actual pressure and the desired or pre-set value, and the goal of the baroreflex system is to eliminate this difference. Cerebral perfusion is therefore maintained and loss of consciousness is prevented. It is a system expressly designed to ensure that all organ systems of the body are adequately perfused despite any postural alterations, such as in going from a lying to a standing position, or when experiencing high +Gz loads (Bevegard et al., 1977; Blomqvist and Stone, 1983; Borst et al., 1982; Downing, 1983; Fulco et al., 1985; Hainsworth and Al-Shamma, 1988; Harrison et al., 1986; Howard, 1965; Kircheim, 1976; Mancia and Mark, 1983; Sagawa, 1983; Sprangers et al., 1991; Tuckman and Shillingford, 1966; Ward et al., 1966; Weiss and Baker, 1933).

The operation of the baroreflexes is relatively simplistic. Increases in mean distending pressure cause a stretching of the walls of the major arteries and cardiac chambers, which in turn stimulates stretch receptors located within these structures. These stretch receptors (or mechanoreceptors, as they are also perhaps more appropriately known) transmit electrical signals to the vasomotor centre in the medulla oblongata region of the brainstem. In accordance with the normal operation of such proprioceptive reflex arcs, signals are then transmitted via effector nerves to the heart (to decrease HR) and blood vessels (to vasodilate) which eventually result in a lowering of arterial pressure. The converse applies when pressure decreases. This reflex is physiologically very important, as it produces a generally stable arterial pressure level despite wide-ranging external influences (Blomqvist and Stone, 1983; Downing, 1983; Hainsworth and Al-Shamma, 1988; Mancia and Mark, 1983; Weiss and Baker, 1933).

Anatomical Structure of the Baroreflexes

The arterial baroreflexes have been by far the most widely studied. Details of the role and function of the arterial baroreflexes began to emerge in 1900 through the work of two Italian physiologists, Pagano and Siciliano, who discovered that the pressor effect of common carotid artery occlusion in dogs depended on certain nervous structures within the neck (Mancia and Mark, 1983). The German physiologists Hering and Koch discovered in the 1920s that these structures were branches of the glossopharyngeal nerve (Mancia and Mark, 1983). A significant amount of research since that time has established that these reflexes are of paramount importance in the regulation of the human circulatory system.

There are two principal arterial baroreflex arcs, named after the anatomical locations of their receptors: the carotid sinus baroreflex and the aortic baroreflex. The carotid sinus baroreceptors are, as the name suggests, located in the carotid sinus (Downing, 1983; Guyton and Hall, 1996; Mancia and Mark, 1983; Weiss and Baker, 1933). The carotid sinus is a segmental fusiform dilatation of the upper part of the common carotid and the adjacent part of the internal carotid arteries. The walls of the sinus are much more elastic, due largely to the significantly higher collagen and elastin content of the sinus wall compared with that of adjoining segments of the carotid system (Downing, 1983). Within the walls of the carotid sinus are found a multitude of spray-type nerve endings that function as stretch receptors. These stretch receptors are predominantly located in the adventitia of the sinus wall next to the media. The nerve terminals or sensory fibres are unmyelinated, 2–4 micrometres in size, and quite morphologically variable (Downing, 1983). The aortic baroreceptors are located in the arch of the aorta, and consist of the same form of spray-type stretch receptor nerve endings, located within the artery walls at the medial–adventitial interface in great numbers. There is less morphological variation in the nerve endings in the aortic receptors than in the carotid receptors (Downing, 1983).

The cardiopulmonary baroreceptors have not been as extensively investigated due to significant methodological and practical limitations (Folkow et al., 1965). These mechanoreceptors are similar functionally and morphologically to the high-pressure arterial receptors (Guyton and Hall, 1996). They are concentrated within the walls of the pulmonary arteries, near the bifurcation of the main pulmonary artery into right and left branches, and in the sub-endocardial part of the atria near the venoatrial junctions (Hainsworth, 1991; Tanaka et al., 1996).

Afferent impulses are transmitted from the various baroreceptors to the nucleus of the tractus solitarius (NTS) in the posterolateral medulla and lower pons (Guyton and Hall, 1996; Seagard et al., 2000). The carotid sinus impulses are transmitted along a small branch of the glossopharyngeal nerve (Cranial Nerve IX) known as the sinus nerve (or Hering's nerve, for it was originally described by him in 1923), while afferent impulses from the remaining baroreceptors travel via the vagus nerves (Downing, 1983). From the NTS, secondary fibres communicate with vasodilator and vasoconstrictor areas in the rostral and caudal parts of the ventrolateral medulla (Sasaki and Dampney, 1990). These three areas constitute the vasomotor centre (Guyton and Hall, 1996), which lies close to the dorsal motor nucleus of the vagus (the vagal centre). Secondary impulses from the NTS also travel to this latter centre.

Efferent sympathetic impulses from the vasomotor centre are then transmitted to the heart and blood vessels via the paravertebral sympathetic chain, while efferent parasympathetic impulses are conducted along the vagus nerves (Cranial Nerve X) via the vagal centre. The vasomotor centre thus receives afferent inputs from several sources and integrates this information before dispatching the appropriate efferent impulses via common output arms.

Function of the Baroreflexes

Baroreceptor inputs maintain both a tonic inhibitory influence on the vasomotor centre, that tends to limit vasoconstriction, and a tonic excitatory influence on the vagal centre, that tends to produce the parasympathetically-mediated decreases in HR and cardiac contractility. This set of circumstances represents the normal balance between sympathetic and parasympathetic tone in the cardiovascular system that results in a certain resting HR and resting arterial BP in a given individual (Bishop and Sanderford, 2000; Guyton and Hall, 1996; Mancia and Mark, 1983).

If arterial pressure falls, the arterial baroreceptor input decreases. It loses its normal inhibitory effect on the medullary vasomotor centre, allowing this centre to produce a degree of peripheral vasoconstriction mediated by the sympathetic nervous system. Efferent sympathetic impulses to the heart increase atrial and ventricular contractility, sino-atrial node frequency and atrio-ventricular node conduction. The reduced excitation of the vagal centre results in less parasympathetic influence. The tone of the circulatory system has thus shifted to be more in favour of the sympathetic system, resulting in an increase in both HR and cardiac contractility. These measures tend to return arterial pressure to its normal level (Borst et al., 1982; Cooke et al., 1999; Downing, 1983; Eckberg et al., 1988; Fritsch et al., 1991; Guyton and Hall, 1996; Mancia and Mark, 1983; Seidel et al., 1997; Smith et al., 1994; Sprangers et al., 1991; Ward et al., 1966; Weiss and Baker, 1933). This outcome is shown in Figure 3.2.

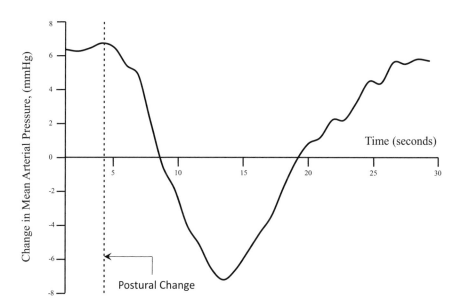

Figure 3.2   Arterial blood pressure (BP) response to upright postural change

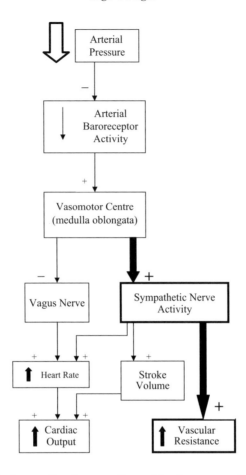

Figure 3.3   The baroreflex in operation – blood pressure (BP) decrease

Conversely, any increase in arterial pressure will cause activation of the baroreceptors and an increase in the degree of vasomotor inhibition and vagal excitation. The parasympathetic system assumes the dominant position in this situation. The efferent vagal cholinergic impulses depress sino-atrial node activity, atrial contractility and transmission through the atrio-ventricular node. These effects will lead to vasodilatation, bradycardia and a relative reduction in cardiac contractility, thereby resulting in a reduction in arterial pressure until the normal BP level is restored.

Various research techniques have been developed in order to study the baroreflexes in both humans and animals. Simple blockade of the vagus nerves, either pharmacologically or surgically, allows study of the aortic baroreceptors.

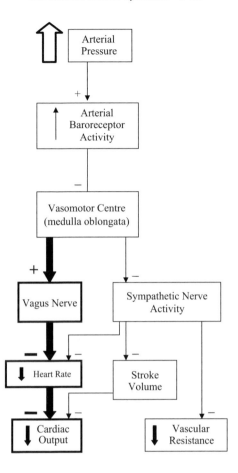

Figure 3.4   The baroreflex in operation – blood pressure (BP) increase

The variable pressure neck chamber has proved to be a useful tool for studying the carotid baroreflexes, as it allows various incremental increases and decreases in transmural pressure to be applied externally to the carotid sinus. A major limitation of this technique, however, is that carotid sinus baroreflex-mediated BP responses may be modified by the action of the aortic baroreflex, which tends to produce an opposite effect. Despite the technical and methodological limitations of these research tools, a significant amount of information has been developed over the years in terms of the role and function of the arterial baroreflexes.

The general function of the arterial baroreflexes is summarised in Figure 3.3 (pressure fall) and Figure 3.4 (pressure rise).

Heart Rate Effects

The baroreflex effect on HR can develop rapidly and effectively modulate the cardiac pacemaker on a beat-to-beat basis (Mancia and Mark, 1983; Smith et al., 1994). However, the latency of HR response (the time from the onset of a change in baroreceptor activity levels to the first alteration of the R-R interval, which is the interval from the peak of one heart beat to the peak of the next on an electrocardiogram trace) varies between deactivation and stimulation of the reflex. Latencies have been measured in the order of 200–600 milliseconds for baroreceptor stimulation, with slightly longer periods for deactivation. This difference in latencies of the arterial baroreflexes is thought to be a function of asymmetric central integrating processes (Mancia and Mark, 1983). Baroreceptor modulation of the atrio-ventricular node maintains a constant time interval between atrial and ventricular events during HR changes (Mancia and Mark, 1983).

Blood Pressure Effects

The arterial baroreflex system exerts a profound influence on control of BP. In addition to mean distending pressure, PP appears to be an important factor in activation of the baroreflexes, particularly the carotid system (Downing, 1983; Gauer and Thron, 1965). Arterial pressure regulation is influenced by two additional characteristics of the system. The first relates to an inherent degree of physiological inertia (Mancia and Mark, 1983). Changes in vascular resistance and cardiac contractility are mediated by the slower-responding sympathetic nervous system, while changes in HR are vagally mediated (and thus faster-responding). The latency period for arterial pressure decrease with baroreceptor stimulation is about 3 seconds, but that for arterial pressure increase with baroreceptor deactivation is greater (in the order of several seconds) (Mancia and Mark, 1983). If the stimulus is maintained, a peak fall in pressure is reached after 10–20 seconds for baroreflex stimulation, compared with 20–30 seconds for peak rise in pressure for baroreflex deactivation (Mancia and Mark, 1983). The inertia (due to the long latencies and slowly developing responses) of the baroreflex system helps to promote a stable arterial pressure despite phasic changes in baroreceptor stimulation (such as occur with respiration).

The second characteristic is an asymmetric pattern of response to arterial pressure changes. Baroreflex responses to sustained arterial pressure decreases (deactivation) are greater than those for arterial pressure increases (stimulation). Indeed, studies of baroreflex sensitivity suggest a 48 per cent increase in sensitivity when deactivation is compared with stimulation (Mancia and Mark, 1983). It would appear that this is a natural, inherent function of the arterial baroreflex system. This asymmetry of response has been verified experimentally by several investigators. Neck chamber studies have shown that the carotid baroreflex can buffer approximately two-thirds of the pressure change that reduces baroreceptor activity (that is, reduced arterial pressure), and about one-half of the pressure change that increases activity (that is, increased arterial pressure) (Mancia and Mark, 1983).

This buffering effect may, however, be underestimated, due to the fact that changes in neck pressure can produce opposing effects on aortic and carotid baroreflexes. Nonetheless, this asymmetry of response is an important operating characteristic of the arterial baroreflexes. It translates in practical terms into the fact that the system is much better able to buffer a decrease in arterial pressure than an increase (Downing, 1983; Mancia and Mark, 1983). It is functionally skewed towards defending the cardiovascular system against a potentially disastrous fall in arterial perfusing pressure.

The modulation of TPR is dependent on the relative tone of the sympathetic nervous system, and as such is influenced by arterial baroreflex activity. This influence is important in determining the magnitude of the baroreceptor–blood pressure response. The arterial baroreflexes exert a degree of control over regional circulations, such as the skin, skeletal muscle and splanchnic region. While the role of arterial baroreflexes in the control of cutaneous circulation remains inconclusive, they do appear to significantly influence resistance vessels in the splanchnic circulation. Current research findings suggest that while the overall role of arterial baroreflexes in the control of limb vascular resistance is minor, the possibility exists that they exert a highly dynamic influence over the skeletal muscle circulation. It has been speculated that arterial baroreceptor control of skeletal muscle circulation is suited to rapid, short-term arterial pressure changes, while longer-term changes are mediated by baroreflex effects on splanchnic and other vascular regions (Mancia and Mark, 1983).

In terms of baroreflex control of venous circulation, studies revealing that no change in central venous pressure occurs after either arterial baroreflex stimulation or deactivation suggest that, as in animals, these baroreflexes do not have any influence over the venous circulation in humans. Indeed, current evidence favours vasoconstriction rather than venoconstriction as the major adjustment to upright posture (Rowell, 1986). In general terms, the action of the baroreflexes on cardiovascular dynamics on assuming an upright posture results in a headward shift in the location of the HIP. This new position has been described as the regulated HIP (Gauer and Thron, 1965).

Regulation of Blood Pressure

The arterial baroreflex system has little function in terms of the long-term regulation of BP. It is a system designed to counter short-term perturbations in BP and to thereby maintain a relatively constant perfusion pressure. In this sense it is an effective system of cardiovascular control. Cowley's experiments on dogs that had undergone sino-aortic denervation (Guyton and Hall, 1996) and later studies by other researchers (Mancia and Mark, 1983) support the notion that the primary function of the baroreflexes is to buffer and protect against transient deviations from the normal pre-set BP level, rather than to mediate long-term regulation of arterial pressure.

The reflexes produced by the cardiopulmonary baroreceptors are in parallel with those of the arterial baroreceptors. While they do not detect systemic pressure, they respond to small pressure differences in the low-pressure side of the circulation, thereby minimising the effect of central blood volume changes (due to postural changes, for example) (Bevegard et al., 1977; Churchill and Bungo, 1997; Mack et al., 1991; Zoller et al., 1972). The combination of high- and low-pressure baroreceptors results in a significantly more powerful system for regulation of arterial pressure (Guyton and Hall, 1996). This is well illustrated by an experiment in which dogs were infused with a bolus of 300 mls of blood. With all reflexes intact, arterial pressure rose by 15 mmHg. With the arterial baroreceptors denervated, pressure rose by 50 mmHg, but rose by 120 mmHg with denervation of the cardiopulmonary receptors as well (Guyton and Hall, 1996).

The Role of the Vestibular System

There are good theoretical grounds for the existence of a neural control link between the vestibular and cardiovascular systems. Postural changes are accurately transduced by the vestibular system in order to derive an accurate internal model of spatial orientation, and also to maintain balance. It seems logical that vestibular inputs could be used to assist in the maintenance of an adequate cerebral perfusing pressure during orthostatic stress.

There is experimental evidence supporting the existence of a link between the vestibular system and cardiovascular control. Some of the earliest work was performed by Spiegel and Demetriades (Yates, 1996) in the 1900s. Using both electrical and caloric stimulation of vestibular afferents they demonstrated increases in BP in a variety of animals such as cats and dogs. Subsequent experiments have determined that vestibular stimulation results in increased sympathetic activity, and that this mediates the cardiovascular changes (Yates, 1996). Furthermore, this increase in sympathetic outflow can be abolished by experimental lesions in the vestibular nuclei (Yates, 1996). Woodring et al. (1997) demonstrated increased sympathetic nerve activity and a consequent pressor response (manifested by BP increases without corresponding HR increases) following nose-up vestibular stimulation in cats. This response was abolished in cats with transected vestibular nerves. Other researchers have reported similar findings (Jian et al., 1999). Doba and Reis (1974) found that cats with bilaterally transected vestibular nerves were unable to compensate for the orthostatic hypotension produced by head-up tilt (HUT), whereas normal cats with intact vestibular nerves fared much better.

Studies in human subjects have also pointed to the existence of a link between the vestibular system and cardiovascular control (Yates and Miller, 1998). Shortt and Ray (1997) found that head-down neck flexion (HDNF) in human subjects promoted an increase in muscle sympathetic nerve activity that caused subsequent rises in calf vascular resistance. Essandoh et al. (1988) reported similar increases in forearm and calf vascular resistance. Skin sympathetic nerve activity, however, does not seem to be affected by HDNF (Ray et al., 1997).

Based on these findings, the suggested link between the vestibular system and cardiovascular control has become known as the vestibulosympathetic reflex, VSR (Jáuregui-Renaud et al., 2006; Schlegel et al., 1998; Woodring et al., 1997; Yates, 1992, 1996; Yates and Miller, 1994). The efferent output of the reflex appears to be an increase in peripheral vascular resistance, which is sympathetically-mediated (Ray et al., 1997; Shortt and Ray, 1997; Woodring et al., 1997). There is little evidence that the parasympathetic system is influenced by the vestibular system (Woodring et al., 1997; Yates, 1992). HR changes have not been consistently shown as a result of vestibular stimulation (Ray et al., 1997; Woodring et al., 1997).

Experimental findings suggest that the VSR is primarily the result of otolith activation, as the changes in sympathetic outflow are limited to pitch inputs rather than roll or yaw (Yates, 1996). Furthermore, the response characteristics and gain of the VSR to sinusoidal pitch inputs are similar to otolith afferents (Yates, 1996). Researchers have concluded that a specific group of vestibular receptors (otolithic pitch responders) is responsible for vestibulosympathetic responses, and that these responses are appropriate to offset hydrostatic challenges to the circulation, such as postural changes and exposure to the high +Gz environment (Yates, 1996).

Furthermore, the vestibular system may have a role as a feed-forward mechanism in the regulation of arterial pressure. Woodring et al. (1997) commented on the likelihood that vestibular signals could provide feed-forward adjustment of arterial pressure during unexpected postural change. Via the vestibulo-ocular neural pathways, inputs from the visual system during postural change will supplement the vestibular information, and may augment this feed-forward mechanism. Ray et al. (1997) postulated that the vestibular system could signal postural changes (and the attendant cardiovascular consequences) before the baroreflexes become active. The interesting question is where do the feed-forward pathways project? Does the vestibular information feed forward to the baroreflex system, or independently to the peripheral vasculature? Or does it send parallel inputs to both? These questions remain largely unanswered.

Conclusion

The heart is effectively at the mercy of the hydrostatic force, as it can only pump out what it receives from the dependent regions of the body in terms of VR, which due to peripheral pooling is often less than required. For these reasons, upright posture represents a significant challenge to the human circulation.

The importance of the cardiovascular control mechanisms is only truly realised when they fail. Such failure can occur either as a consequence of some pathological condition or disease state, or during changes in applied hydrostatic force due to a change in the gravitational field. In all of these situations, regulatory and controlling ability over the circulatory system is lost, and the hydrostatic effects of the ambient gravitational field are left unchecked. The result is somewhat inevitable: the individual with such an impairment will experience syncope on assuming (or attempting to assume) the upright posture. This can be totally disabling. Pathological conditions or disease states that can result in such autonomic insufficiency vary from diabetes mellitus to rare conditions involving autonomic failure such as multiple system atrophy (MSA), formerly known as Shy-Drager syndrome (Brook, 1994; Kaufmann, 1996; Shy and Drager, 1960; Wenning et al., 2004). This latter syndrome is characterised by severe orthostatic hypotension and Parkinsonian features such as akinesia and rigidity.

Changes in the gravitational field result in the circulatory system experiencing an altered hydrostatic force, which can render the baroreflex system ineffective in its attempt to restore normal perfusion pressure if the change in hydrostatic force is too great. This latter situation will be addressed in the next chapter, which deals with the cardiovascular system's behaviour when exposed to high G forces.

Chapter 4
The Cardiovascular System at High Gz

The previous chapter examined the function and responses of the cardiovascular system under normal conditions of +1 Gz. However, the cardiovascular system can be subjected to accelerations well in excess of the normal level of +1 Gz, as occurs in modern high-performance fighter aircraft, civilian aerobatic aircraft and the launch phase of spaceflight, as seen in Chapter 2. These accelerations impose significant stress on the humans subjected to them. In this chapter the cardiovascular consequences of exposure to high levels of G are examined.

From a cardiovascular perspective, the effects of G represent a continuum. The cardiovascular system's inherent difficulties in ensuring adequate supply of blood to the eyes and brain in a high G environment leads to several significant issues such as visual impairment and ultimately loss of consciousness. These issues are all a result of the impact of hydrostatic force, considered in the previous chapter. Due to its orientation in the long axis of the body, the cardiovascular system is by far and away the system most affected by exposure to G-induced HP increases.

Effects of Acceleration on the Circulation

The physiological problems inherent in exposure to accelerations beyond +1 Gz are simply accentuations of the same problems encountered by humans when they assume upright posture, which is essentially an applied acceleration of +1 G in the z axis. The hydrostatic effects of this force have been well described (Armstrong and Heim, 1938; Blomqvist and Stone, 1983; Fong and Fan, 1997; Gauer and Thron, 1965; Green, 2006a; Green and Miller, 1973; Howard, 1965; Ludwig and Convertino, 1994; Peterson et al., 1975; Rowell, 1986, 1993; Stewart, 1945). These same hydrostatic forces are at work when the human is subjected to +2, +4 or +9 Gz, but are obviously several orders of magnitude greater. The physiological consequences are thus magnifications of what occurs at +1 Gz. Indeed, the cardiovascular system endeavours to cope with these effects in much the same way, albeit with differing results in many cases.

Exposure to high levels of applied +Gz causes considerable fluid shifts and redistribution throughout the body. Plasma volume is lost to the interstitial space, with a sustained exposure to +4 Gz leading to a fluid loss of 200 mls/min in the lower limbs (Blomqvist and Stone, 1983; Green, 2006a). The heart is vulnerable to +Gz acceleration, and some centrifuge studies have shown that systolic and diastolic chamber volumes were reduced under +Gz, which also tended to force the heart downwards. The mechanical effects of applied +Gz on the heart have been implicated in the development of cardiac arrhythmias, as discussed in Chapter 7.

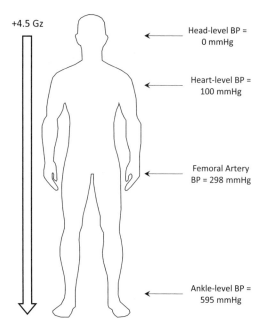

Figure 4.1   Blood pressure (BP) changes with high +Gz exposure

As seen in Chapter 3, the arterial pressure of the human in the upright posture varies in accordance with the magnitude of the hydrostatic force. The effect of high +Gz exposure on the BP gradient throughout the body is shown in Figure 4.1. Arterial pressure at head level is reduced under high +Gz, while arterial pressures below the heart increase with distance from the heart, such that pressure at the ankle is markedly increased.

Assuming a MAP of 100 mmHg, the arterial pressure above the heart at the base of the brain is about 78 mmHg. There is therefore a pressure differential between the heart and the brain of 22 mmHg at an applied acceleration of +1 Gz (Green, 2006a; McKinley et al., 2005). This pressure differential is increased by a factor proportional to the magnitude of the applied acceleration. Thus, at +2 Gz, the pressure differential will be 44 mmHg, and at +4 Gz it will be 88 mmHg. From this analysis, it can be determined that if the MAP remains at a level of 100 mmHg, blood flow to the brain will cease at an applied acceleration of +4.5 Gz. This would then result in a G-LOC. Indeed, it was von Diringshofen who originally described human tolerance to +Gz as being within the range of +4.5 to +5.5 Gz (Von Beckh, 1981).

In practical terms, cerebral blood flow does not actually cease at the hydrostatically-predicted +Gz level. The hydrostatic forces involved in +Gz exposure are applied equally to the venous system and the cerebrospinal fluid, as well as the arterial system. An arteriovenous pressure gradient is maintained under gravitational stress, even when arterial pressure falls to zero (Henry et al., 1950; Rushmer et al., 1947).

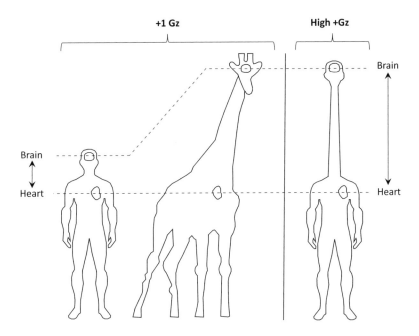

Figure 4.2   Rushmer's human–giraffe comparison

In this situation, provided the veins do not collapse due to the negative internal pressure (values of -60 mmHg at the jugular bulb have been recorded), cerebral blood flow will be maintained by the 'jugular siphon' effect (Henry et al., 1950). Cerebral autoregulation is also an important factor in this 'perfusion without pressure' concept, which was first postulated by Ranke in 1937 (Wood, 1990). Cerebral blood flow thus continues beyond the level of gravitational force that hydrostatic considerations would predict. However, at approximately +5 Gz (for a relaxed healthy subject) cerebral perfusion cannot be sustained any longer and unconsciousness then results (Blomqvist and Stone, 1983; Burns, 1992; Burton et al., 1974; Fong and Fan, 1997; Howard, 1965; Parkhurst et al., 1972; Werchan, 1991).

This increasing pressure differential between heart and brain during exposure to +Gz acceleration has been compared with the cardiovascular dynamics of the giraffe (Guggisberg, 1969; Schmidt-Neilsen, 1991; Warren, 1974). Rushmer (1947) described the effect of applied acceleration on human cardiovascular dynamics as the physiological equivalent of being transformed into a giraffe. This analogy makes quite a deal of sense. At an acceleration of +4 Gz, the pressure differential is 88 mmHg. This same pressure differential could be generated at +1 Gz, *inter alia*, if the human neck was extended by a proportional amount, that is, by assuming the form of a giraffe. This is shown in Figure 4.2. Rushmer's analogy allows a good understanding of the basic cardiovascular effects of applied acceleration.

Effect of Acceleration on Vision

As the human cardiovascular system is exposed to acceleration, the increasing hydrostatic force is well tolerated up to a certain point. Then, a number of well-defined changes occur. The most significant of these affects the visual system, particularly the retina (Jaeger et al., 1964). The human eye has an internal pressure of 15–20 mmHg (Bayer et al., 2004; Green, 2006a). As the G load increases, so too does HP, which in turn accentuates the head-to-heart pressure differential. This results in a proportional reduction in BP in the region of the eye. This will affect the delivery of blood and oxygen to the retina, resulting in two well-known +Gz visual phenomena: grey-out and black-out.

As the pressure differential continues to increase with acceleration, there comes a point when the perfusing arterial pressure is less than the internal ocular pressure. At this point, the level of function of the eye becomes impaired due to retinal ischaemia arising through lack of the appropriate level of blood flow. The changes that occur in the vision of the accelerating human subject are well documented (Blomqvist and Stone, 1983; Burton et al., 1974; Burton and Whinnery, 1996; Gillingham et al., 1977; Green, 2006a; Howard, 1965; Jaeger et al., 1964; Weeks et al., 1964; Wood and Sturm, 1989).

Grey-out

At a level of +3 to +4 Gz, retinal blood flow diminishes as arterial pressure approaches the level of internal ocular pressure (Burton and Whinnery, 1996; Green, 2006a). The retinal periphery is first affected, essentially as a function of distance from the blood supply entering the retina (Burton and Whinnery, 1996; Green, 2006a; Jaeger et al., 1964). The delivery BP is not sufficient enough to supply blood and oxygen to the outer edge of the retina. Peripheral vision therefore becomes impaired, and this phenomenon is known as 'grey-out'. This loss of peripheral vision manifests itself as a general greying of vision, sometimes with a tunnel vision effect. The visual field may appear to sparkle, while at the same time being severely degraded. It may also occur in an asymmetric fashion, especially if the head is tilted under high +Gz (with the uppermost eye being affected more). It is the first sign to a pilot that they are experiencing a degree of G-induced cardiovascular compromise. It is a very common symptom, familiar to almost every military pilot. In a survey of RAAF fighter pilots, 98 per cent reported experiencing grey-out (Rickards and Newman, 2005).

Black-out

At a slightly higher level of acceleration, in the order of +4 to +4.5 Gz, blood flow into the retina is prevented by the higher internal ocular pressure relative to the driving arterial pressure (Burton and Whinnery, 1996; Green, 2006a; Whitton, 1992). Complete loss of vision occurs. This is termed 'black-out'.

This term should not be confused with loss of consciousness, with which it is popularly associated. This complete loss of vision typically occurs with the pilot still fully conscious. They are still able to manoeuvre their aircraft, receive radio transmissions, communicate, and so on. There is no mental impairment or motor skill incapacity, and their higher cognitive functions are all still essentially intact. It is only their visual input that has been lost. There is an interval of approximately 4–6 seconds between arterial pressure falling below the critical level of 20 mmHg and complete loss of vision (Green, 2006a). This is due to the existence of a small, short-term reserve oxygen store within the extravascular fluid of the retina which must be exhausted first before loss of vision is apparent (Blomqvist and Stone, 1983; Burton et al., 1974; Green, 2006a; Howard, 1965).

Black-out is more significant a symptom than grey-out, as it is an indication to the pilot that they are approaching the physiological limits of their individual G tolerance. It is, however, less common than grey-out: 29 per cent of RAAF fighter pilots reported experiencing black-out (Rickards and Newman, 2005). Importantly, the symptoms of grey-out and black-out should be considered a visual warning to the pilot of impending loss of consciousness if the G load is maintained or increased.

Almost Loss of Consciousness (A-LOC)

A-LOC (Almost Loss of Consciousness) is a relatively newly described G-related phenomenon that has gained some prominence in recent years. It represents one point on the continuum of G effects, and can be considered to lie between visual symptoms and frank loss of consciousness. According to Shender et al. (2003), the use of the term A-LOC was originally coined at the Naval Air Development Center, Warminster, PA, at some time in the 1980s and subsequently entered the aviation training curriculum. It is a term that aircrew (at least in the United States Navy, USN) have become familiar with.

However, it was for a time a term that was not without controversy in the scientific community. It has been the subject of debate at various meetings, including the International Acceleration Research Workshop. The debate centres on the appropriateness of the term A-LOC. Shender et al. (2003) made the following comment in relation to this debate:

> To be more consistent with the medical literature, the phenomenon should be termed 'Near-Loss of Consciousness', or N-LOC (analogous to the clinical term near-syncope).

However, Shender et al. (2003) advocate continuing with the use of the term A-LOC, given that it has already entered the common parlance of tactical aircrews, and that continuing to use a term accepted by the target audience will help avoid any confusion. A-LOC has subsequently been the subject of several papers, thus ensuring that it remains the commonly used and generally accepted term (Rickards and Newman, 2005).

A-LOC is defined as +Gz-induced impairment of cerebral function with no corresponding loss of consciousness (McGowan, 1997; Morrissette and McGowan, 2000; Shender et al., 2003). It occurs with short duration, rapid onset +Gz exposures, such as 3 seconds at +6 Gz. An episode of A-LOC generally only lasts a short time, in the order of approximately 5 seconds, but the incapacity can extend beyond this time to about 10–15 seconds. If the G load is backed off and adequate blood flow is allowed to return to the brain, the symptoms of A-LOC will resolve quite quickly.

The physiological consequences of a short-term +Gz pulse have attracted some research attention over the years. Beckman et al. (1954) found that a rapid onset, high +Gz pulse of only 4.25 seconds in duration was enough to precipitate G-LOC in subjects. Later centrifuge-based work by Cammarota et al. (1997a, 1997b) duplicated Beckman's +Gz pulse profiles with a view to examining the central nervous system's ability to tolerate acute loss of blood flow. They found that there is a critical balance between oxygen supply and demand. Once this balance is disturbed beyond a critical point, subsequent loss of consciousness is inevitable, as seen by a number of G-LOC events that occurred after a +Gz pulse but after the centrifuge had returned to baseline.

Typically, the pilot with an episode of A-LOC will experience mental impairment, often with a loss of situational awareness (SA). The symptoms are many and varied, and are said to depend on which part of the brain is affected. Cognitive, physical, emotional, and physiological signs and symptoms have all been described, including sensory abnormalities (twitching of the hands, immobility, numbness and tingling), euphoria, amnesia, apathy, loss of short-term memory, and reduced auditory acuity (McGowan, 1997; Morrissette and McGowan, 2000; Shender et al., 2003).

Often A-LOC is said to be associated with the disconnection between the desire and the ability to perform an action (Morrissette and McGowan, 2000; Shender et al., 2003). In one study, an inability to speak or form words was seen in eight out of 66 (12 per cent) A-LOC events (Shender et al., 2003). The subjects apparently knew what they wanted to say but were unable to form and enunciate the words. This difficulty persisted for several seconds after full vision had returned. Such a disconnection between cognition and the ability to act is also evidenced by subjects being able to generally see and hear, but not caring about or adequately attending to what they are seeing and hearing.

A-LOC is an insidious and potentially very serious G-related problem. The effects of A-LOC persist beyond the end of the Gz exposure. From an operational perspective, A-LOC can be a significant in-flight risk if pilots do not realise that A-LOC has occurred. In this situation, pilots may misinterpret their state of awareness, leading to errors, loss of SA, spatial disorientation and potentially a catastrophic outcome. Indeed, as some authors suggest there is a fine line between A-LOC and G-LOC (Shender et al., 2003).

Prevalence of A-LOC

In a survey of A-LOC symptoms in operational fighter pilots, Morrissette and McGowan (2000) reported that 14 per cent of fighter pilots (from the US Air Force, US Navy and US Marines) had experienced A-LOC symptoms including motor, sensory and cognitive abnormalities. In a study involving fighter pilots from the RAAF, at least one A-LOC symptom (not associated with G-LOC) was reported by 52 per cent of the pilots (Rickards and Newman, 2005). In a controlled centrifuge study, Shender et al. (2003) reported 66 A-LOC incidents out of a total of 161 +Gz pulse exposures, a rate of 41 per cent. Clearly, A-LOC is a significant in-flight operational hazard.

The operational hazards associated with pilots experiencing A-LOC can be as dangerous as a complete loss of consciousness. The short-term loss of SA and cognitive impairment, especially if they occur during a critical phase of flight, represent a significant flying safety hazard.

G-Induced Loss of Consciousness (G-LOC)

The principal problem faced by the human cardiovascular system when exposed to a force environment greater than +1 Gz is that the hydrostatic effects of the applied acceleration may overwhelm the system's ability to maintain the required level of cerebral perfusion. When this occurs, G-LOC is the end result. It typically occurs (for a relaxed, unprotected subject) at +4.5 to +5.5 Gz. Such G-induced unconsciousness is clearly a significant life-threatening hazard for a pilot in a high-performance aircraft.

G-LOC has been formally defined (Burton, 1988a) as:

> A state of altered perception wherein (one's) awareness of reality is absent as a result of sudden, critical reduction of cerebral blood circulation caused by increased G force.

G-LOC can be regarded as the most dire consequence of exposure to accelerations greater than +1 Gz.

Historical Aspects of G-LOC

G-LOC is not a new problem. Indeed, it has been a challenge to pilots for many years, almost since humans first took to the skies in powered aircraft. Episodes of 'fainting in the air' were first described during and after the First World War by several authors (Armstrong and Heim, 1938; Burton, 1988a; Livingston, 1939; Von Beckh, 1981). In 1922 the winner of the Pulitzer Air Race is said to have experienced unconsciousness during turns, and the 1923 winner apparently flew an extra lap of the course as a result of being dazed and only partly conscious (Von Beckh, 1981).

In 1924, Lieutenant (later Lieutenant-General) James Doolittle studied the accelerations inherent in aerobatic manoeuvres, concluding that lack of blood flow to the brain and therefore lack of oxygen was responsible for the pilot's resultant 'loss of faculties' (Von Beckh, 1981). Other researchers during the 1930s, such as Dobrotvorskii and Andre Louis Flamme, pointed to the importance of hydrostatic forces in the development of pilot impairment during aerial manoeuvring (Nelson, 1987; Von Beckh, 1981). Flamme in fact theorised that under significant +Gz acceleration the circulation in the internal carotid arteries would slow, then stop and might actually reverse (so-called 'circulation contrarie') (Von Beckh, 1981).

In 1938 Livingston carried out significant research in England into this problem, using modified aircraft to examine human response to acceleration (Livingston, 1939). He accurately reported the time of incapacitation, and also described the attendant event amnesia as well as some of the psychophysiological aspects of G-LOC.

Working in Germany in the 1930s, Dr Heinz von Diringshofen (1900–1967) proposed the hydrostatic theory of tolerance to +Gz, based on elegant experiments he carried out on pilots flying an aircraft instrumented for data collection (Harsch, 2000; Von Beckh, 1981). His hydrostatic theory has contributed significantly to acceleration research, and it has undergone little change since it was first put forward and remains valid today. Much of what is known about the effects of acceleration on the human cardiovascular system is based on von Diringshofen's work, as it generally explains the effects of applied acceleration in a satisfactory way. His experimental work enabled him to identify the limits of human tolerance to acceleration. Indeed, he was arguably the first researcher to accurately describe the BP changes occurring under acceleration stress and the cardiovascular compensations brought to bear as a result. He also showed that reclining the pilot's seat would improve tolerance to +Gz (discussed later in Chapter 8).

By the Second World War, the problem of 'aviator's vertigo' was receiving a lot of attention in many countries, including the United Kingdom, the United States and Canada (Armstrong and Heim, 1938; Burton, 1988a; Lambert and Wood, 1946; Rook, 1938; Stewart, 1945; Vinake, 1948; Von Beckh, 1981). The relatively high-performance aircraft being produced and operated during this conflict were causing physiological problems in the pilots. This 'aviator's vertigo' involved pilots experiencing transient cognitive deficits or impairments not necessarily due to vestibular problems. As knowledge of this problem grew, it became apparent that the accelerations generated by the aircraft were compromising the cardiovascular systems of the aircrew. The body of knowledge concerning G-LOC was beginning to take shape.

Human centrifuges became increasingly popular as research tools, as they were able to generate the same level of acceleration as the aircraft but in a safe and reliable manner. In 1934, von Diringshofen established the world's first human centrifuge for aerospace medicine research at the Aeromedical Research Institute in Berlin, based on plans created by himself and his brother Bernd, a mechanical engineer (Harsch, 2000; Von Beckh, 1981). It had a diameter of 5.4 metres, and a maximum performance of 20 Gz with an onset rate of 1.5 Gs^{-1}. It was used extensively during the Second World War (Harsch, 2000; Von Beckh, 1981). During and immediately after the Second World War, the Allied forces had six such centrifuges which were conducting G-related research, including the Mayo Clinic Centrifuge established in 1942, and the US Navy centrifuge at Warminster, Pennsylvania, established in 1951 (Burton, 1988a; Von Beckh, 1981).

As aircraft became more powerful and manoeuvrable, G-LOC assumed a position of even greater significance. Modern materials technology has allowed fighter aircraft to be developed and produced that are remarkably strong and certainly capable of generating levels of acceleration well beyond the tolerance of the human occupant. The introduction of the F-15 and F-16 fighter aircraft in the mid 1970s illustrates this point quite well. Experience with these new high-performance aircraft led to a resurgence of interest in the problem of G-LOC, which had not received much research attention since the mid 1950s (Beckman et al., 1954; Burton, 1988a; Edelberg et al., 1956; Lyons et al., 1992; Powell et al., 1957; Rayman, 1973a, 1973b; Rayman and McNaughton, 1983; Stewart, 1945; Zuidema et al., 1956). These aircraft were involved in a significant number of accidents, many of which were fatal (Burton, 1988a). A disturbing proportion of these accidents were attributed to pilot incapacitation as a result of G-LOC (Burton, 1988a).

It became apparent that the acceleration envelopes of these aircraft were greater than had previously been experienced, and existing countermeasures were not providing the necessary margin of safety for the pilots. Once again G-LOC became a serious problem in the high-performance aircraft community, and has resulted in the loss of many aircraft and pilots over the last several decades. While the prevalence of G-LOC is considered in a later section, recent surveys of fighter pilots indicate that the problem of G-LOC is certainly still present and still responsible for significant losses of both expensive materiel and highly trained personnel (Alvim, 1995; Hickman, 1991; Johanson and Pheeny, 1988; Lyons et al., 2004; Pluta, 1984; Rickards and Newman, 2005; Ross, 1990). G-LOC thus remains a challenging problem for both researchers and pilots (Cirovic et al., 2000; Hickman, 1991; Rickards and Newman, 2005).

Characteristics of a G-LOC Episode

As discussed earlier, when the applied acceleration is greater than +4.5 to +5.5 Gz, the driving pressure generated by the heart is insufficient to overcome the magnitude of the hydrostatic force. Cerebral blood flow ceases and unconsciousness (G-LOC) results.

It can be seen that G-LOC ultimately represents the failure of the cardiovascular system to tolerate a high-applied acceleration.

An episode of G-LOC has several features that have been well described in the aerospace medicine literature (Burton and Whinnery, 1985; Cammarota, 1991; Forster and Cammarota, 1993; Gillingham, 1988; Green, 2006a; Houghton et al.,

1985; Howard, 1965; Werchan and Shahed, 1992; Whinnery, 1986, 1988, 1989; Whinnery and Burton, 1987; Whinnery and Jones, 1987; Whinnery and Shaffstall, 1979; Whinnery and Whinnery, 1990; Whinnery et al., 1987, 1989; Wilson et al., 2005; Wood, 1947). In simple terms, a G-LOC episode will result in a period of unconsciousness followed by a period of disorientation and confusion.

In operational terms, the total amount of time that the pilot is not in control of their aircraft is termed the total incapacitation period. This period consists of an absolute incapacitation period and a relative incapacitation period (Houghton et al., 1985; Gillingham, 1988; Ross, 1990; Whinnery, 1986, 1988, 1989; Whinnery and Jones, 1987; Whinnery and Shaffstall, 1979; Whinnery et al., 1987, 1989). The absolute incapacitation period represents complete incapacitation or true unconsciousness, which usually lasts for about 15 seconds (Whinnery and Shaffstall, 1979; Whinnery et al., 1987). In experimental terms, it is defined as the time from the subject's head dropping at the moment of unconsciousness to the raising of the subject's head as consciousness is restored (Houghton et al., 1985).

This absolute incapacitation period is then followed by a period of relative incapacitation with a duration of approximately 10–15 seconds (Whinnery et al., 1987; Whinnery and Shaffstall, 1979). This period is defined as the time interval from raising of the head to the first voluntary, purposeful limb movement (Houghton et al., 1985). During the relative incapacitation period, the pilot is once again conscious, but only in a technical sense. That is, while cerebral blood flow has been restored, the pilot is somewhat dissociated from their situation and unable to function appropriately. The pilot is disoriented and confused, with significant cognitive slowing, and their higher cortical centres are largely dysfunctional (Gillingham, 1988; Howard, 1965; Whinnery, 1986, 1988, 1989; Whinnery and Burton, 1987; Whinnery and Jones, 1987; Whinnery et al., 1987, 1989; Whinnery and Shaffstall, 1979).

As a result, the pilot is incapable of appropriately assessing their situation and thus perceiving danger. Fine motor control is absent, and often only gross motor acts are carried out. The pilot is thus still incapacitated inasmuch as they are unable to save themselves or correct their situation. The pilot is still recovering from the major ischaemic insult that their brain has sustained as a result of inadequate blood and oxygen delivery. Obviously, in a high-performance aircraft pulling high +Gz levels at low altitudes, the potential for disaster in such a situation is enormous (Lamb et al., 1960). It has been reported that some pilots in such situations have watched in fascination as their altimeters have registered their rapid descent towards subsequent ground impact, the pilot not appreciating the significance of what they are seeing and therefore not reacting to it appropriately.

There is also a characteristic recovery process from an episode of G-LOC. Tingling in the extremities and perioral numbness have been reported (Whinnery, 1988). Myoclonic convulsions and flailing of the arms commonly occur, generally coinciding with the re-establishment of effective cerebral blood flow. Typically these convulsions occur in the latter third of the absolute incapacitation period, generally in the last four seconds of this so-called convulsion-prone period, and are not associated with any underlying structural abnormalities of the brain (Whinnery, 1989). Whinnery (1989) has proposed that these convulsions occur as a result of a functional caudal reticular formation becoming disinhibited by a non-functional cerebral cortex.

In addition, cognitive distortions of a dream-like nature are said to occur towards the very end of the absolute incapacitation period (Forster and Whinnery, 1988; Whinnery, 1989). These dreams can often incorporate the myoclonic convulsions which typically occur in the same phase of the G-LOC event. No link has been established between these dreams and REM sleep, but they are akin to the hypnopompic dreams which can occur at the end of a normal sleep cycle, in that they tend to be associated with the terminal phases of unconsciousness (Whinnery, 1989).

G-LOC also has a number of neuropsychological effects, which are accentuated by repeated G-LOC episodes. These include denial, euphoria, irritation, embarrassment, confusion, dissociation and anxiety, among others (Forster and Cammarota, 1993; Whinnery and Jones, 1987). It has been reported that G-LOC has the potential to 'exert a temporary psychologically crippling effect' on the combat effectiveness of tactical aircrew, who may have altered judgement, and a loss of aggressiveness and motivation to carry out their mission (Whinnery and Jones, 1987). In the post-G-LOC period, psychological mechanisms often result in suppression and denial of the actual G-LOC event. In approximately 50 per cent of cases, recovery from G-LOC is associated with event amnesia, with the pilot not recollecting having had a period of unconsciousness at all (Green, 2006a). As far as they are aware, they have been conscious and in control of their aircraft for the whole flight. These post-G-LOC psychological reactions can have a detrimental impact on flight safety. Full psychophysiological recovery from an episode of G-LOC is only reached after a complete sleep cycle.

G-LOC should not be considered as an abnormal event. Rather, it is a normal physiological response to an abnormal stimulus, that is, high +Gz acceleration. It is also not a form of seizure or syncope (Jones, 1991). It is best defined as a sudden, orderly and progressive shut-down of the brain, largely thought to occur as a self-protective mechanism. It reflects the end-point on the continuum of +Gz effects from consciousness to unconsciousness.

There is an important period from the onset of high +Gz during which the brain is able to still function despite the absence of any effective cerebral blood flow. This has been described as the functional buffer period, and has in several studies been shown to have a duration of approximately six seconds (Burns et al., 1991; Gillingham, 1988). This buffer period is due to stored oxygen and metabolic substrate supplies within the brain (Whinnery, 1989). This buffer period is generally considered to have a protective role, in that it allows for large scale accelerations to be tolerated as long as they are not sustained beyond the critical six-second mark (Gillingham, 1988). At the end of this buffer period, consciousness is said to terminate abruptly with complete cerebral shut-down.

Prevalence of G-LOC

Many nations have reported their G-LOC prevalence rates in military operations. The observed rate of G-LOC in published international studies ranges from 8–19 per cent (Alvim, 1995; Green and Ford, 2006; Rickards and Newman, 2005; Sevilla and Gardner, 2005; Yilmaz et al., 1999). In the UK, 19 per cent of Royal Air Force (RAF) pilots surveyed had experienced a G-LOC event during their flying career (Green and Ford, 2006). In the RAAF, a survey involving F/A-18 and Hawk 127 pilots revealed a 9 per cent rate of G-LOC, and in 50 per cent of cases these involved the flying pilot (Rickards and Newman, 2005).

In the USAF, G-LOC events by aircraft type showed that the higher the G capability of the aircraft, the higher the reported G-LOC rate. Twelve per cent of USAF tactical pilots have had a G-LOC event (Pluta, 1984). Twenty-eight per cent of F-16 G-LOC events result in the loss of the aircraft and/or the pilot. In another USAF study covering the years 1982–2002, a total of 559 G-LOC events were reported, giving a rate per million sorties of 25.9 (Lyons et al., 2004). Additionally, their data suggested that ground attack missions were the most at-risk of a fatal outcome, largely due to the low altitude at which they operate giving insufficient time to recover from a G-LOC event (Lyons et al., 2004). In the US Navy, 12 per cent of pilots admit to experiencing a G-LOC event (Johanson and Pheeny, 1988). In the civilian aerobatic environment, the prevalence of G-LOC is not well known. However, a number of accidents involving aerobatic aircraft have been reported as being attributed to possible G-LOC (Kirkham et al., 1982).

These prevalence figures may only represent 50 per cent of actual G-LOC events due to the lack of recall when pilots regain consciousness and the possible reluctance to admit these symptoms for fear of being removed from flight status and issues of self-esteem (Whinnery et al., 1987). For all the reported G-LOC events from current surviving pilots, many more probably go unreported and a number of fatal accidents may be the result of G-LOC, but cannot be definitively classified as such. Clearly, then, G-LOC is still a major ongoing hazard for pilots of high-performance military and civilian aerobatic aircraft.

The Effect of Rate of Change of +Gz

The rate of onset and offset of high +Gz has been shown to affect the nature of the subsequent G-LOC episode. Gradual onset of +Gz results in longer absolute and relative incapacitation periods (Houghton et al., 1985; Whinnery, 1989; Whinnery and Burton, 1987). This is due to the longer period of absent or reduced cerebral perfusion during gradual onset exposure. Gradual onset thus produces a greater perfusion deficit and hence greater embarrassment to the central nervous system than rapid onset.

In terms of the rate of recovery from an episode of G-LOC, studies have shown that there is considerable individual variation. Indeed, it appears that a particular subject's G tolerance and their rate of recovery from an episode of G-LOC are not related. They are, in fact, independent variables (Houghton et al., 1985). Burns et al. (1991) showed that recovery times become shorter after multiple G-LOC episodes, and become longer with longer periods of unconsciousness.

Several centrifuge studies have shown that gradual onset runs (GORs) consistently produce prolonged incapacitation times (Houghton et al., 1985). Rapid onset runs (RORs), on the other hand, typically produce shorter incapacitation periods. In one centrifuge study, for example, incapacitation following rapid onset was 23.7 seconds, compared with 32.3 seconds for gradual onset (Houghton et al., 1985).

Gradual offset of +Gz tends to prolong the time of incapacitation in much the same way as gradual onset, as it prolongs the period of overall cerebral hypoperfusion and delays re-establishment of full cerebral blood flow. Centrifuge studies involve offset rates in the region of 0.5 to 0.9 Gs^{-1}, while in-flight G offset rates have been found to be approximately 0.5 Gs^{-1} (Whinnery and Burton, 1987; Whinnery et al., 1989). A centrifuge ROR usually takes nine seconds to return to +1 Gz from a peak of +9 Gz (Burton et al., 1988). Obviously the quicker the G offset, the quicker cerebral blood flow will be returned to normal, and the shorter the resultant incapacitation time.

Rapid onset of +Gz is often not associated with myoclonic convulsions or dreams. This is thought to be due to the rapid onset of +Gz disabling the reticular formation just as quickly as it does the cerebral cortex (Whinnery, 1989). This prevents myoclonic convulsions from occurring.

The unconsciousness resulting from G-LOC has been compared with that resulting from acute arrest of the cerebral circulation via a cervical occlusion cuff (Rossen et al., 1943; Whinnery and Burton, 1987). Important facts emerge as a result of this comparison. The times of incapacitation are different between the two types of unconsciousness. G-LOC results in longer incapacitation times than acute arrest of the cerebral circulation. This is related to onset and offset rates. Both onset and offset of an applied +Gz load tend to take at least several seconds. On the other hand, acute arrest of the cerebral circulation can be achieved almost instantaneously, and can be reversed just as quickly. Higher onset and offset rates produce less overall incapacitation.

However, the two types of unconsciousness are strikingly similar in one important aspect. The time from application of the stress (high +Gz load or acute arrest) to onset of unconsciousness is virtually the same in both cases, being 6–7 seconds. Rossen et al. (1943) found that the induction time to achieve loss of consciousness after acute arrest of the cerebral circulation was 6–6.5 seconds. These findings were subsequently replicated ion a much later study by Cammarota (1994). This time interval represents the functional buffer period, which as has been discussed earlier is the period of time that the central nervous system can function after the blood supply has become inadequate (Whinnery, 1989). Once this critical time period has elapsed unconsciousness results (Whinnery, 1989).

The physiological consequences of exposure to high +Gz forces as shown above represent a cardiovascular spectrum. This spectrum is dependent on the rate of application of the +Gz force. As discussed previously, the onset and offset rates of applied +Gz can affect the time of incapacitation if G-LOC results. The rate of +Gz application is also important in terms of the appearance of symptoms prior to the occurrence of G-LOC. The critical G onset rate in this context is 2 Gs^{-1}. If the rate of application of G is less than this critical value, then the cardiovascular system will experience the entire spectrum of +Gz effects. That is, grey-out will occur at +3 to +4 Gz, followed by black-out at +4 to +4.5 Gz and G-LOC at +4.5 to +5 Gz (Green, 2006a). If the rate of onset is higher than this value, loss of consciousness is too rapid for the other effects to be experienced. The pilot may thus bypass the earlier signs of cardiovascular compromise and proceed straight to G-LOC.

In modern high-performance fighter aircraft engaged in ACM, Gz onset rates can often be at the design limits of the aircraft, resulting in onset rates as high as +15 Gs^{-1}. At lower rates the visual symptoms can be used as an early warning or premonitory sign to alert the pilot to the approaching danger of G-LOC. In practical terms, however, this does not often occur, for the fighter pilot typically needs to manoeuvre their aircraft quickly and forcefully during an ACM engagement, resulting in high G onset rates with consequently no visual warning signs. G-LOC is thus an ever-present threat to the fighter pilot. Similarly, a competition aerobatic pilot needs high onset rates to deliver a very tight, crisp corner, for example, also therefore increasing their risk of G-LOC if the G peak is too high or sustained for too long. The importance of G onset rate in terms of tolerance to +Gz is considered in further detail in Chapter 8.

A Word on Negative Gz

Negative Gz (–Gz) is the end result of a manoeuvre where the pilot's head is on the outside of the circular path of motion (opposite to that of a normal loop, for example). Such manoeuvres include an outside loop (see Figure 4.3) or a push-over, where the pilot simply pushes the control column forward in order to quickly descend. The centripetal and centrifugal forces develop in exactly the same way as seen in Chapters 1 and 2, except that the centrifugal force directs blood flow to the head, rather than to the feet (due to the orientation of the body with respect to the G vector).

While military fast jet pilots do not tend to be exposed to high levels of –Gz, since they can simply roll and pull in order to keep the G vector predominantly in the more tolerable +Gz axis, civilian aerobatic pilots do routinely experience high levels of –Gz. An outside loop (as seen in Figure 4.2) in an advanced competition aerobatic aircraft can generate –Gz levels well in excess of –6 Gz. Indeed, the performance envelope for such advanced aircraft includes significant ±Gz onset and offset rates – it can take no more than 3 seconds to transition from +5 Gz to –5 Gz (Burton and Whinnery, 1996).

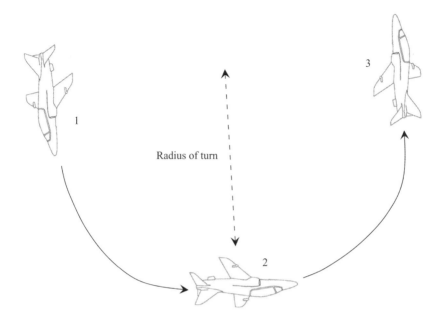

Figure 4.3   The outside loop as an example of a –Gz flight manoeuvre

From a cardiovascular perspective, the redistribution of blood flow and the resultant cardiovascular countermeasures are opposite to those seen in +Gz exposures. Head-level BP increases due to the hydrostatic force developed, and the baroreflexes become increasingly activated, in an attempt to drive BP back to the normal level. As far as the cardiovascular system is concerned, the system is basically overfilled and there is too much cerebral perfusion. The baroreflexes and other countermeasures try to reverse this overperfusion problem.

The hydrostatically-mediated increase in head-level arterial pressure tends to be counterbalanced somewhat by corresponding increases in both venous pressure and the cerebrospinal fluid pressure. The end result of these increases is that transmural pressures tend to remain constant, such that a tendency for blood vessels to rupture due to overfilling is minimised (Gauer and Henry, 1964). Whether this is true at extremely high levels of –Gz, or at very high –Gz onset rates, remains to be determined. However, what is clear is that after several seconds the cerebral circulation becomes sufficiently compromised as the arteriovenous pressure differential narrows. Altered cognitive states such as confusion can result, and ultimately loss of consciousness may occur (Green, 2006a).

In general, negative Gz is poorly tolerated due to the unpleasant subjective sensations that it generates. Feelings of increased head and neck congestion, headache, subconjunctival haemorrhage, facial puffiness and eye distension tend to be uncomfortable enough as to limit deliberate exposure, with these symptoms becoming particularly unpleasant at –3 Gz. The HR changes during –Gz exposure are dramatic, mediated by the cardiovascular countermeasures brought to bear such as the baroreflexes. At a –Gz level of –3.8 Gz, HR has been recorded at 38 beats per minute, down from over 110 prior to the –Gz exposure (Bloodwell and Whinnery, 1982; Burton and Whinnery, 1996). Loss of consciousness can occur with sustained exposure to –Gz. This is usually attributed to baroreflex-mediated HR reductions ultimately resulting in cardiac asystole (Green, 2006a).

So-called 'red out' is a visual concomitant of high –Gz exposure. The underlying mechanism responsible for this apparent reddening of vision remains unclear. Initial thoughts were that it was due to hydrostatically-mediated internal ocular bleeding, but this has now been somewhat discounted. The current belief is that red-out is due to the –Gz forcing the lower eyelid (which may be engorged due to the extent of head-level BP increase) to enter the visual field. The mechanism of red-out in –Gz exposure remains an unresolved area of G research.

Conclusion

The spectrum of adverse cardiovascular consequences which occur under high +Gz have thus been well described. These consequences range from the visual symptoms of grey-out (loss of peripheral vision) and black-out (complete loss of vision) to G-LOC. G-LOC occurs when either the magnitude of the applied acceleration, or its rate of application, is greater than the cardiovascular system's ability to maintain cerebral perfusion. The consequences of G-LOC are potentially catastrophic: the pilot of a single-seat aircraft may not regain consciousness before the aircraft impacts the ground.

As this chapter has shown, the cardiovascular system is most affected by exposure to high levels of applied Gz. However, the effects of G force exposure are not restricted to the cardiovascular system alone. All parts and functions of the body are potentially affected, including the respiratory system, the musculoskeletal system and various other systems. These are considered in the next several chapters.

Chapter 5
Respiratory Effects of G

The previous chapter demonstrated that the cardiovascular system, as a closed-loop column of fluid, is particularly sensitive to acceleration in the longitudinal or Gz axis. The respiratory system, by contrast, is essentially an air-filled system, which accounts for its sensitivity to acceleration in all three axes – Gx, Gy and Gz. This now warrants some consideration, which is the purpose of this chapter.

It is important to bear in mind, as Chapter 2 explained, that aircraft flight generates predominantly acceleration in the Gz axis, while the launch and re-entry phase of spaceflight generates high levels of Gx acceleration. There is little opportunity in these settings for physiologically significant lateral G to be generated, but for the sake of completeness the respiratory effects of exposure to high G in all three axes will be examined.

Some of the important countermeasures for high G exposure, such as the anti-G straining manoeuvre (AGSM), the G-suit and PBG, have significant respiratory effects. These are covered in more detail in Chapters 10, 11 and 12 respectively.

The Respiratory System at +1 Gz

In order to appreciate the effects of G exposure on the respiratory system, it is useful to first understand the normal situation in the lungs at +1 Gz. This gives a baseline picture of lung function, from which an understanding of the effects of high G exposure can be developed. The normal situation can be considered as upright posture, with a constant +Gz level of +1.

The lungs under normal, resting conditions contain around 6 l of air. This volume is known as total lung capacity (TLC). The amount of air expelled each breath is known as the tidal volume (TV), which is around 500 ml during non-exercising conditions. With a maximum inspiration and then a maximum exhalation, a total of around 4.5 l of air can be expelled from the lungs. This volume is known as the vital capacity (VC). The gas remaining in the lungs after such maximal breathing effort is thus around 1.5 l, and this volume is known as the residual volume (RV). This volume is important, as it helps ensure ongoing inflation of the air spaces in order to prevent collapse of the lungs, despite maximum expiratory efforts as might occur during maximal exercise.

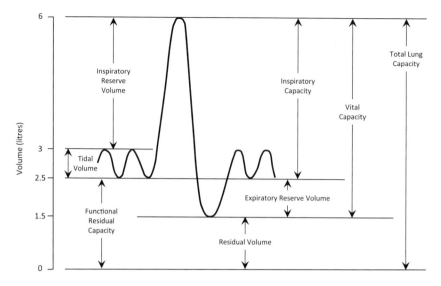

Figure 5.1   Lung volumes and capacities under normal resting conditions

The other lung capacity that is often described is functional residual capacity (FRC), which is the RV plus the expiratory reserve volume (ERV). The ERV is the volume of gas that could be expelled from the lungs following an additional forceful expiratory effort that could be made if required, and is around 1 litre. FRC is around 2.5 l or so. The inspiratory reserve volume (IRV) is the additional volume of air that could be inspired beyond TV if required, and is around 3 l. Inspiratory capacity (IC) is the sum of TV and IRV. The combined sum of IRV, TV and ERV gives VC. These lung volumes and capacities are shown in Figure 5.1.

In terms of perfusion, blood supply to and from the lungs is via a low pressure circuit driven by the right-side of the heart, compared with the high-pressure circuit driven by the left-side of the heart that delivers oxygenated blood to the rest of the body. Pulmonary artery pressure is around 25 mmHg (systolic) and 8 mmHg (diastolic). These pressures are those that occur during rest conditions – during maximal exercise pulmonary artery pressure increases in proportion to the exercise-driven metabolic demands for additional oxygen.

HP exerts a well-known effect on BP and flow through the lung when in the upright posture. BP at the top of the lung is thus lower than that at the base of the lung. Moreover, there are regional differences in blood flow from the top of the lung to the bottom, as a result of this HP effect. The very top few centimetres of the lung may not be significantly perfused at all under +1 Gz conditions. In general, blood flow per unit of lung increases with distance from the lung apex when in the upright posture, reaching a maximum value at the base of the lung. At the same time, there are regional differences in ventilation across the lungs while in the upright posture. The air spaces at the apices of the lungs tend to be relatively distended, due to the weight of the lung effectively dragging itself downwards, putting traction on the upper part of the lung and stretching the apical air spaces open. At the bottom of the lungs, however, the weight of the lungs (due to the effect of gravity at +1 Gz) and the splinting effect of the diaphragm (which limits further descent of the lungs) combine to reduce the relative size of the airspaces.

As a result, there are ventilation–perfusion inequalities throughout the lung. At a certain point, ventilation will match perfusion, but in general there is relatively more perfusion and less ventilation at the bases, and more ventilation and less perfusion at the apices. The effect is more pronounced for perfusion than ventilation – as such, the ventilation–perfusion (V/Q) ratio decreases overall with increasing distance from the apex of the lung. In general, this results in a V/Q ratio around three to four at the apices, decreasing to around 0.5 at the bases. Under normal conditions, these differences in ventilation and perfusion across the lungs are not reflected in adverse symptoms or performance for the average fit and well person.

There is a certain degree of work associated with the breathing task. Under normal conditions, inspiration is an active process in which the respiratory muscles (such as the intercostal muscles and the diaphragm) contract, causing elevation of the rib cage and descent of the diaphragm. This creates a small pressure differential (relative to atmospheric pressure), which encourages air flow into the lungs. In contrast, expiration is a passive process, in which the muscles relax and the rib cage and diaphragm return to their normal positions, effectively pushing the air out of the lungs. The normal respiratory rate is around 12 breaths per minute. This rate, with a TV of around 500 mls, results in a minute respiratory volume (the total amount of gas expelled from the lungs per minute) of around 6 l per minute.

Under resting conditions, then, the work of breathing is basically due to the inspiration phase. There are three components to this work. The major element of this is compliance work, which is the work needed to expand the lungs, against the natural tendency of the lungs to collapse (known as elastic recoil). This collapsing tendency is due to the high content of elastic fibres throughout the lung, which are routinely stretched during inflation, and the surface tension of the lipoprotein-rich fluid lining the alveoli (known as surfactant). The surface tension component accounts for approximately two-thirds of the elastic recoil potential, with the remainder being due to the elastic fibre content. A small negative intrapleural pressure (approximately 4 mmHg) helps counter this elastic recoil tendency in order to maintain stable lung inflation.

The other components of inspiratory work are known as tissue resistance work (to overcome the viscosity of the thoracic structures, including the lungs and the rib cage) and airway resistance work (to overcome the resistance to movement of air in the airways). Under rest conditions, the majority of work is compliance. With increased respiratory demand (as with exercise), the increased breathing rate and depth leads to a greater role for airway resistance work.

The situation under +1 Gz conditions is clearly well tolerated by most people, and represents an entirely normal situation which humans have adapted to over generations of regular exposure to upright posture. The situation only changes when the background level of acceleration changes from the usual +1 Gz to a higher level of G that might also be in an entirely different axis.

Respiratory Effects of High Gz Exposure

In general, the effects of exposure to high levels of +Gz are basically exaggerations of what is seen under the normal +1 Gz situation, as discussed above. The pleural pressure gradient that normally exists at +1 Gz is increased by around 0.2 cm H_2O per centimetre of lung per unit of +Gz (Green 2006a). Apical air space widening and basilar airspace narrowing are both accentuated due to this +Gz-mediated pressure gradient increase, itself a function of the increased weight of the lung under high +Gz loads.

What is clear from most of the scientific evidence is that in overall terms respiratory function in most people is well preserved with little ill-effect at +Gz levels of up to +5. However, several changes in the lung volumes have been described as a result of high +Gz exposure, and these are shown in Figure 5.2. These changes reverse extremely quickly and revert back to normal once the high +Gz loads have been released. Importantly, no pathologic changes or physical damage to the lungs such as spontaneous pneumothorax have been described at +Gz levels up to +10 Gz (Burton and Whinnery, 1996).

TLC and VC remain effectively unchanged at +3 Gz, but at +5 Gz there is a noticeable reduction in these volumes, amounting to approximately 15 per cent. TV decreases, but respiratory rate often increases. The end result on minute volume is a net reduction. In addition, +Gz exposure causes an increase in FRC, due to a concomitant increase in the +Gz-induced descent of the diaphragm. Indeed, at +4 Gz the diaphragm can undergo an approximately 2 cm downward displacement. FRC is around 500 ml greater at around +3 Gz (Green, 2006a; Lombard et al., 1948). This effect on FRC can be reduced or even eliminated by the use of a G-suit, which effectively splints the diaphragm and prevents its downward displacement (discussed in detail in Chapter 11).

As discussed above, increases in the level of +Gz leads to the lungs becoming progressively heavier, and the pressure gradient down the pleural cavity increases in accordance. The upper air spaces are opened even more, due to the traction of the heavier lung mass below and the intrinsically elastic structure of the lung in general. For similar reasons, the air spaces at the bases of the lungs tend to be reduced still further. With increasing +Gz loads, alveoli at the base of the lung can attain their minimum volume with subsequent airway collapse. This can lead to a degree of basal atelectasis. At the same time, the applied +Gz causes an exaggerated perfusion gradient down the lungs, with progressively more blood going to the bases and less to the apices,

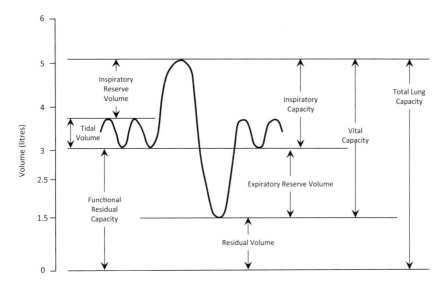

Figure 5.2   Lung volumes and capacities under +5 Gz conditions

mediated by the +Gz-induced increase in the hydrostatic force (Glaister, 1970; Pendergast et al., 2012). At +4 to +5 Gz the upper half of the lungs may not be perfused at all (Green, 2006a).

The combination of these ventilation and perfusion changes under +Gz leads to a considerable ventilation–perfusion (V/Q) mismatch, involving a right-to-left shunt in the lower lungs (Burton and Whinnery, 1996; Dowell et al., 1968; Green, 2006a). The right-to-left shunt can result in around 50 per cent of the blood in the lungs not being involved in gaseous exchange at +7 Gz (Burton and Whinnery, 1996). The V/Q ratio at the top of the lungs (where there is ventilation but no perfusion) is by definition infinite, whereas at the base of the lungs (where there is perfusion but no ventilation, as seen in the next section on atelectasis) the V/Q ratio is zero. Such V/Q mismatches can lead to an overall reduction in arterial oxyhaemoglobin saturation, which can be approximately 85 per cent at +5 Gz, compared with the normal 98 per cent at +1 Gz (Green, 2006a). This relative hypoxic effect can be offset by the pilot breathing a higher oxygen concentration (up to 100 per cent). Indeed, in many air forces the use of 100 per cent oxygen during all phases of flight is standard operating procedure (Burton and Whinnery, 1996).

High +Gz also increases the physical work of breathing (Armstrong and Heim, 1938; Burton and Whinnery, 1996; Green, 2006a; Gronkvist et al., 2003, 2005, 2008; Howard, 1965). The +Gz acceleration forces the diaphragm and abdominal contents downward, and the chest wall becomes proportionally heavier, requiring more effort. The respiratory rate tends to undergo a modest increase, and TV also increases at +5 Gz (Armstrong and Heim, 1938; Lombard et al., 1948).

Up to about +3 Gz there is little adverse effect. At higher levels, the work of breathing increases due to reduced lung compliance (Burton and Whinnery, 1996). An increase in respiratory work of some 55 per cent at +3 Gz has been reported (Burton and Whinnery, 1996).

The discussion so far has centred on the respiratory effects of +Gz. Exposure to –Gz results in opposite effects to those seen with +Gz (Burton and Whinnery, 1996; Green, 2006a). Blood is preferentially directed to the apices of the lung, while the basilar air spaces of the lung are relatively more distended due to the increased weight of the lung. These effects are not as directly opposite to +Gz as might have been imagined. –Gz results in a more uniform lung perfusion than that seen at +Gz, particularly at –1 Gz. Lung volume changes at –3 Gz have involved reductions of 150 ml in TLC, 400 ml in FRC and 1 l in VC (Burton and Whinnery, 1996). These reductions are largely due to the –Gz-induced headward shift of the diaphragm and abdominal contents (Green, 2006a).

Acceleration Atelectasis

As mentioned above, the effect of increasing +Gz on the alveoli at the base of the lung can be significant, with airway collapse being the end result. This particular +Gz-induced respiratory condition is known as acceleration atelectasis, and is a very specific form of +Gz-related respiratory effect. It requires certain conditions to be met before it can occur: the pilot needs to be breathing 100 per cent oxygen, have been exposed to at least +3 Gz and should be wearing a G-suit (Burton and Whinnery, 1996; Green, 2006a; Howard, 1965; Tacker et al., 1987).

Under the application of high +Gz (at least +3), the increased pleural pressure gradient and weight of the lung (as discussed above) can lead to airway collapse in the basilar parts of the lung. This collapse is accentuated by the use of a G-suit, where the abdominal bladder applies pressure over the abdomen and lower thorax, splints the diaphragm preventing its descent and increases the pressure over the airways in the lung bases. Once the airways have collapsed, the alveoli become closed air spaces, and the 100 per cent oxygen that they contain is rapidly absorbed. Once this occurs, the air sacs collapse, and +Gz-induced atelectasis is achieved.

It should be noted that such atelectasis can also be achieved under –Gz conditions, for the same fundamental reasons. It can also be achieved with ±Gx and ±Gy exposures. In the Gz axis, atelectasis is said to be more readily achieved under –Gz loads than +Gz loads, due to the –Gz-induced reduction in FRC (Green, 2006a). Furthermore, under –Gz conditions the G-suit no longer tends to be a precursor condition, given the significant changes in FRC.

In terms of symptoms, the pilot with acceleration atelectasis may experience some shortness of breath and coughing, and pain on deep inspiration (which ultimately reinflates the lower lung and fixes the problem after flight). There are several possible countermeasures that can be adopted so as to prevent this problem in pilots. Dilution of the inspired oxygen concentration by an inert gas (for example, nitrogen), which is not as rapidly absorbed from the air sacs in the lung bases as oxygen, will help prevent the collapse of the air sacs. It has been shown that the use of around 30 per cent nitrogen in a breathing gas mix can prevent the development of acceleration atelectasis (Haswell et al., 1986. The use of PBG (discussed in Chapter 12) can also help prevent atelectasis, as the increased breathing pressure tends to hold open the airways despite the application of high +Gz and the use of the G-suit. However, this picture is complicated somewhat by the concurrent use of a chest counterpressure garment (CCPG), discussed further in Chapter 12. Performing an AGSM (discussed in Chapter 10) will increase intrathoracic pressure and similarly offset the tendency for the airways to collapse under high +Gz (Tacker et al., 1987).

Respiratory Effects of High Gx Exposure

High Gx exposure tends to occur predominantly during the launch phase of spaceflight, and for some operations it is also important for re-entry and landing, as discussed in Chapter 2. It is rare for high Gx to be a physiologically significant factor in conventional aircraft operations, due to the lack of sufficient linear acceleration. However, as indicated in Chapter 2, super-agile fighter aircraft may impose some Gx on the occupants, which may be violent but is generally not sustained for enough time to have any adverse effect. In this section, the emphasis is on the respiratory effects of launch and re-entry exposure to high Gx in commercial spaceflight operations.

As seen in Chapter 2, commercial spaceflight operations may expose the occupants to +Gx levels in the order of +4 Gx. In this axis, the person exposed to the Gx is facing the direction of acceleration. The G thus acts (in an inertial sense) from front-to-back. In general, the application of high +Gx will increase the difficulty of raising the chest wall during inspiration, as the chest wall will effectively weigh more due to the +Gx load, but the inspiratory muscles will not be correspondingly stronger.

Similarly, Gx loads will tend to exaggerate the expiratory phase of breathing. This is usually a passive process, and the increased weight of the chest wall will result in it collapsing once the inspiratory muscles relax. This will result in an accentuated, rapid exhalation. This could be significant in those individuals who have pre-existing medical conditions, particularly respiratory illnesses. This has led to some recent work in terms of defining appropriate medical guidelines for such commercial spaceflight participants (Rayman et al., 2002). Although quite rare, traumatic injuries due to Gx exposure have been reported. Wood (1992) reported the case of a centrifuge subject who developed significant and incapacitating mediastinal emphysema during sustained exposure to +5.5 Gx.

Difficulty in breathing has been observed at modest Gx levels, in the order of +3 Gx, with pain in the chest at +5 Gx (Green, 2006a). Breathing frequency has been reported to be as high as 30 breaths per minute at +8 Gx (Burton and

Whinnery, 1996). Once the +Gx level reaches +12 Gx, the chest pain is quite strong (worse on inspiration) and the breathing pattern is shallow and rapid. The limit of tolerance for human exposure to Gx is approximately +15 Gx (Burton and Whinnery, 1996; Green, 2006a). Beyond +15 Gx, the difficulty in breathing is extremely pronounced.

The anatomical arrangement of the thorax is clearly different from front to back. At the back of the thorax, the various spinal structures can restrict lung volumes in the +Gx axis. The infero-posterior part of the thoracic cavity is also impinged upon by the abdominal contents when in the +Gx axis. The front of the thorax is not restricted by such anatomical arrangements. The result of this difference in structure is reflected in lung volume changes seen at +Gx and –Gx. At +6 Gx, VC is reduced by up to 75 per cent compared with normal values, whereas at –6 Gx the reduction in VC is only 15 per cent (Burton and Whinnery, 1996). At +12 Gx, VC becomes the same as TV. At +5 Gx, FRC is reduced by half, and compliance of the lung is also known to reduce significantly, by up to 40 per cent at +4 Gx (Burton and Whinnery, 1996). FRC reductions are not seen under –Gx conditions, due again to the difference in the anatomical structure of the thorax. Under –Gx, FRC may actually increase.

Acceleration atelectasis is possible with +Gx exposure, for the same fundamental reasons as discussed above for Gz exposure. However, the site of atelectasis will be the back or front of the lung (depending on the direction of Gx) rather than the top or bottom of the lung as seen in Gz exposure. Acceleration atelectasis has been reported in individuals breathing 100 per cent oxygen and exposed to +Gx levels of around +5.5 to 6.5 Gx. As with –Gz exposure, a G-suit is not necessary as a precursor condition for +Gx-induced atelectasis.

Furthermore, as noted above, there is a difference between –Gx and +Gx in terms of restriction of lung volume changes due to the anatomical structure of the thorax. This means that atelectasis is not seen equally in –Gx and +Gx exposure. –Gx exposure is not affected by such anatomically-induced lung volume restriction, and as a result, acceleration atelectasis is rarely seen with –Gx exposure. Indeed, the inertial forces associated with –Gx tend to lift the abdominal contents away from the infero-posterior part of the thoracic cavity, thus reducing pressure on that part of the lungs.

Unlike Gz exposure, the predominant vector in Gx exposure is horizontal (front-to-back, or back-to-front) rather than vertical. This results in similar variations in the ventilation–perfusion ratio across the lung as seen in Gz exposure, except that instead of being from apex to base, it will be from front of the lung to the back, for example. The distance involved is less than with Gz exposure, so these regional differences in V/Q ratio do not tend to be as physiologically significant with Gx exposure as they can be with ±Gz. The right-to-left shunt observed at +6 Gx can be around 40 per cent of total lung blood volume, leading to a fall in arterial oxyhaemoglobin saturation to 90 per cent after 2 minutes at +4 Gx (Burton and Whinnery, 1996). No reduction in arterial oxygen saturation is generally seen with –Gx, at levels up to –6 Gx.

By and large, it is the increased weight of the chest wall interfering with the normal breathing pattern and increasing the work of breathing that tends to be the major issue with Gx exposure. In spaceflight operations, as mentioned in Chapter 2, the peak values of Gx and exposure times tend to be well within the maximum tolerable limit for humans.

Respiratory Effects of High Gy Exposure

Exposure to lateral G (±Gy) can lead to similar ventilation and perfusion changes in the lungs as are seen with Gx and Gz exposure. The vector is left-to-right, or right-to-left. Since this distance is much less than that in Gz axis from top of the lung to the bottom, these V/A changes under lateral G are for the most part not physiologically significant. Furthermore, as Chapter 2 demonstrated, there is very little opportunity in aviation and spaceflight operations for meaningful amounts of lateral G to be developed or experienced. Indeed, any lateral G that might be developed (as might conceivably occur during a violent departure from controlled flight or during some form of super-agile manoeuvre) is unlikely to be sustained for long enough to create adverse physiological issues.

However, one problem that could occur with lateral G (from a theoretical if not a practical perspective) is Gy-induced mediastinal shifting. The increased weight of the heart and mediastinal contents will result in movement in the direction of the applied Gy (which could potentially adversely affect the normal function of the heart itself, particularly if the Gy is sufficiently high and sustained for long enough). This shifting of the mediastinum will impinge on the space occupied by the so-called dependent lung. This lung is thus at higher risk of collapse and the development of a significant right-to-left shunt, decreasing overall oxygenation levels. The other lung tends to be uniformly stretched open. This effect tends to be dramatic at a Gy level of 3 to 4 (Green, 2006a).

Conclusion

The respiratory system is potentially affected in an adverse manner by exposure to both high levels of +Gz and ±Gx. Arguably it is the only physiological system of the body that is so sensitive to these two axes. The reasons are clearly anatomical in nature – the lungs are both air-filled and blood-filled spaces. The blood-filled spaces are sensitive to +Gz, while the air-filled spaces are sensitive to ±Gx. Either one of these G axes can affect the ventilation–perfusion ratio, the output of which is the main reason for the work of the lungs in the first place. Any deterioration in the ventilation–perfusion ratio will have an adverse impact on the oxygenation of the blood, which in turn can have adverse consequences on cerebral perfusion and oxygenation. Clearly the interplay between the cardiovascular and respiratory systems is of vital importance when considering the physiological consequences of high G exposure. However, other body systems can also be affected by high levels of G exposure, as the next chapters will show.

Chapter 6

Musculoskeletal Effects of G

Under high applied +Gz loads, the increased weight of the body is borne by the skeletal structures. These can potentially be injured as result of the applied +Gz, either through sustained weight-bearing exceeding the structural integrity of the bones, muscles or ligaments, or through an acute traumatic effect of rapid high +Gz application.

In this chapter, the significant effects of high +Gz on the musculoskeletal system are explored. The emphasis is on injuries to the neck and spine of the pilot exposed to high +Gz, as these two issues have received significant research attention and are common issues for pilots in the high +Gz environment.

+Gz-Induced Neck Injuries

+Gz-induced neck injuries are a common problem for military fast jet aircrew regularly exposed to the high +Gz environment (Albano and Stanford, 1998; Andersen, 1988; Averty and Green, 2005; Coakwell et al., 2004; De Loose et al., 2008; Green, 2003; Hamalainen et al., 1994a, 1994b; Hamalainen and Vanharanta, 1992; Jones, 2000; Kang et al., 2011; Kikukawa et al., 1994; Lange et al., 2011, 2014; Netto and Burnett, 2006; Netto et al., 2007; Newman, 1996, 1997a; Petren-Mallmin and Linder, 2001; Schall, 1989; Tolga Aydog et al., 2004; Vallejo Desviat et al., 2007; Vanderbeek, 1988; Wagstaff et al., 2012; Yacavone and Bason, 1992). Wearing a helmet and oxygen mask increases the weight of the pilot's head, and the neck muscles thus have to do much more work during ACM in order to maintain visual contact with the adversary aircraft. As a result, neck injuries are common in this environment. Far less is known about the prevalence of these injuries in pilots of civilian aerobatic aircraft.

Prevalence

Many air forces have over the years reported on the prevalence of these +Gz-induced injuries in their fast jet aircrew populations (Albano and Stanford, 1998; Averty and Green, 2005; Hamalainen et al., 1994a; Jones, 2000; Kikukawa et al., 1994; Knudson et al., 1988; Newman, 1997a; Vanderbeek, 1988; Wagstaff et al., 2012; Yacavone and Bason, 1992). Yacavone and Bason (1992) reported a period prevalence among US Naval aviators with G-induced neck pain of 26.8 per cent. A prospective study of student fighter pilots in Finland produced a cumulative incidence of 37.9 per cent (Hamalainen et al., 1994a), while a survey of Japanese F-15 pilots revealed a rate of 89.1 per cent (Kikukawa et al., 1994). Studies in the RAF show a prevalence rate of up to 70 per cent (Averty and Green, 2005; Wickes and Greeves, 2005). A similar rate (72 per cent) has been found in the Royal Norwegian Air Force (Wagstaff et al., 2012).

Knudson et al. (1988) reported that 74 per cent of surveyed F/A-18 pilots had experienced neck pain with high +Gz. Vanderbeek (1988) reported a period prevalence (for the preceding three-month period) for this injury of 50.6 per cent among a large number of USAF fighter pilots. In an F-16 pilot survey, the results showed that the one-year prevalence of neck injuries was 56.6 per cent, and for an entire career as an F-16 pilot the prevalence was 85.4 per cent (Albano and Stanford, 1998). This is consistent with a RAAF study, where the career prevalence of G-induced neck injuries in RAAF fighter pilots was 85 per cent (Newman, 1997a). Four per cent of the RAAF fighter pilot population surveyed reported some degree of neck pain with every flight, while 12 per cent said that they experienced neck pain with every high G flight or during every squadron ACM programme.

The findings shown above clearly indicate that +Gz-induced neck injuries are a very common problem in military fast jet aircrew. The wide variation in prevalence rates is almost certainly due to methodological differences between studies, as well as differences in reporting within a given air force. Also, the studies represent different populations of pilots, with different ages, physical fitness levels and flying experience across a variety of different aircraft types.

It should be remembered that neck pain is also very common in the general (non-flying) population; up to two-thirds of all adults experience neck pain at some time in their lives (Bovim et al., 1994; Côté et al., 1998, 2004; Fejer et al., 2006; Guez et al., 2002; Makela et al., 1991). Overall, the consensus of opinion in the scientific literature is that the prevalence of lifetime neck pain in the general population is around 50 per cent, with an annual neck pain prevalence of around 37 per cent (Fejer et al., 2006). The corresponding prevalence rates in the fast jet aircrew community are significantly higher than these general population rates, despite the various methodological differences between studies. +Gz-induced neck injuries are therefore a significant aerospace medicine problem.

Risk Factors

While +Gz-induced neck injuries are multi-factorial in origin, there are several factors that have been strongly linked with the development of a neck injury. The nature of the high +Gz environment is clearly of primary importance. In the very dynamic environment of ACM, the neck of a fast jet pilot is subjected to variable and repetitive high +Gz loads. ACM (involving high G air-to-air sorties) has been identified as the most common mission type associated with development of a neck injury (Averty and Green, 2005; Newman, 1997a). The performance limits and manoeuvrability of the aircraft, particularly the rate of onset of +Gz, the peak +Gz levels attained and the period of time that these +Gz loads are sustained for, are important determinants of the potential for neck injuries. To illustrate the extent of these +Gz loads, Hamalainen et al. (1996) found that after 40 minutes of ACM, the height of a pilot decreased by around 5 mm.

Several studies have indicated that the number of pilots developing neck injuries increases in direct proportion with the +Gz capability of their aircraft (Andersen, 1988; Hamalainen et al., 1993a; Knudson et al., 1988; Newman, 1997a; Schall, 1989; Vanderbeek, 1988). In several studies, pilots of the F/A-18 were found to have a greater rate of neck injury than pilots of aircraft with lower performance, such as the A-4 and A-7 (Knudson et al., 1988; Newman, 1997a; Yacavone and Bason, 1992).

The cervical spine can tolerate the highest +Gz loads when in the neutral, vertically aligned position (Helleur et al., 1984). In the ACM environment, the pilot must maintain a visually-based SA, which requires significant amounts of head movement while under high +Gz loads. During ACM, the pilot's neck typically spends most of its time in an unfavourable position, where it is less able to tolerate the applied +Gz loads. Such positions involve significant deviation from the normal axial alignment of the cervical spine, such as maximum lateral rotation, hyperextension or various combinations. These less than optimal head positions can exceed the ability of the cervical muscles and ligaments to support the cervical spine, leading to injury. In extreme cases, the eccentric head position under high +Gz loads can lead to failure of the vertebral bodies in the cervical spine itself.

Directly behind the aircraft is the most vulnerable sector of airspace and the one most susceptible to attack, since it is by nature the most difficult to observe. This area is known as the 'six' position (using positions on a clock-face), and in order to maintain SA fast jet pilots must manoeuvre their heads to 'check six', often under high +Gz loads (as seen in Figure 6.1). The 'check six' head position represents an extreme form of deviation from the normal axial alignment of the cervical spine. It often combines maximum lateral rotation with a degree of lateral flexion and extension. This position has been identified in many studies as the most likely head position for a +Gz-induced neck injury to occur (Averty and Green, 2005; Knudson et al., 1988; Lange et al., 2011; Newman, 1997a, 1997b; Wagstaff et al., 2012).

Complicating the situation further is the head-borne equipment used by the fast jet pilot. The nature, design, weight, size and position relative to the centre of gravity of the pilot's head of the helmet, oxygen mask, oxygen hose and any helmet-mounted equipment such as helmet-mounted displays (HMD) and night vision goggles (NVG) all have implications in terms of the development of +Gz-induced neck injuries. The flight helmet and oxygen mask assembly increase the overall weight of the head, giving the neck muscles an even bigger challenge in terms of their important role as supporting structures for the cervical spine (Andersen, 1988; Coakwell et al., 2004; Hamalainen, 1993; Lange et al., 2014; Newman, 1997b, 2002, 2006, 2014; Wagstaff et al., 2012). While lighter helmets have affected a reduction in the rate of neck injuries (Hamalainen and Vanharanta, 1992; Hamalainen et al., 1993a; Newman, 1996; Schall, 1989), the increasing complexity of helmets and the addition of various helmet-mounted sighting and display systems (such as the Joint Helmet-Mounted Cueing System, JHMCS) mean that reducing helmet weight further is unlikely to be possible (Newman, 2002, 2014).

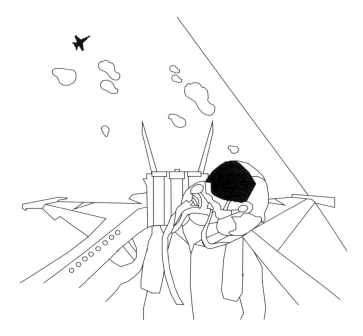

Figure 6.1   The 'Check 6' head position during air combat manoeuvring (ACM)

Under normal circumstances, at +1 Gz, the pilot's head weighs on average around 5 kg. A typical helmet and oxygen mask might weigh an average of 2 kg, giving a total of 7 kg at +1 Gz. At +9 Gz, the neck muscles and cervical spine are required to deal with a 63 kg head-borne mass, but are not inherently any stronger than they were at +1 Gz. Interestingly, there is some evidence that bone mass increases over time as a result of repetitive exposure to high +Gz loads, especially in the cervical spine (Naumann et al., 2001, 2004), but the effect of this on the likelihood of +Gz-induced neck injuries is not clear.

This situation is compounded further by any head movements that are required by the tactical situation, as discussed above, as well as the forward shifting of the centre of gravity of the head/helmet complex by the oxygen mask assembly (Newman, 1997b, 2002; Phillips and Petrofsky, 1983). The addition of helmet-mounted sighting and display systems complicates the situation even more, by increasing total head-borne mass and affecting the centre of gravity position (Äng and Kristoffersson, 2013; Knight and Baber, 2004; Lange et al., 2011; Manoogian et al., 2006; Newman, 1997b, 1998, 2002, 2006, 2014; Sovelius et al., 2008a; Wagstaff et al., 2012). This frontal loading of the head-helmet complex results in much greater neck extensor muscle activation in order to support the increased mass and forward centre of gravity (Knight and Baber, 2004).

Several other risk factors are worth mentioning. A positive association between total flight time (a marker of overall exposure to the high +Gz environment) and prevalence of neck pain has been documented in some studies (Albano and Stanford, 1998; Averty and Green, 2005; Hamalainen et al., 1994a; Hermes et al., 2010). Age is also linked (Hermes et al., 2010; Landau et al., 2006; Vanderbeek, 1988), but it is difficult to determine whether the neck injuries seen are due to increased age itself, or the greater cumulative experience of the high +Gz environment that occurs with increasing age in a fast jet pilot, or some combination of the two. Other studies have highlighted the potential contribution of various physical and psychosocial factors to the development of neck pain in F-16 pilots (De Loose et al., 2008).

Seating position in the aircraft has also been considered as a potential risk factor, especially an increased seat-back angle as seen in the F-16 aircraft (discussed in Chapter 8). The F-16 seat creates a posture with sustained forward neck flexion and decreased cervical lordosis (Coakwell et al., 2005; Hoek van Dijke et al., 1993). However, the F-16 can also achieve sustained +Gz loads greater than many other fast jets. The results of such ergonomic examinations have so far been equivocal (Coakwell et al., 2005; Drew, 2000; Jones, 2000; Vanderbeek, 1988; Wagstaff et al., 2012; Yacavone and Bason, 1992).

One study found no difference in neck pain prevalence between F-16 pilots and F-15 pilots flying in a more upright seat (Drew, 2000), while another study showed a higher prevalence in F-16 pilots compared with F-15 pilots (Vanderbeek, 1988). A study of cervical muscle morphology using magnetic resonance imaging (MRI) in F-16 pilots found a larger relative cross-sectional area in those pilots with neck pain (De Loose et al., 2009b). The authors speculated that this might be due to activation of deep cervical muscles to help stabilise the cervical spine in the presence of pain or injury due to +Gz. They also found that this increase was asymmetric, with a greater increase on the right side. They attributed this to the nature of flight operations in the F-16, with the right hand constantly on the right-sided control side-stick.

The advent of increasingly +Gz-capable super-agile aircraft are likely to increase the prevalence of +Gz-induced neck injuries in the future (Coakwell et al., 2004; Newman, 1998, 2014; Newman and Ostler, 2011). These aircraft are designed with improved flight control systems and control laws, against extremely relaxed stability criteria, and often make use of vectored thrust technology. They are able to operate in the post-stall regime of the flight envelope, at very low speeds and high AOA with full flight control authority (Alcorn et al., 1996; Boyum et al., 1995; Ericsson, 1995).

The manoeuvrability envelope of a super-agile fast jet is extremely complex. While conventional fighter aircraft have a +Gz environment predominantly in the Gz axis (Newman and Callister, 1999), super-agile aircraft are capable of generating high multi-axial Gx, Gy and Gz loads, high rates of G change, rapid transitions and rotational motions. This environment has significant implications for the aircrew, and the potentially adverse nature of this multi-axial G environment has been recognised by several authors (Albery, 2004; Coakwell et al., 2004; Frazier et al., 1982; Newman, 2006).

The multi-axial force environment of the super-agile fast jet can increase the likelihood of neck injury, given that the unrestrained head–neck complex will bear the brunt of these forces. In a study that mathematically modelled the geometry of super-agile flight manoeuvres, Newman and Ostler (2011) found that high AOA velocity vector rolls would lead to significant lateral G loads being imposed on the head and neck of the pilot, up to 6.7 Gy at an AOA of 70° and a roll rate of 200°/sec. These lateral G loads have significant potential to increase the prevalence of neck injuries in super-agile aircraft pilots. While there are obvious tactical benefits in achieving this level of enhanced performance capability, the cervical spine of the pilot flying such an aircraft may well suffer an increased risk of injury as a result.

Types of Injury

+Gz-induced neck injuries cover a varied spectrum of clinical pathology, from simple muscle strains involving pain and neck stiffness to intervertebral disc protrusions and even cervical vertebrae displacement (Andersen, 1988; Averty and Green, 2005; Hamalainen et al., 1994b; Newman, 1996; Schall, 1989; Vallejo Desviat et al., 2007; Wagstaff et al., 2012). Acute compression fracture of the cervical vertebrae is extremely rare, but has been reported (Andersen, 1988; Schall, 1989). Injury to the cervical muscles is the most commonly reported +Gz-induced neck injury (De Loose et al., 2009a; Newman, 1997a; Vanderbeek, 1988; Wagstaff et al., 2012; Yacavone and Bason, 1992).

Several case reports have been published which detail particular +Gz-induced neck injuries in pilots of high-performance fighter aircraft (Andersen, 1988; Newman, 1996; Schall, 1989). One report involved a Danish Air Force flight surgeon flying as the rear-seat occupant of an F-16B. Following an acute exposure to a violent +8 Gz manoeuvre, the flight surgeon developed a significant ligamentous injury in the cervical spine leading to a relative displacement of the C6 vertebral body relative to the C5 body above. Radiological opinion was divided as to whether a compression fracture of C6 was present or not (Andersen, 1988).

Another case report involved the pilot of a RAAF F-111C aircraft who developed a right-sided protrusion of the C6-C7 intervertebral disc, with displacement of both the anterior and posterior longitudinal ligaments (Newman, 1996). The pilot had significant neurological symptoms arising from this injury, including weakness and pain in the right arm. He ultimately made a full recovery and returned to operational flying. What is interesting in this case is that the +Gz environment of the F-111C was not particularly high, rarely going above +4 Gz. Despite this relatively benign +Gz environment, the pilot still suffered a serious cervical spine injury with no other apparent causal factors. This case highlights the importance of individual variation in the development of +Gz-induced neck injuries.

Degenerative changes in the cervical spine of fighter pilots have been the subject of much research attention (Hamalainen et al., 1993b, 1994b, 1999; Hendriksen and Holewijn, 1999; Landau et al., 2006; Petren-Mallmin and Linder, 1999, 2001; Sovelius et al., 2008c). It has proven difficult to establish whether the degenerative changes seen were due to chronic +Gz exposure or non-G factors such as ageing. Some studies have shown degenerative changes in the cervical spine at younger ages than in matched control groups (Hamalainen et al., 1993b, 1994b; Petren-Mallmin and Linder, 1999, 2001).

However, a study in Finland found no statistical difference in the frequency of degenerative changes in the cervical spine between a group of fighter pilots and a matched non-pilot control group over a 13-year period (Sovelius et al., 2008c). Some studies have also shown a high prevalence of degenerative changes in the cervical spine in otherwise asymptomatic individuals, including pilots exposed to high +Gz loads (Burns et al., 1996; Landau et al., 2006). The link between degenerative cervical spine changes, neck pain and exposure to the high +G environment remains to be clearly established. The research effort so far has been hindered by small group effects and the fact that symptomatic degenerative changes in the cervical spine are very common in the general population.

The aeromedical disposition of the aviator with a demonstrated +Gz-induced cervical spine injury is important. Permanent removal from flight duty is generally the exception rather than the rule (Newman, 1996). Conservative treatment is generally recommended, such as rest, heat, physiotherapy and anti-inflammatory medication. This approach generally is successful in returning the pilot to flight status as quickly as possible (Albano and Stanford, 1998; Coakwell et al., 2004; Drew, 2000; Newman, 1996). Surgery generally imposes a far longer period of time away from flying, but nonetheless if successful will allow the aviator to return to flying high-performance aircraft (Newman, 1996; Schall, 1989; Vallejo Desviat et al., 2007). In all cases, careful and thorough investigation of the pilot with such an injury is important.

Operational Impact

+Gz-induced neck injuries can have a potentially significant operational impact. Several studies have shown that the development of a neck injury in-flight can compromise the ability of the pilot to either satisfactorily complete their mission or be available for missions in the first place (Newman, 1997a; Wickes and Greeves, 2005).

Studies have shown that most aircrew who develop a +Gz-induced neck injury do not seek help (Averty and Green, 2005; Newman, 1997a; Wagstaff et al., 2012). In a RAAF survey, only 27 per cent of pilots sought medical attention, with 17 per cent being temporarily taken off flying duties as a result (Newman, 1997a). The average duration of restriction from flying was two weeks, but in one case involved a three-month period of grounding. Wickes and Greeves (2005) reported that 31 per cent of the fast jet pilots surveyed were grounded with neck pain for an average period of eight days. In a RAF survey involving 82 Hawk T1 fast jet instructors and students, three aircrew were permanently restricted from fast jet flying (Averty and Green, 2005). Such groundings due to +Gz-induced neck injuries can adversely affect the operational combat readiness of a fast jet squadron, through the non-availability of experienced aircrew.

The operational significance of these injuries is well demonstrated by a RAAF study which found that 38 per cent of pilots surveyed reported their neck injury as having interfered with their ability to complete their assigned mission (Newman, 1997a). This interference usually consisted of either early termination of the sortie, limited manoeuvring under G after developing the injury, and decreased tactical performance during the sortie.

Preventive Measures

+Gz-induced neck injuries are a significant aerospace medicine problem, and a lot of research attention has been directed at preventing such prevalent injuries. There are two fundamental ways to try to prevent +Gz-induced neck injuries: neck muscle conditioning for increased strength, and in-flight head positioning strategies.

Neck muscle conditioning programmes have been recommended by several researchers, as a way of improving the neck muscles' ability to better support the head and therefore to withstand the high +Gz environment (Albano and Stanford, 1998; Burnett et al., 2004; Coakwell et al., 2004; Drew, 2000; Green and Brown, 2004; Hamalainen et al., 1993a; Kikukawa et al., 1994; Knudson et al., 1988; Lange et al., 2013b; Newman, 1996, 1997a, 1997b; Schall, 1989; Vanderbeek, 1988; Yacavone and Bason, 1992). The case for neck muscle conditioning is based on the premise that any deviation from the normal axial alignment of the neck will predispose to injury, particularly if this occurs under high +Gz loading (as occurs during ACM and aerobatic flight). Stronger neck muscles should theoretically be able to tolerate high +Gz loads without injury and in so doing confer some degree of protection to the cervical spine. Stronger neck muscles should also take longer to fatigue, increasing the protection time in the high +Gz environment (Oksa et al., 1999).

Despite these theoretical advantages, the ideal neck muscle conditioning programme has yet to be defined. Furthermore, neck muscle conditioning programmes tend to be deployed on a somewhat ad hoc basis. No two programmes in use by air forces are the same. Some programmes make use of standard gymnasium equipment, while others use more novel techniques, such as elasticated bands (Netto et al., 2007), specially weighted helmets (Alricsson et al., 2004) and even a trampoline (Sovelius et al., 2006, 2007, 2008a). Indeed, not all fast jet aircrew even perform any neck muscle conditioning exercises. In a RAAF study, only 23 per cent of the fighter pilots surveyed reported doing any specific neck strengthening exercises (Newman, 1997a). Similarly, in a study of F-16 pilots, only 30 per cent reported participation in neck strengthening exercises (Albano and Stanford, 1998).

The search for the definitive link between neck muscle conditioning and a reduction in +Gz-induced neck injuries remains problematic, and is hampered by methodological differences in study design and also small group numbers. Some studies show that pilots that have conducted neck muscle conditioning programs have a lower prevalence of +Gz-induced neck injuries (Albano and Stanford, 1998; Jones, 2000; Lange et al., 2013b). Other studies have shown that even though neck muscle conditioning leads to greater neck muscle strength, this does not appear to translate into a lower prevalence of Gz-induced neck injuries (Alricsson et al., 2004; Averty and Green, 2005; Hamalainen et al., 1994a; Jones, 2000; Newman, 1997a; Taylor et al., 2006; Wickes and Greeves, 2005). However, most of these researchers noted the small sample sizes involved. Furthermore, the nature of the exercise programmes varied significantly between these studies, with many of them not being a standardised exercise programme, and in several of the studies there was a lack of appropriate matched control groups.

It has been argued that a well-designed and methodologically sound study of the effect of a specific neck muscle conditioning programme on the prevalence of +Gz-induced neck injuries is warranted (Newman, 1997a). The various methodological limitations in the studies conducted to date need to be recognised and addressed, such that a true picture of the role of neck strengthening as a protective countermeasure might emerge.

The effect of exposure to the high +Gz environment on the cervical muscles has been examined by some authors (Alricsson et al., 2001; Äng et al., 2005; Burnett et al., 2004; De Loose et al., 2009a; Lecompte et al., 2008; Seng et al., 2003). This relationship tends to look at the problem of +Gz-induced neck injuries from effectively the opposite direction. The interest here seems to be on determining whether exposure to high +Gz on a regular basis improves the strength of the cervical muscles, via a forced training effect. The results of these endeavours are mixed at best, and tend to suffer from similar methodological limitations to those described above.

Seng et al. (2003) did not show any strength increases associated with flying, when comparing a pilot group with a control group of non-pilots. Other studies have shown increases in cervical muscle strength with exposure to the high +Gz flying environment (Alricsson et al., 2001; Burnett et al., 2004). The impact of these changes on the prevalence of +Gz-induced neck injuries is not clear.

Other studies have shown relative decreases in neck muscle strength in pilots with a history of neck pain. The overall clinical implications of these findings, however, as noted by the authors, remain to be elucidated. In one study, neck extensor strength in fighter pilots with a reported history of neck pain was shown to be less than that in a matched control group of fighter pilots with no history of neck pain (Äng et al., 2005). However, whether this finding reflected the cause or the effect was not able to be established. A similar study comparing symptomatic pilots with pain-free pilots found some differences in cervical muscle strength. Symptomatic pilots had less lateral bending strength, and some muscular adaptations in asymptomatic pilots appeared to have occurred as a result of flight exposure (Lecompte et al., 2008). In a study involving F-16 pilots, no significant differences in neck muscle strength or neck position sense were found in a comparison between pain-free pilots and those with a history of neck pain (De Loose et al., 2009a). However, the neck pain pilots were found to have a limited range of movement of the cervical spine compared with the pain-free pilots. The authors felt that this could be overcome by stretching exercises, which might prove protective in the high +Gz environment.

While regular neck muscle conditioning is not universal for fast jet pilots, there is evidence that many pilots voluntarily perform some form of pre-flight neck exercise, generally as a warm-up immediately prior to a high G sortie (Albano and Stanford, 1998; Coakwell et al., 2004; Newman, 1997a; Schall, 1989; Vanderbeek, 1988). In a RAAF study, 63 per cent of surveyed fighter pilots reported that they usually performed such a pre-flight neck warm-up exercise (Newman, 1997a). These pre-exposure neck exercises usually consisted of a series of stretching, rotation and limbering up motions, combined with stretching of their necks in all axes. The 'check six' position was invariably emphasised by the pilots. In general these exercises were performed either immediately before walking to their aircraft or in the cockpit prior to take-off.

It seems eminently reasonable to suggest that both long-term neck muscle strength training and pre-flight stretching are important in minimising the rate of neck injury in fighter pilots exposed to high +Gz loads. Strength training would ensure that the pilot's neck is regularly conditioned to meet the +Gz challenge, while pre-flight stretching would make sure that these stronger neck muscles are prepared for each particular flight. It is analogous to many sporting activities, in which the athlete trains regularly for strength and endurance, and then immediately prior to the event completes a stretching or warm-up routine. However, the evidence base for this remains outstanding, as discussed above.

The other preventive strategy is the use of in-flight head positioning strategies. The evidence shows that fast jet aircrew who are regularly exposed to high +Gz forces do over time develop some form of individualised approach to protecting their cervical spines from +Gz-induced injury via a head positioning strategy (Albano and Stanford, 1998; Drew, 2000; Green and Brown, 2004; Newman, 1997b; Schall, 1989; Yacavone and Bason, 1992). In a RAAF study, 69 per cent of F/A-18 pilots surveyed reported using some form of head positioning strategy (Newman 1997b). Such head positioning strategies have been shown to reduce neck injuries in the high +Gz environment (Albano and Stanford, 1998).

The basic underlying principle of these head positioning strategies is to reduce the level of applied +Gz force endured solely by the neck muscles. There are several different strategies used by fast jet pilots. In a comprehensive study of head positioning strategies employed by RAAF F/A-18 pilots, it was found that aircraft structures such as the ejection seat and/or canopy structures were used to share the +Gz load otherwise faced solely by the neck muscles (Newman, 1997b). The strategy involved positioning the head in advance of the high +Gz application, bracing it against the head-box of the ejection seat and/or the canopy.

In doing so the head and its helmet assembly were well supported and not totally dependent on the neck muscles alone for support. Similar findings have been reached by other researchers (Schall, 1989).

Using the shoulders and upper body to assist in any turning manoeuvres required under +Gz also resulted in a load distribution effect that tended to reduce the strain taken by the neck muscles on their own (Newman, 1997b). Indeed, the level of neck muscle activation under applied +Gz has been shown to be less when the head is braced against a supporting structure (Green and Brown, 2004).

This strategy of positioning the head prior to the onset of high +Gz was the most commonly reported strategy (20 per cent of respondents) in the RAAF study (Newman, 1997b). In this strategy, the head was kept in position throughout the +Gz application, and only moved to a new position once the +Gz had eased off to a more comfortable level before reapplying the +Gz. The beneficial effect of this strategy is to reduce the overall workload of the supporting neck muscles. It is clearly easier for them to move the head and its helmet assembly under +1 Gz than under +7.5 Gz.

Another reported strategy is to move the head in only one plane at a time, rather than in two planes simultaneously (Newman, 1997b). Fourteen per cent of RAAF F/A-18 pilots reported using this strategy, which was described as moving the head either left or right, then up or down rather than moving the head straight to the rotated, up/down position. Several pilots in the RAAF study reported that failure to move their heads according to this particular technique almost invariably resulted in them developing a neck injury (Newman, 1997b). Such a strategy appears to result in relatively slower, more calculated head movements which are in only one direction at a time. This would seem to offer protection to the neck muscles from the obvious effects of a single rapid head movement in a complex, multiaxial direction under high accelerative loads (Newman, 1997b).

Pilots often employ a combination of strategies, depending on the circumstances of the tactical encounter (Newman, 1997b). In a RAAF study, several pilots reported that while they had developed personal head positioning strategies, they were sometimes not able to use them, as the rapid development of the ACM engagement gave them little time to consciously adopt their neck-protective strategies. In many instances this failure to use a protective strategy subsequently resulted in the development of a +Gz-induced neck injury.

Schall (1989) reported that some pilots were able to move their head around in a high +Gz environment with no difficulty. A similar finding was documented by Newman (1997b), who found that 17 per cent of RAAF F/A-18 pilots did not use a particular strategy or technique for head positioning, as they were generally able to move their heads around with apparent impunity under whatever +Gz loads the tactical situation called for. These findings highlight the level of individual variation in the aetiology of +Gz-induced neck injuries.

It has been argued that the best approach to minimising +Gz-induced neck injuries is probably a combination of preventative neck muscle conditioning for strength and in-flight protective head positioning strategies to reduce the exposure of the cervical spine to high and potentially damaging +Gz loads (Newman, 1997b). This makes intuitive sense, despite the current lack of supporting case-control evidence. More research is required to examine the effects of +Gz on the cervical spine and its supporting structures in greater detail, particularly given the increasing use of helmet-mounted display and sighting systems. Attention needs to be directed to the role of specific neck muscle training programs, including pre-high-+Gz mission warm-up exercises. Extended epidemiologic studies, including prospective cohort studies, are needed to more fully analyse and understand the multi-factorial risk determinants of +Gz-related neck injuries in pilots of high-performance aircraft. Only in this way can appropriate countermeasures be developed.

Spine Injuries

In this section, injuries to the spine (other than the cervical spine) due to +Gz exposure will be considered. These injuries are not quite as prevalent as +Gz-induced neck injuries, and as a result have attracted less research attention. Furthermore, the incidence of and mechanisms responsible for spinal disorders in helicopter pilots have drawn most of the research attention in terms of spinal disorders in pilots. In general terms, +Gz-induced injuries to the thoracic and lumbar spine in fast jet aircrew are most often associated with the high applied +Gz forces (peak and onset rates) involved with ejection from the aircraft. These ejection-related spinal injuries are beyond the scope of this book, and are considered in detail elsewhere (Newman, 2014). The injuries to be considered here in this section involve those due to regular exposure to the high +Gz environment of ACM and aerobatics, rather than assisted escape under emergency conditions.

Prevalence

As with +Gz-induced neck injuries, the issue of thoracolumbar injuries in pilots exposed to the high +Gz environment is complicated by the fact that thoracolumbar pain is common in the general population. There are few reports in the scientific literature dealing with non-cervical spine injuries in pilots exposed to the high +Gz environment. A Finnish study compared 320 fighter pilots with 283 non-flying controls (matched for age and gender), and found a greater incidence of pain in the thoracolumbar spine in the pilot group (Hamalainen, 1999). This greater prevalence of spinal pain was attributed to the high +Gz exposure of the pilots. A Turkish study found 10 per cent of F-16 pilots had degenerative changes in the lumbar spine (Tolga Aydog et al., 2004).

An Israeli study found that while the prevalence of low back pain was similar in fighter, transport and helicopter pilots, fighter pilots had nearly twice the prevalence of chronic pain compared with transport and helicopter pilots (Froom et al., 1986). Other authors have also suggested that lumbar spine symptoms are an important clinical issue in military fast jet pilots (Vallejo Desviat et al., 2007).

Risk Factors

There are numerous potential risk factors that have been identified for lumbar spine symptoms in fast jet pilots. These include exposure to the high +Gz environment, with the high compressive forces involved (Hamalainen et al., 1996), as well as prolonged sitting on a relatively hard ejection seat and the vibration of the aircraft during turbulence and low-level flight (Tolga Aydog et al., 2004). Increasing age, flight experience and tall stature have been linked with an increased prevalence of vertebral degenerative changes in fast jet pilots (Hermes et al., 2010; Tolga Aydog et al., 2004). Hermes et al. (2010) found that the risk of lumbar spine problems was significantly increased for those pilots who were older and had accumulated over 2,000 flying hours. While recognising the multi-factorial origin of lumbar spine disorders, they argued that age was likely to be the major influence (Hermes et al., 2010). Thus, as with cervical injuries, the relationship between +Gz exposure, flying experience, age and lumbar spine injuries is complicated.

Interestingly, repetitive exposure to the high +Gz environment results in quantifiable increases in bone mineral density and content in pilots (Naumann et al., 2001). This change is not universal: some parts of the skeleton are affected more than others. In terms of the spinal column, the changes are seen in the thoracic spine rather than the lumbar spine.

Types of Injury

The types of spinal injury seen are similar to those described in the section dealing with cervical injuries. These range from simple pain and muscle strains through to ligamentous injuries and even vertebral fractures. As with cervical injuries, the most common injury is muscular in origin.

There have been some interesting cases reported of spinal issues in pilots. In one case, a 25-year-old male F-16 pilot experienced G-LOC at +9 Gz while undergoing centrifuge training (Lange et al., 2013a). The pilot subsequently recovered, but soon after reported increasing pain in the upper part of the thoracic spine. This pain continued during the next eight years of operational flying. MRI investigation revealed disc degeneration in most of the thoracic spine.

In a Finnish study, pilots showed a non-statistically significant tendency towards more degenerative changes in discs in the lumbar spine (Sovelius et al., 2008c). The authors concluded that based on their findings exposure to acceleration in fast jet aircraft did not cause significant radiological changes in the spinal column of a fast jet pilot compared with non-flying controls.

The Republic of Singapore Air Force reported the case of an F-16 pilot who suffered a compression fracture of the fifth lumbar vertebral body during a rapid onset centrifuge training run (Low et al., 2008). Subsequent investigation revealed that the pilot had osteopenia (a low bone mineral density, often considered to be a precursor to osteoporosis). He recovered from this fracture, but was removed from fast jet flying operations and transferred to transport aircraft operations.

Preventive Measures

Little is published about preventive measures for thoracolumbar spinal injuries in fast jet pilots. The emphasis tends to be on treatment should such an injury occur, given that they are less common than cervical spine injuries. Lumbar supports have been investigated as one way of improving the comfort of fast jet aircrew and therefore in preventing the development of thoracolumbar spine injuries (Sovelius et al., 2008b; Winfield, 1999). In a Finnish study, the use of a lumbar support appeared to subjectively relieve in-flight symptoms and reduce the level of fatigue in the muscles of the lower back (Sovelius et al., 2008b). The apparent benefits of the lumbar support were not universal, however, with some subjects reporting that it made no difference.

Conclusion

Exposure to the high +Gz environment imposes significant stresses on the musculoskeletal system of the pilot of a military fast jet or civilian aerobatic aircraft. Due to the dynamic nature of the manoeuvring environment, the cervical spine is most at risk of injury. Such +Gz-induced neck injuries are a significant occupational hazard and aerospace medicine challenge. Neck muscle conditioning, pre-flight stretching and head positioning strategies have all been suggested as preventive measures. Given the rapidly evolving developments in military aircraft agility, and the increasing use of the head as a mounting platform for sighting and display systems, these injuries are likely to be an ongoing issue that needs to be adequately understood and dealt with, in order to protect the pilot from significant injury.

Chapter 7
Miscellaneous Clinical Effects of G

In previous chapters the effects of G exposure on the cardiovascular, respiratory and musculoskeletal systems have been considered in detail. This largely reflects the importance of these systems in terms of the adverse consequences of G exposure. However, it must be remembered that the entire human body can be subjected to these high levels of G force. All systems of the body are therefore potentially affected, albeit to different extents. In this chapter, the effects of G exposure on some of the other body systems are considered.

Cardiac Effects

The human heart is designed to operate in a constant +1 Gz environment. Its response to this environment was considered in detail in Chapter 3. However, the way in which the heart responds to and deals with the effects of high applied +Gz loads is of considerable interest to acceleration physiology researchers. The need to understand the possible long-term health implications in individuals exposed to a dynamic high +Gz environment, and to use this understanding to develop appropriate countermeasures, has driven much of the subsequent research.

Arrhythmias

It is well recognised that cardiac arrhythmias are a common accompaniment of high +Gz exposure (Balldin et al., 1999; Bartok et al., 1968; Blomqvist and Stone, 1983; Burton and Whinnery, 1996; Chung and Lee, 2001; Comens et al., 1987; Green, 2006a; Hanada et al., 2004; Krol and Holewijn, 1995; McKenzie and Gillingham, 1993; Newman, 1999; Skyttä et al., 1994; Tachibana et al., 1994; Whinnery et al., 1990; Wood, 1992; Zawadzka-Bartczak and Kopka, 2004, 2011; Zuidema et al., 1956). The available evidence overwhelmingly suggests that these arrhythmias tend to be clinically non-significant, not typically representative of any underlying cardiac pathology and generally only transient in duration (Chung and Lee, 2001). They tend to occur during and after +Gz exposure.

These cardiac rhythm disturbances tend to reflect a physiological response to a variety of +Gz-induced changes. These include the release of catecholamines and increased sympathetic drive, which tend to drive HR upwards. In addition, the heart is mechanically deformed by exposure to high +Gz, in common with all other organ systems. The heart will experience an increase in its apparent weight with +Gz exposure, leading to a caudad displacement of the heart.

Since the heart is fixed at its top, the heart will undergo a degree of +Gz-induced stretch as it reacts to the applied +Gz. This degree of mechanical deformation can stress or even damage the electrical circuitry of the heart, triggering +Gz-induced arrhythmias (Blomqvist and Stone, 1983; Burton and Whinnery, 1996; Chung and Lee, 2001).

In general, the types of arrhythmia seen include premature ventricular contractions (PVC) and supraventricular premature beats (SVPB). Other more serious rhythm disturbances such as ventricular tachycardia and sino-atrial block have been reported in various centrifuge studies, often coinciding with G-induced loss of consciousness (Sekiguchi et al., 1986; Tachibana et al., 1994; Whinnery, 1982b, 1990; Whinnery et al., 1979, 1980). The ventricular tachycardia is generally attributed to the autonomic imbalance produced by increased sympathetic drive due to the significant hydrostatic challenge experienced at high +Gz (Tachibana et al., 1994; Whinnery et al., 1980). These arrhythmias tend to resolve once the high +Gz application has ended.

Some researchers have attempted to document the arrhythmias produced by in-flight +Gz applications rather than centrifuge-based +Gz applications. In one study involving F-16 pilots of the Republic of Korea Air Force undergoing air combat manoeuvring sorties, cardiac arrhythmias were seen in 49 per cent of pilots (Chung and Lee, 2001). None of the rhythm disturbances were significant in a clinical sense. These findings were similar to those of other researchers. Skyttä et al (1994) found no haemodynamically significant or subjectively troubling arrhythmias in any of the 24 pilots they examined during air combat manoeuvring at +Gz levels up to +7.5. Krol and Holewijn (1995) also found no clinically significant arrhythmias in their study population of F-16 pilots.

The consensus of opinion, therefore, is that the arrhythmias seen under high +Gz conditions are clinically benign and effectively normal physiological responses to the high +Gz environment. Chung and Lee (2001) have argued that the autonomic imbalance developed as a result of acute high +Gz exposure could potentially lead to serious arrhythmias, which could jeopardise G tolerance and help precipitate loss of consciousness. They argue that if the autonomic balance is shifted too far then serious arrhythmias could result. Too much sympathetic activity could lead to ventricular tachycardia and even ventricular fibrillation, while a marked parasympathetic bias could lead to sinus arrest or sino-atrial block. Despite these acknowledged possibilities, the evidence as reported does suggest a rather benign view of the observed +Gz-induced cardiac arrhythmias.

Morphologic Changes

Researchers have also examined the effect of high +Gz loads on the morphology of the heart, both in terms of acute changes and also the long-term health implications of occupational high +Gz exposure. Cardiac volumes have been studied under various high +Gz conditions (Albery, 1999; Burton and McKenzie, 1975; Carter et al., 2006, 2010; Grossman et al., 2011; Laughlin, 1982;

Lu et al., 2008; Tripp et al., 1994; Whinnery, 1982b, 1990). A two-dimensional echocardiographic study showed that end-diastolic volume (EDV) and SV decreased during exposure up to +7 Gz, which was partly compensated for by the use of a G-suit (Tripp et al., 1994). Those findings essentially just confirm the hydrostatic challenge involved in maintaining appropriate VR under high +Gz conditions.

Carter et al. (2010) found no significant differences in cardiac dimensions between pilots exposed to high +Gz loads and pilots who were not. They speculated that anti-G countermeasures might play a protective role. In a long-term prospective study, 96 fighter pilots underwent echocardiographic assessment before and several years after repetitive high +Gz exposure, and found no significant changes had occurred in either cardiac or aortic morphology (Assa et al., 2011).

Another prospective study followed a group of military pilots flying to high +Gz over an average 12 years (Carter et al., 2006). These pilots were also diagnosed with a congenital cardiac valve abnormality (bicuspid aortic valve). The follow-up revealed no worsening of their cardiac or valve function, and there were no complications arising from the interaction of their high +Gz exposure and their valve abnormality. A large multi-nation study by the North Atlantic Treaty Organisation (NATO) also used echocardiography to determine whether long-term occupational exposure to high +Gz loads causes cardiac damage. Almost 300 pilots were studied and compared with a non-+Gz exposed control group, and no clinically significant differences were found in 16 echocardiographic variables (AGARD, 1997).

However, other reports have shown that in some individuals (and even animals such as the swine and baboon) repetitive high +Gz exposure can cause some cardiac changes. Exposure to +Gz levels up to +8 was found to be associated with myocardial ischaemia in swine and baboon subjects (Burns et al., 2008). A French study compared Mirage 2000 pilots with transport aircraft pilots, and found that the Mirage 2000 pilots had echocardiographically-demonstrated increases in right ventricular diameter of approximately 3mm (Ille et al., 1985). Another echocardiographic study showed that pilots of high +Gz aircraft had a higher prevalence of valvular abnormalities, particularly the pulmonary valve and the tricuspid valve (Martin et al., 1999). The clinical significance of these findings in the subject pilots was not addressed.

This issue of clinical significance is important. Detailed investigations may well reveal cardiac changes in pilots exposed repetitively to high +Gz loads, but if those changes do not appreciably alter cardiac function, do not reduce G tolerance and do not threaten the long-term health of the pilot, then they may be regarded as clinically trivial. Indeed, after full and comprehensive clinical evaluations, pilots with a history of ECG abnormalities and arrhythmias have been permitted to return to the high +Gz environment and even undertake spaceflight with no ill-effects (Jennings et al., 2010; Newman, 1999). It therefore seems fair enough to conclude that the weight of the combined evidence suggests that the human heart does not appear to develop any long-term clinically significant morphologic changes as a result of repetitive high +Gz exposure.

Cognitive Changes

The ultimate cognitive change that occurs as a result of +Gz exposure can be considered to be G-LOC, as discussed in Chapter 4. G-LOC has been extensively investigated. However, there has also been considerable interest over the years in the cognitive changes that might be present before G-LOC occurs. +Gz-induced cognitive impairments in the conscious pilot may be just as much a threat to the safety of the flight and the outcome of the mission as either A-LOC or G-LOC. These cognitive changes now warrant some attention.

A centrifuge study examining the mood of subjects after their +Gz exposure showed some interesting results (Biernacki et al., 2012). The study showed that arousal increased as a result of being centrifuged to high +Gz, mainly before and during the centrifuge run. Interestingly, perhaps, subjective enjoyment did not change. The adverse effect of +Gz on mood has been seen by several researchers (Dern et al., 2014; Schneider et al., 2008). Dern et al. (2014) examined the utility of a single bout of high +Gz as a long-duration spaceflight 'holistic countermeasure'. They were interested in whether such an exposure would have any impact on psychophysiological and cognitive performance. They found that while an intermittent +Gz exposure profile (five cycles of three minutes at +2 Gz and three minutes at rest) produced no psychophysiological changes, a sustained 30-minute exposure to +3 Gz had a negative impact on the mood of the subjects. These results call into question the use of high +Gz as a therapy for psychiatric illness, as was apparently promoted in 1818 by Dr Ernst Horn (1774–1848) of the Charité-Hospital in Berlin who used a primitive centrifuge device to 'treat' hysteria (Harsch, 2006)!

Another study examined executive functions (Biernacki et al., 2013). They found that exposure to applied +Gz loads in the centrifuge significantly improved attention switching (due to heightened arousal), but also led to an impaired visuospatial working memory. They argued that situational awareness (SA, a key element of flight safety) might be adversely affected by +Gz exposure, since attention and memory are affected by +Gz. The main memory effect seems to be the loss of a memory trace, rather than a change in processing time. The authors attributed these results to the hydrostatic effects of +Gz exposure, leading to a degree of cerebral ischaemia. Executive-level functions have also been observed to change after prolonged bed-rest (Lipnicki et al., 2009).

In another memory-based study, a word-based continuous recognition task was used under different +Gz conditions (Levin et al., 2007). Their results also showed an impairment of memory function. Specifically, they found that words encoded under +1 Gz conditions were recognised under sustained high +Gz loads, suggesting that retrieval was not affected by high +Gz exposure. However, words encoded under high +Gz conditions were not recognised as well, suggesting that sustained high +Gz affects the encoding process but not retrieval.

Various cognitive and psychomotor tasks have been examined under high +Gz conditions, including before and after G-LOC (Forster and Cammarota, 1993; Frazier et al., 1982; McKinley and Gallimore, 2013). Performance on a multiplication task and the ability to concentrate were impaired during a sustained exposure to +3 Gz (Frankenhauser 1958). In a reaction time study, the simple response time of a group of centrifuge subjects at a sustained level of +4.5 Gz was significantly increased (Truszczynski et al., 2013).

Motor performance under +Gz has also received considerable attention, and impairment in motor performance under high +Gz conditions has been seen by many researchers (Burton and Jaggars, 1974; Cohen, 1970; Dalecki et al., 2010; Frazier et al., 1982; Göbel et al., 2006; Guardiera et al., 2007a, 2007b, 2008, 2010; Sand et al., 2003). In one study, tracking performance (using a manual tracking task) at +3 Gz was impaired by about 50 per cent compared with values at +1 Gz (Guardiera et al., 2008). The performance impairment was in relation to accuracy of tracking. No influence on motor learning was observed at +3 Gz. The authors attributed the reduced tracking performance to vestibulospinal effects and/or the stressful nature of the +3 Gz exposure, a view supported by others (Frazier et al., 1982; Girgenrath et al., 2005; Göbel et al., 2006; Schneider et al., 2008).

Interestingly, other researchers have found that practice tends to reduce the motor performance impairment (Göbel et al., 2006; Guardiera et al., 2007a). Other researchers have found that the ability to control isometric force produced during movement is impaired by applied +Gz loads, potentially impacting upon flight safety (Sand et al., 2003). Alcohol intake has been shown to potentiate the deterioration in task tracking performance in the high +Gz environment (Burton and Jaggars, 1974).

Vestibular Effects

G-induced impairment of the vestibular system (the inner ear balance organs) as a result of either aerobatic flight or centrifuge exposure has been described in the scientific literature in recent years (Anton et al., 1994; Cheung, 2004; Davis et al., 1991; Jia et al., 2009; Muller, 2002; Williams et al., 1998). Supporting evidence of such G-induced vestibular impairment has been seen in participants in a number of human as well as animal studies (Anton et al., 1994; Cheung, 2004; Davis et al., 1991; Jia et al., 2009; Lim et al., 1974; Muller, 2002; Ohashi and Igarashi, 1985; Ostrowski and Bojrab, 2005; Parker et al., 1968; Sondag et al., 1996; Williams et al., 1998). The symptoms of this impairment include vertigo, balance problems, gait disturbance and even spatial disorientation.

This impairment has been termed 'G-induced vestibular dysfunction' (GIVD), but is also known by the colloquial term 'the wobblies' due to the unsteady post-flight gait reported by aerobatic pilots (Cheung, 2004; Muller, 2002). It is predominantly seen in civilian aerobatic pilots, particularly those participating at the highest levels of competition where the G environment is highly dynamic. Indeed, some 75 per cent of aerobatic pilots from several countries participating at the 1998 World Aerobatic Championships reported having experienced at least one episode of GIVD (Muller, 2002).

Muller (2002) reported the case of a 41-year-old aerobatic pilot who suffered from several episodes of GIVD involving vertigo and nausea, all of which resolved spontaneously following avoidance of aerobatic flight. The subject pilot's most recent episode occurred during practice for the World Aerobatic Championships, after a flight manoeuvre involving an exposure to -7 Gz. The diagnosis of benign paroxysmal positional vertigo (BPPV) was made after post-flight evaluations, which confirmed some ongoing vestibular dysfunction (predominantly an unsteady gait).

While commonly reported in civilian aerobatic pilots, there have been cases of GIVD reported in the military fast jet community. As an example, there was the case of an F-16 pilot who developed sudden onset of vertigo in a high $+$Gz turn (up to $+8$ Gz) and turned his head to look behind the aircraft in the 'Check 6' position (Williams et al., 1998). This particular pilot was also diagnosed initially with BPPV. Indeed, quite often these cases are diagnosed as BPPV (Davis et al., 1991; Muller, 2002; Williams et al., 1998), but increasingly they are being recognised as GIVD, since exposure to a high $-$Gz or $+$Gz load (alone or in combination) is intimately involved in the development of symptoms. The two conditions share much in common, clearly – according to some reports, traumatic head injury (involving high mechanical $+$Gz loads) is involved in more than half of BPPV cases (Ostrowski and Bojrab, 2005).

The $\pm$Gz threshold for developing GIVD has been examined. In a study by Jia et al. (2009), 11 pilots were exposed to $+9$ Gz for 10 seconds. No significant effect on vestibular function was detected after this high Gz exposure. They concluded that while a short-term (10 seconds) exposure to high $+$Gz ($+9$ Gz) does not appear to lead to GIVD, the role of more sustained high $+$Gz exposure needs to be considered. Most of the case reports of GIVD are based on civilian aerobatic flight with significant $-$Gz exposures (Muller, 2002). Indeed, aerobatic flight (whether civilian or military) involves frequent and repetitive exposures to various high $+$Gz and $-$Gz levels, representing a far more complex dynamic acceleration environment than that used in the study by Jia et al. (2009). Given the increasing multi-axial agility of both competition aerobatic aircraft and military fighter aircraft, the problem of GIVD in pilots will continue to be an issue that warrants ongoing research (Cheung, 2004).

It is increasingly recognised that head positioning under applied $+$Gz appears to be a contributing factor to the development of GIVD (Cheung, 2004; Jia et al., 2009; Williams et al., 1998). Both military fast jet crews and civilian aerobatic pilots often turn their heads while under high $+$Gz, in order to check their position relative to the ground or horizon, or to track an opponent aircraft

(Green and Brown, 2004; Newman, 1997b). Such head movements while under a high applied +Gz load complicate the operating environment for the vestibular system. Dizziness in pilots undergoing repetitive sustained high +Gz exposure in a centrifuge was reported in one study, where the dizziness was found to be more severe with head turning and which persisted for several weeks (Anton et al., 1994).

The underlying pathophysiological mechanism for GIVD appears to involve traumatic injury to the otolith organs, where the high $\pm$Gz load can overwhelm the structural integrity of the otoconia, leading to damage and thus the vestibular symptoms of vertigo and dizziness. Such damage to the otoconia has been seen in various animal studies (Lim et al., 1974; Ohashi and Igarashi, 1985; Parker et al., 1968; Sondag et al., 1996). This situation is similar to that for post-traumatic BPPV, where the blunt force trauma leads directly to otoconial damage (Ostrowski and Bojrab, 2005). Head movement and/or eccentric head positioning is thought to magnify the shearing effects of the applied +Gz (Jia et al., 2009; Ostrowski and Bojrab, 2005).

GIVD is an important issue for pilots exposed to high applied +Gz loads. The vestibular impairment can potentially lead to difficulties in controlling the aircraft, and any deterioration in spatial or SA due to GIVD can lead to a potentially catastrophic outcome. While GIVD can be considered to be an acute flight safety hazard for the high G pilot, the long-term health implications of multiple episodes of GIVD due to high G exposure remain to be determined.

Auditory Function

Several authors have looked at the question of whether auditory function is altered by exposure to the high +Gz environment. Given the increasing use of auditory warnings in the modern fast jet cockpit, particularly in a three-dimensional modality (Newman, 2014), this is a question of more than simply academic interest. Sandor et al. (2004) found that exposure to acceleration up to +4 Gz did not lead to a rise in the hearing threshold. Nelson et al. (1998) looked at the accuracy of a pilot's ability to localise auditory cues in the high +Gz environment. They found no increase in error up to a +Gz level of +5.6, however there was some impairment in accuracy seen at +7 Gz. They concluded that auditory cues are not compromised at moderate Gz levels. Similar findings were reported by Sandor et al. (2005), where acceleration up to +4 Gz did not significantly affect the accuracy of sound localisation ability.

Interestingly, one study has looked at whether the characteristics of a pilot's voice change under conditions of high +Gz exposure (Murbe et al., 2004). The results of this small study (with only four subjects) showed some non-significant changes in certain characteristics of the voice under high +Gz (including fundamental frequency). The practical implications of these apparent changes in voice characteristics under high +Gz conditions remain to be determined.

Visual Function

The human eye is particularly sensitive to low oxygen levels, and so +Gz-induced reductions in arterial delivery pressure to the eye can result in symptoms of visual impairment. While the emphasis of G-related visual impairment research has been around grey-out and black-out (as described in Chapter 4) there has also been a significant amount of work done in more subtle forms of G-induced visual impairment (Allnutt et al., 1999; Allnutt and Tripp, 1998; Braunstein and White, 1962; Cheung, 2004; Cheung and Hofer, 1999, 2003; Chou et al., 2003; Frankenhaeuser, 1958; Howard, 1965; McCloskey et al., 1992).

At a sustained level of +3 Gz, visual pursuit ability was seen to deteriorate (Cheung and Hofer, 1999). In a subsequent study, exposure to sustained +3 Gz resulted in immediate and significant papillary constriction (Cheung and Hofer, 2003). The authors attributed this finding to parasympathetic reflex activity involving the vestibular system (specifically, the otoliths).

Visual acuity and light perception have been observed to deteriorate under conditions of high applied +Gz loads (Braunstein and White, 1962; Frankenhaeuser, 1958; Howard, 1965; McCloskey et al., 1992). In a study of brightness discrimination under high +Gz, it was found that the contrast required to detect a change in illumination increased with acceleration: 16 per cent contrast was required at +5 Gz compared with only 9 per cent at +1 Gz at the same foot-Lambert level of luminance (Braunstein and White, 1962). Contrast sensitivity was evaluated in a number of subjects undergoing a centrifuge exposure (Chou et al., 2003). The results of this study showed a deterioration in contrast sensitivity after high +Gz exposure, which persisted for some time (over 20 minutes) after the centrifuge run.

Colour perception under high +Gz conditions has been evaluated by several researchers (Allnutt et al., 1999; Allnutt and Tripp, 1998; Balldin et al., 2003a; Chelette, 1999). This is of practical importance, given the increased and extensive use of colour in the primary flight displays (PFD) and multi-function displays (MFD) in modern high-performance aircraft (Newman, 2014). G-induced impairment of colour perception may potentially have an adverse impact on flight safety and mission performance.

In one centrifuge study, while almost all exposures to various Gz loads did not involve errors in identifying colours, some changes in hue perception were noted (Balldin et al., 2003a). These hue shifts were mainly noted at high +Gz-levels (up to +9 Gz). The hue most frequently perceived as changed was yellow. Rapid +Gz onset rates did not appear to affect colour recognition, up to and including +9 Gz. Similarly, Derefeldt et al. (2000) did not show any change in colour perception up to +4.6 Gz, which corresponded with 70 per cent relaxed G tolerance for the subjects involved.

Problems with the correct perception of chromatic colour (in terms of both hue and saturation) have been reported by several authors, however. Howard (1965) documented that at high levels of +Gz colours can be wrongly identified – red can be perceived as either orange or yellow. More recent experimental studies have also shown acceleration-induced difficulties with colour perception (Allnutt et al., 1998, 1999; Chelette et al., 1999). In one study subjects found it difficult to distinguish cyan from white, and green from yellow (Allnutt et al., 1999). These colour perception changes seen at +Gz levels approaching the individual's limit of tolerance have been used in other studies as training tools for improving +Gz tolerance (Borchart et al., 2000).

The results of studies examining the effects of +Gz on colour perception are not consistent, however. In many cases this reflects methodological differences between studies (G levels used, G onset rates used, relaxed G tolerance thresholds used, and so on). The true state of the relationship between colour perception and high +Gz exposure remains to be fully determined. Given the rise of multi-colour MFDs in modern fast jet cockpits, and the requirement to operate in varying luminance levels (day versus night and so on), this work remains of some practical importance.

Endocrine and Biochemical Changes

There is a well-documented stress response to high +Gz exposure. This response involves the release of several hormones and biochemical markers, ADH, adrenalin and cortisol (Comens et al., 1987, 1998; Obminski et al., 1997; Schneider et al., 2008; Tarui and Nakamura, 1987).

Obminski et al. (1997) found that 15 minutes after a centrifuge run (to approximately +6 Gz) the subjects demonstrated a significant increase in both salivary and serum cortisol levels, compared with the levels before +Gz exposure. Testosterone levels were also seen to increase. The findings suggest, according to the authors, that acceleration stress is a potent stimulant for endocrinological responses. Similar findings were seen in another centrifuge-based study, where cortisol levels were significantly elevated by +Gz exposure (Tarui and Nakamura, 1987). The authors of this study argued that salivary cortisol was a simple and effective marker for acceleration stress.

In another centrifuge study, various biochemical and endocrinological markers were seen to dramatically increase following 15 minutes at +3 Gz (Schneider et al., 2008). Relative to their levels before the centrifuge exposure, serum cortisol increased by 70 per cent, adrenocorticotropic hormone (ACTH) increased by a factor of three, prolactin by a factor of two, epinephrine by 70 per cent and norepinephrine by 45 per cent. At the same time, the perceived physical well-being of the subjects reportedly decreased. Acceleration thus clearly stresses the human body, as consistently shown by these responses.

On a related note, a significant level of protein in the urine has been reported after exposure to moderate +Gz levels (up to +5.5 Gz) in a centrifuge (Noddeland et al., 1986). This +Gz-induced proteinuria has been attributed to severely reduced renal blood flow as a result of the elevated hydrostatic forces involved in the centrifuge run. Such +Gz-induced proteinuria is important to be aware of from a clinical perspective. A pilot undergoing a routine medical evaluation may be incorrectly assumed to have kidney disease worthy of further clinical investigation if such +Gz-induced proteinuria is discovered and the link to recent +Gz exposure is not considered. Repeat urine testing some 24–48 hours later will reveal no ongoing proteinuria.

Trauma

Since G is a force, it stands to reason that high levels of applied +Gz might result in a direct physical injury to various parts of the body. While this has already been extensively described in Chapter 6 dealing with musculoskeletal effects of +Gz exposure, other body systems and organs have also been seen to suffer direct physical trauma from such +Gz exposure. These types of injuries are relatively rare (especially relative to +Gz-induced spinal injuries), but have been well described in a series of published cases. These now deserve some attention, for the sake of completeness.

Vascular Effects

Direct +Gz-induced trauma to the blood vessels, while uncommon, has been described. In one case, a 55-year-old civilian aerobatic pilot developed abdominal pain immediately after an aerobatic flight in an Extra 300 aircraft (Beyer and Daily, 2004). He had undertaken aerobatic flights on five of the six preceding days. His ±Gz exposure was quite significant – it was estimated that each flight involved approximately 50 manoeuvres with a ±Gz range from +8 Gz to –6 Gz. Subsequent investigation revealed that he had experienced a dissection (a delamination effect, involving separation of the layers of a blood vessel wall) of the right renal artery. He eventually made a full recovery and returned to aerobatic flight. The authors attributed the trauma to the artery as being due (most likely) to the rapid G onset, the high G peak, and the age of the pilot, among other factors.

A similar but potentially more serious case involved a carotid artery dissection (Adler et al., 2013). The pilot involved was a 38-year-old civilian aerobatic pilot, who had undergone four practice aerobatic sorties of 25 minutes each in a Sukhoi Su-31 aircraft. The ±Gz range experienced in these sorties was from –6 Gz to +8 Gz. Some four days later, during the airshow display, he developed significant neurologic impairment while in a high G manoeuvre. This impairment included confusion, an inability to talk and some right-sided paralysis. Subsequent investigations showed a dissection of the left internal carotid artery. The pilot went on to make a full recovery. The authors attributed the event to an embolic stroke during the airshow routine, caused by the arterial dissection some four days prior. This dissection they in turn attributed to the combination of neck rotation and flexion, a rapid –Gz-to-+Gz transition and a sustained high level of –Gz, which led to stretching of the artery and resultant internal dissection.

Respiratory System

The pulmonary and respiratory effects of high +Gz exposure have been considered at length in Chapter 5. However, some interesting cases involving damage and trauma to the respiratory system as a result of +Gz exposure have been described (Cui et al., 2012; Gan et al., 2008; Maningas et al., 1983).

Cui et al. (2012) reported the case of a fighter pilot who was found to have a rare congenital abnormality known as pulmonary sequestration. This involves a segment of non-functioning lung tissue with its own systemic arterial supply. The pathogenesis of this aberrant condition is unclear. Although not due to +Gz exposure, the case is of interest in that the authors noted that the effect of repetitive +Gz exposure on such a condition is also unclear. However, the subject pilot's condition was not discovered as a result of his flight experience, and after successful treatment he returned to full flight duties and had no further issues due to the condition in the subsequent five years.

Direct respiratory trauma is a more significant +Gz effect. Rupture of the diaphragm was reported in a case involving an aircrew member in a T-33 jet (Maningas et al., 1983). The subject underwent several high +Gz manoeuvres and developed nausea and vomiting as a result of the significant dynamic motion. After landing, severe epigastric pain was reported. Post-flight medical evaluation revealed a diaphragmatic rupture, which was subsequently repaired successfully. The authors attributed this event to the combination of vomiting and high +Gz exposure.

The Republic of Singapore Air Force reported six cases of pneumomediastinum in subjects undergoing centrifuge training in the period 1995–2006 (Gan et al., 2008). This condition involves the presence of air in the central compartment of the thorax, particularly around the heart. The authors of this report were of the view that these centrifuge-derived events were due to excessive or incorrectly performed AGSMs in trainees naive to the high +Gz environment. Such cases highlight the importance of correctly used anti-G countermeasures.

Abdominal Trauma

Although relatively rare, traumatic injuries to the abdominal area have also been reported due to exposure to a high +Gz environment (Hatton and Harford, 1985; Snyder and Kearney, 2002). A flight surgeon flying in an F-16 during 2 v 2 ACM exercise developed left inguinal pain after a +6.8 Gz manoeuvre. This pain was subsequently found to be due to a left inguinal hernia, caused by the combination of high +Gz exposure and the vigorous AGSM employed by the subject. This anti-G strain significantly elevates intra-abdominal pressure (discussed in Chapter 10) and as a result can contribute to the development of a hernia (Snyder and Kearney, 2002).

An unusual +Gz-related abdominal issue was reported in a fast jet test pilot (Hatton and Harford, 1985). This particular pilot was found to have a calcified haematoma of the greater omentum, which is the large peritoneal fold overlying the abdominal organs. The authors of the case report argued that exposure to the high +Gz forces involved in fast jet flying might increase the risk of haemorrhage in the omentum, which the subject pilot had apparently sustained in the past. The clinical significance of this type of injury is not likely to be major, but does reflect the potential for high +Gz forces to cause rupture of blood vessels in relatively delicate tissues.

Orthopaedic Issues

Most of these issues relate to the more common G-induced trauma to the cervical and lumbar spine, as discussed at length in Chapter 6. However, there have been some interesting cases reported on which are somewhat rarer and worthy of mention. One of these involved an avulsion of the triceps tendon in a pilot (Blumberg et al., 2002). In this case, the pilot was an F-16 pilot who underwent several weeks of intense and repetitive +Gz exposure, following a period of some months away from such flying. After a flight involving repetitive peaks to +5 Gz, the pilot developed pain in his left elbow after around 1 minute at +5 Gz. Subsequent medical investigations revealed the presence of a left triceps tendon avulsion. The pilot made a full recovery from this relatively rare type of traumatic injury (Blumberg et al., 2002).

Less significant but perhaps equally troubling is the case of a pilot who developed a significant swelling of the external ear, known as an othematoma (Aghina, 1984). The trauma and damage to the external ear was attributed to the combination of a helmet which was not fitted correctly (leading to direct pressure) and the concomitant exposure of the pilot to high applied +Gz loads. This case illustrates the importance of correctly fitted flight equipment in the high +Gz environment.

Skin Effects

High +Gz exposure can lead to rupture of skin capillaries in dependent, unprotected (that is, not covered by a G-suit) parts of the body. This results in cutaneous petechiae formation (known colloquially as 'G measles'), which can be spectacular and widespread. It does, however, resolve quickly over a few days, with no apparent ongoing clinical implications. It is quite a common sequelae of exposure to high +Gz levels. Cutaneous petechiae begin to develop once the +Gz level exceeds around +5 Gz (Ganse et al., 2013; Whinnery, 1987). It has also been described with high levels of Gx exposure, as would occur with the launch and re-entry phases of spaceflight operations (Wu et al., 2012). In this setting the petechiae tend to most commonly occur on the back of the thorax, mainly due to the Gx involved in the launch phase.

The exact mechanism for the formation of such petechiae as a result of high +Gz exposure is not fully understood (Gerzer, 2009). External counterpressure (as provided by an inflated G-suit) prevents the petechiae from developing, presumably by keeping the transmural pressure in the capillaries at a more tolerable level. Capillaries in areas of the body with no external counterpressure applied do not have this protection from internal pressure increases, such that the transmural pressure rises to a level that ultimately leads to capillary rupture. What is interesting is that some research suggests that regular exposure to high +Gz (as might occur in a centrifuge) can lead to some form of adaptation of the vascular to the hydrostatically-mediated pressure increase, resulting in petechiae formation occurring at a higher +Gz threshold than might otherwise be the case (Gustaffson et al., 2013).

Conclusion

The effects of +Gz can clearly be widespread. Almost no part or system of the human body is exempt from the potentially deleterious effects of high +Gz. With that in mind, the practical application of this knowledge is in how best to protect those exposed to the high G environment from these particular adverse effects. What factors affect how an individual will tolerate a given high +Gz load, and what countermeasures can be deployed to augment tolerance and ensure a safe outcome for the flight are important questions. The next parts of this book will explore the issues of G tolerance and countermeasures in detail.

PART III
Tolerance and Adaptation

Chapter 8
Tolerance to High G

A given pilot's ability to tolerate an applied G load is a function of many different factors. These include a variety of individual factors, such as dehydration and physical conditioning, for example, as well as a host of flight-related factors such as frequency of exposure and the nature of the specific flight manoeuvre being undertaken. It is important to remember that improving tolerance to G remains an ongoing task, particularly as the G ability of aerobatic and military fast jet aircraft continues to expand.

The purpose of this chapter is to examine all of the various individual and flight-related factors that can affect a given pilot's tolerance to high applied +Gz.

Defining and Measuring G Tolerance

Firstly, it is useful to consider what is meant by the term G tolerance, and how it might be measured. While the term G tolerance is used somewhat liberally in the scientific literature, it is important to note that tolerance to +Gz can be defined in several different ways, depending on the physiological end-point chosen (Burton and Whinnery, 1996; Coburn, 1970; Green, 2006a). It is thus essential to specify which end-point is being used when describing +Gz tolerance, in order to prevent confusion and to allow meaningful and valid comparisons to be made between research findings. This is particularly imperative when comparing the effectiveness of different anti-G protective systems.

G tolerance can refer to either how much G can be achieved while the pilot remains conscious, or for how long a pilot can sustain a given G level. How much absolute G can be achieved has been referred to as peak G or G intensity tolerance (Burton, 2000a). It relates to the absolute level of G that a pilot can tolerate without losing consciousness. How long a pilot can sustain a given G level is known as G duration tolerance (Burton, 2000b). This might involve ongoing exposure to a specific G level, or a series of alternating G loads repeated over time.

The next issue is one of measuring tolerance to G, in either intensity or duration terms. The adverse visual symptoms of high +Gz exposure as described in detail in Chapter 4 have long been used as physiological end-points in research designed to establish tolerance limits for human exposure to +Gz (Burton and Whinnery, 1996; Coburn, 1970; Green, 2006a; Krutz et al., 1975). Much of this work has been, and is still, performed in human-carrying centrifuges. Use of these devices allows several types of acceleration profile to be used for the assessment of G tolerance. These include the gradual onset run (GOR) which applies G at an incremental rate (often 0.1 Gs^{-1}), the ROR at a higher rate (often 6 Gs^{-1}) and the simulated air combat manoeuvring

(SACM) profile. The SACM involves repetitive excursions to high +Gz levels (typically, +4.5 Gz for 15 seconds and +7 Gz (or +9 Gz) for 15 seconds, repetitively), and is designed as an approximation for the G environment which occurs during ACM (Bain et al., 1994; Burton et al., 1987; Burton and Shaffstall, 1980; Lalande and Buick, 2009; Tong et al., 1998a; Weigman et al., 1995). In experimental use, the SACM functions as a tolerance end-point tool for measuring the effectiveness of new anti-G countermeasures (Burton and Shaffstall, 1980). The SACM is illustrated in Figure 8.1.

The most commonly used physiological end-point in acceleration research for determining G intensity tolerance is 100 per cent peripheral light loss, PLL (Burton et al., 1974; Burton and Whinnery, 1996; Howard, 1965; Parkhurst et al., 1972). In the centrifuge, this is achieved via a series of lights positioned within the centrifuge gondola in front of the subject and extending to the periphery of vision. +Gz tolerance is then expressed as the +Gz level that resulted in PLL. Both relaxed and straining +Gz tolerances can be defined using this method (Burton and Shaffstall, 1980; Burton and Whinnery, 1996; Gillingham, 1988; Parkhurst et al., 1972). Relaxed +Gz tolerance is the +Gz level at which a relaxed subject experiences PLL, while straining tolerance refers to that level of +Gz at which PLL occurs despite the subject using an AGSM (discussed in Chapter 10). Black-out (complete loss of visual function) occurs when there is central light loss (CLL).

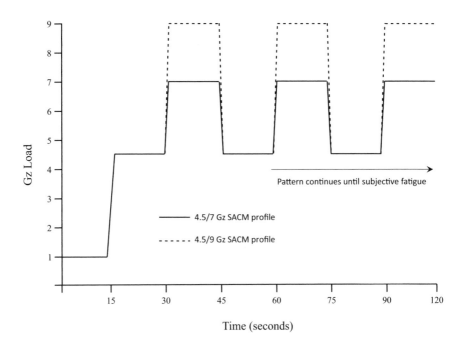

Figure 8.1   The simulated air combat manoeuvring (SACM) centrifuge profile

For assessing G endurance tolerance, subjective fatigue is the physiological end-point most commonly used (Green, 2006a). The tolerance metric is the length of time (in seconds or minutes) that the subject was able to endure a given +Gz profile, which might be either a specific constantly-held G level or an alternating sequence such as the SACM profile (Burton and Shaffstall, 1980; Burton and Whinnery, 1996; Parkhurst et al., 1972; Tong et al., 1988a). The alternating levels are chosen to reflect an ACM profile, but the ability to accurately mirror the performance of the aircraft is directly related to the performance and capabilities of the centrifuge being used.

There are some methodological problems inherent in the use of these measures of +Gz tolerance. They are all subjective, and therefore highly variable, and depend very much on the ability of the subjects to recognise a given end-point (Gillingham, 1987; Ludwig and Krock, 1991). Experienced subjects tend to give more reliable data than naïve subjects, who are often overwhelmed by the sensations involved in the +Gz exposure (Parkhurst et al., 1972). Furthermore, a recognised difficulty with use of PLL is that it will only apply to gradual onset +Gz exposures (Gillingham, 1988; Krutz, 1975). More objective tolerance measures have been proposed by some researchers (Hrebien, 1988), as well as more operationally relevant centrifuge profiles such as the tactical air combat manoeuvring (TACM) profile (Tong et al., 1998a). Currently, a reliable and valid objective measure of +Gz tolerance is yet to be defined.

G-Time Tolerance Curve

The relationship between +Gz level and time in terms of overall G tolerance was first described by Stoll (1956), and has since been well established. The result is the G-time tolerance curve, depicted in Figure 8.2.

Several important aspects of high G physiology are evident in the G-time tolerance curve. Firstly, the metabolic energy reserve, which is the basis of the functional buffer period, is well shown. Even very high levels of +Gz can be tolerated if they are not sustained for more than a few seconds, as the metabolic reserve prevents G-LOC from occurring (Kydd, 1972). If the G level is sustained, however, the risk of sudden G-LOC with no visual premonitory signs becomes much greater. Thus, as magnitude and rate of application increase, the likelihood of experiencing the visual symptoms decreases correspondingly. The effects of different rates of +Gz application are shown in the following version (Figure 8.3) of the G-time tolerance curve.

Slower, gradual rates of onset of +Gz typically result in these visual warning signs, as shown above (Aircraft C and D). The full spectrum of +Gz effects is thus experienced, from consciousness to grey-out, black-out and then G-LOC. It is important to note that these visual symptoms occur about +1 Gz lower than G-LOC, as indicated by the width of the shaded area in the diagram. As the rate of +Gz onset increases, however, this bandwidth decreases, until at high onset rates no visual warning signs occur, and G-LOC is rapid and sudden if the G exposure is prolonged (Aircraft A). If the time at high G is less than the functional buffer period, G-LOC can be avoided (Aircraft B), but clearly the margin for error is very small.

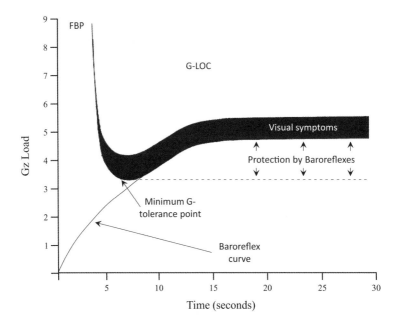

Figure 8.2   The Stoll G-time tolerance curve

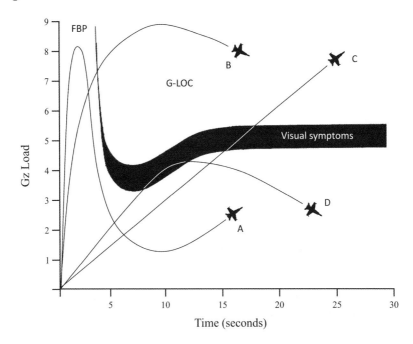

Figure 8.3   The effect of G onset rates on G tolerance

This is the scenario faced by competition aerobatic aircraft, where the G levels reached can be quite high but not sustained for more than a few seconds.

The lower edge of the visual symptom band is formed by the developing action of the baroreceptor reflexes, as discussed in Chapter 3. These take several seconds, (on average around 10 seconds) to become fully activated in response to the application of +Gz stress (Blomqvist and Stone, 1983; Mancia and Mark, 1983). If the onset rate is not too rapid, the threshold for visual disturbance is raised once the baroreflexes are fully operational, as shown in the G-time tolerance curve above (Miller et al., 1959). This increase in visual threshold represents in G tolerance terms an increase of around +1 Gz (Gillingham, 1988). The trough in the curve is due to the temporal intersection of the metabolic energy reserve curve and that of the baroreceptors. It represents minimum effective G tolerance.

The baroreflexes play an integral and vital role in terms of G tolerance. They are the means by which the cardiovascular system responds to an applied +Gz stress. The circulatory effects of exposure to high +Gz are essentially the same as those for assumption of upright posture, as discussed in Chapters 3 and 4, only several orders of magnitude greater. However, the HP increase inherent in such exposure to high +Gz occurs instantaneously with the onset of acceleration, while baroreflex compensation only becomes fully effective after approximately 6 seconds. The baroreflexes thus face a deteriorating cardiovascular situation just as they begin attempts to rectify it. This temporal delay, generally accepted as around 6–10 seconds, results in the baroreflexes having to drive the circulation back to a normal state from a much more compromised starting position than would occur if they were able to react instantaneously.

Once the baroreflexes are fully optimised, however, the cardiovascular situation tends to improve. As seen previously, the increased sympathetic drive mediated by the baroreflexes results in an increase in HR, peripheral vasoconstriction and increased cardiac contractility. This enhances VR and therefore SV and CO. As a result of these compensatory actions, CO falls by only about 20 per cent at +4 Gz (after 30–60 seconds of adjustment to this high +Gz level).

An adequately functional baroreflex system is thus a critical element in the prevention of both orthostatic intolerance and G-LOC. The high gravitoinertial forces experienced by pilots of high performance aircraft represent a major challenge to the cardiovascular system. Failure of the baroreflex in its role as a BP control system to maintain cerebral perfusion in the face of these high +Gz forces results in G-LOC, as seen in Chapter 4.

In summary, then, the physiological consequences of exposure to high +Gz forces as illustrated in Figure 8.3 represent a cardiovascular spectrum. This spectrum is dependent on the rate of application of the +Gz force. The rate of +Gz application is important in terms of the appearance of symptoms prior to the occurrence of G-LOC. The critical G onset rate in this context is around 2 Gs^{-1}. If the rate of application of G is less than this critical value, then the cardiovascular system will experience the entire spectrum of +Gz effects. That is, grey-out will occur at +3 to +4 Gz, followed by black-out at +4 to +4.5 Gz and G-LOC at

+4.5 to +5 Gz. If the rate of onset is higher than this value, loss of consciousness is too rapid for the other effects to be experienced. The pilot may thus bypass the earlier signs of cardiovascular compromise and proceed straight to G-LOC.

Individual Factors Affecting G Tolerance

A pilot's tolerance to +Gz loads is a multi-factorial phenomenon (Galvagno et al., 2004; Hrebien and Hendler, 1985; Newman, 2014; Newman et al., 1999; Whinnery and Parnell, 1987). In the final analysis, increasing a pilot's tolerance to +Gz is the ultimate aim. Arguably the easiest way to do this is to minimise the impact of the known individual factors that reduce a pilot's +Gz tolerance before they step into the cockpit. These factors will now be addressed in this section.

Individual Variation

It is well recognised that there is a degree of individual variation in terms of +Gz tolerance, with some people having better inherent +Gz tolerance than others for no apparent reason. Similarly, it must be remembered that every pilot can have 'good G days' and 'bad G days'. Such variation within an individual may be due to the presence of other individual or flight-related factors, or may have no apparent cause.

Anthropometry and Gender

Attempts have been made by several researchers to relate various anthropometric and physiological variables to +Gz tolerance and the risk of G-LOC. These studies have been largely inconclusive. Indeed, in their review of the subject, Webb et al. (1991) found that in general anthropometric and physiological variables were poor predictors of +Gz tolerance. Other studies have demonstrated a clear lack of a relationship between certain factors and +Gz tolerance. A US Navy study (Johanson and Pheeny, 1988) found that the incidence of G-LOC was not correlated with pilot age, height or weight.

In contrast, a study by Whinnery (1979) documented good correlations between certain individual factors and tolerance to +Gz. For example, short stature (with its concomitant hydrostatically-favourable reduction in effective vertical heart–brain distance) was found to be correlated with improved +Gz tolerance. Whinnery also found that +Gz tolerance was correlated with age, weight, percentage body fat, BP (both resting and during tread-mill exercise), and flying experience (1979). Indeed, the ideal high +Gz tolerant pilot has been described as an individual who is older, shorter, heavier, more experienced (more flying hours and more fighter or high-performance aircraft hours) and with higher BP (Whinnery, 1979).

The gender of the subject or pilot has not been found to be correlated with tolerance to +Gz (Convertino et al., 1998; Dooley et al., 2001; Gillingham et al., 1986; Shender and Heffner, 2001; Zhang, 1999). Female subjects or pilots have demonstrated an equivalent +Gz tolerance to males, especially when countermeasures such as G-suits are correctly fitted (Gillingham et al., 1986).

Blood Volume Changes

A reduction in circulating blood volume will have a negative impact on G tolerance (Burton and Whinnery, 1996; Green, 2006a; Nunneley and Stribley, 1979). Such blood volume changes can arise from dehydration (due to such factors as heat stress or alcohol intake) or blood donation. Heat stress is a well-recognised hazard in military fast jet operations (Nunneley and Myhre, 1976; Nunneley et al., 1981). According to one study, dehydration is associated with a measurable decrease in tolerance time to a sustained +Gz load. A dehydration level of up to 3 per cent of body weight reduced the tolerance time to +7 Gz from 60 seconds to an average of only 35 seconds, a reduction in tolerance time of some 40 per cent (Nunneley and Stribley, 1979). The link between dehydration and reduced +Gz tolerance has been seen in several other studies (Balldin et al., 2002; Balldin and Siegborn, 1992).

The relationship between reduced blood volume and +Gz tolerance is well demonstrated by the orthostatic intolerance seen in astronauts returning to the +1 Gz environment of Earth after prolonged time in orbit. Saline loading prior to re-entry is used as a countermeasure by astronauts to try to offset this intolerance (Bungo et al., 1985). This countermeasure has been shown to be quite effective in reducing the fall in MAP seen in those with orthostatic intolerance. It was used as a standard operational procedure by Space Shuttle crew members (Bungo et al., 1985).

Hypoxia

The hypoxia associated with altitude is another factor that can reduce tolerance to +Gz (Green, 2006a; Howard, 1965). Hypoxia will reduce the functional buffer period, through a reduction in the oxygen stores held in the brain. In one study, exposure to normobaric hypoxia was seen to reduce the subsequent HR response to an orthostatic stress (Rickards and Newman, 2002). It was noted that while the BP responses were unchanged, the changes in the HR response might be more significant when combined with other factors such as heat stress, dehydration and high +Gz loads (Rickards and Newman, 2002).

Caffeine

Caffeine is an extremely commonly used substance, with well-known and understood cardiovascular and central nervous system stimulant properties (Berry et al., 2003; Florence et al., 2005; Walker et al., 2010). There has been some research interest in terms of how caffeine ingestion might affect tolerance to applied +Gz (Berry et al., 2003; Florence et al., 2005; Walker et al., 2010).

In one study (Walker et al., 2010), eight subjects consumed a caffeine-based energy drink and underwent a series of centrifuge exposures (rapid onset, gradual onset and SACM runs). The results showed that relaxed G tolerance was some 13 per cent higher under the influence of caffeine, but significantly SACM duration tolerance was unaffected. There were some adverse consequences of caffeine ingestion seen in the subjects, notably a higher rate of cardiac arrhythmias.

Another study found that caffeine consumption impairs the ability of the cardiovascular system to tolerate an orthostatic challenge (Berry et al., 2003). Specifically, the ability to maintain MAP is compromised by caffeine, which the authors attributed to an adverse effect of caffeine on baroreflex function.

Fatigue

The main effect of fatigue on tolerance to +Gz is in terms of muscular fatigue limiting the ability to perform an appropriate AGSM. This is discussed in more detail in Chapter 10. While fatigue in general has been linked with reduced +Gz tolerance, there is little robust evidence supporting this link. In a recent study, no differences were found in +Gz tolerance terms between subjects undergoing centrifuge testing under various conditions of circadian desynchronosis (Ramsey et al., 2008). However, of interest was the finding (which was statistically significant) that participants in the study reported that performing the AGSM at night was subjectively more difficult than during the day (Ramsey et al., 2008).

Physical Conditioning

Controversy still surrounds the role of physical conditioning in G tolerance. The advantages and disadvantages of both aerobic and anaerobic conditioning have all received significant research attention over the years. In general terms, there are concerns as to the possible adverse effect of aerobic training on a fighter pilot's +Gz tolerance, while anaerobic training is reported as having a beneficial effect on +Gz tolerance (Balldin, 1984; Banta and Grissett, 1985; Bateman et al., 2006; Bulbulian et al., 1994; Burton, 1986b; Burton et al., 1987; Convertino, 1987; Cooper and Leverett, 1966; Epperson et al., 1982, 1985; Jacobs et al., 1987; Newman et al., 1999; Tesch et al., 1983; Whinnery and Parnell, 1987).

Aerobic conditioning involves improving the body's ability to use oxygen by improving cardiovascular efficiency (Banta and Grissett, 1985). Aerobic capacity is generally expressed in terms of maximal oxygen consumption (VO_{2max}) which is given by the amount of oxygen used per kilogram of body weight per minute. Aerobically fit people tend to have higher VO_{2max} values and lower HRs. Highly trained endurance athletes may have VO_{2max} levels exceeding 70 ml O_2/kg/min and resting HRs less than 50 bpm (Dowell, 1983; Stromme et al., 1977). Aerobic activities include running (especially long-distance, endurance running), swimming and distance cycling. Aerobic fitness may translate into the ability to sustain high workloads for longer periods or more repetitions of repetitive activities (as a shorter recovery period is required).

A low resting HR is a well-established indicator of cardiovascular efficiency (Dowell, 1983; Shvartz and Meyerstein, 1972; Stromme et al., 1977). Low HR before and during HUT has been suggested as an indicator of improved orthostatic tolerance (Dikshit et al., 1986; Klein et al., 1969; Shvartz and Meyerstein, 1972). Based on this information, aerobically fit individuals would be expected to have improved orthostatic tolerance. However, this has not been seen. In fact, the research suggests that highly aerobically trained individuals are disadvantaged when orthostatically stressed or subjected to high +Gz loads. Klein et al. (1969) were unable to demonstrate a clear direct relationship between orthostatic tolerance and aerobic fitness due to endurance training. They found similar numbers of fainters among athletes and non-athletes undergoing a HUT challenge, and concluded that 'physical fitness, orthostatic tolerance and the resistance to +Gz forces are almost completely independent qualities of the human body' (Klein et al., 1969). Shvartz and Meyerstein also reported similar numbers of athletes and non-athletes experiencing syncope with HUT (1972). Dikshit et al. (1986) reported a highly aerobically fit individual (VO_{2max} of 60.1) who had an inadequate and widely fluctuating cardiovascular response to HUT and experienced a syncopal episode.

The impact of aerobic conditioning on tolerance to applied +Gz loads has been extensively investigated. A German study found that endurance training tends to reduce the effectiveness of the BP control system, which they argued would be disadvantageous under high +Gz conditions (Stegemann et al., 1974). A centrifuge study which compared the +Gz tolerance of an aerobically trained subject group with a non-exercising group of subjects found no difference in +Gz tolerance between them (Cooper and Leverett, 1966). Another study involving amateur long-distance runners with high aerobic capacities found lower average +Gz tolerances in these individuals compared with a control group (Balldin, 1984). A direct correlation between the aerobic fitness of pilots and an increased total time of incapacitation occurring as a result of G-LOC has also been demonstrated (Houghton et al., 1985). Significantly, a US Navy study found that the chances of experiencing a G-LOC event were higher if the exercise regime of the pilots was aerobic in nature compared with an anaerobic programme (Johanson and Pheeny, 1988).

Other studies have shown a variety of deleterious effects of aerobic conditioning occurring in individuals subjected to +Gz. These effects have included an increased incidence of cardiac arrhythmias and motion sickness (Balldin, 1984; Burton, 1986b; Whinnery and Parnell, 1987). These effects are thought to be due to the increased vagal (parasympathetic) tone which develops in endurance-trained individuals.

A study of the physical activity patterns of a group of current operational fighter pilots found that while they were physically active, most of their training was not targeted specifically at improving their +Gz tolerance (Newman et al., 1999). Rather, their training seemed to be aimed at improving and maintaining a general level of cardiovascular health and physical well-being. While the pilots' aerobic exercise participation was high, the average aerobic fitness levels achieved (VO_{2max} of 50 ± 6 mls 0_2/kg/min) were consistent with values for active healthy males in that age group. The VO_{2max} levels and resting pulse rate data (average of 68 ± 8 bpm) in the pilots did not indicate a high degree of aerobic conditioning. The authors considered this training unlikely to influence their +Gz tolerance, either positively or negatively. Based on the available evidence, many air forces advise restrictions on participation in aerobic activities, such that pilots routinely exposed to the high +Gz environment should have a resting pulse rate no lower than 55 beats per minute in order to prevent excessive vagal tone and its attendant negative effects on +Gz tolerance (Burton, 1986b; Burton and Whinnery, 1996; Green, 2006b).

Anaerobic (or resistance) conditioning involves strength training. Enhanced anaerobic fitness is reflected by the ability to use a lower percentage of maximum muscular force for a given activity, or to sustain a given force for a longer period (increased time-until-exhaustion for a given muscle tension) (Balldin, 1984). Overall muscle power is also increased, so that greater force can be exerted against an object if required (Newman et al., 1999). Anaerobic activities include isometric exercises such as weight-lifting and resistance training activities that provide increases in muscle mass, strength and endurance.

In +Gz tolerance terms, anaerobic training has been advocated as a means of increasing the effectiveness of the AGSM by increasing the strength of the muscle groups involved in this manoeuvre (Burton, 1986b; Epperson et al., 1982, 1985; Burton and Whinnery, 1996; Newman et al., 1999; Tesch et al., 1983; Weigman et al., 1995). Enhanced anaerobic fitness should allow the pilot to strain more effectively against an applied high +Gz load, or to complete more straining cycles during a period of sustained high +Gz exposure. By producing a more effective AGSM, +Gz tolerance should be improved.

The role of anaerobic conditioning in promoting increased +Gz tolerance has been considered by several researchers (Bulbulian et al., 1994; Burton, 1986b; Epperson et al., 1982, 1985; Burton and Whinnery, 1996; Newman et al., 1999; Weigman et al., 1995). Epperson et al. (1982) examined 24 subjects divided into a control group (no physical training), a weight-lifting (anaerobic) group and a running (aerobic) group. A 12-week conditioning programme was followed by centrifuge testing using a SACM profile. Subject fatigue was used as the +Gz tolerance end-point. They found that while the +Gz tolerance of the running group and the control group were similar (with the running group demonstrating no increase in +Gz tolerance), the weight-training group had a significant increase in +Gz tolerance, taking longer to reach the fatigue end-point than the other two groups. SACM tolerance time for the weight-training group increased 53 per cent. A follow-on study by the same researchers found a high degree of correlation between increases in abdominal and biceps muscle strengths of 99 per cent and 26 per cent respectively and SACM tolerance times (Epperson et al., 1985).

A similar Swedish study showed a 39 per cent increase in SACM tolerance time in a group of 11 fighter pilots that had undergone an 11-week strength-training programme (Tesch et al., 1983). Muscle strength in this group increased by up to 59 per cent, while anaerobic power increased by 14 per cent. Subsequent studies have also confirmed the highly correlated relationship between anaerobic power and SACM tolerance times (Bulbulian et al., 1994; Weigman et al., 1995). In a study involving USN aviators undergoing a 10-week weight-training programme, an interesting result was found (Bulbulian et al., 1994). In those pilots with an initial SACM tolerance time above 300 seconds, no improvement in tolerance was noted. However, in those pilots with an initial SACM tolerance time below 300 seconds, the weight-trained group demonstrated a statistically significant increase in tolerance times when compared with the non-weight-trained control group. The researchers speculated that weight-training may be beneficial for only specific subsets of the pilot population. Their results suggest that as a method of improving tolerance to +Gz, weight training may be beneficial for pilots with +Gz tolerance below a certain threshold.

Resistance training of the neck muscles has also been promoted as a means of preventing +Gz-induced cervical spine injuries (Albano and Stanford, 1998; Alricsson et al., 2001, 2004; Green and Brown, 2004; Newman, 1997a, 1997b; Sovelius et al., 2006). This issue was discussed in detail in Chapter 6.

The general consensus in the scientific literature, then, appears to be that resistance training may improve tolerance to +Gz, especially in terms of enhancing the overall duration time in the high +Gz environment. Despite the potential benefits for +Gz tolerance of resistance training, there is no universally applied recommendation for aircrew to undertake such training. In a study involving RAAF fighter pilots, only 26 per cent reported undertaking resistance activities as part of their exercise regimes (Newman et al., 1999). In contrast, the Canadian Forces (CF) have instituted strength-training programmes at all bases operating high-performance fighter aircraft (Jacobs et al., 1987).

So, the question remains as to what is the ideal form of exercise programme for the pilot exposed to the high +Gz environment. This is an ongoing debate, and the appropriate nature, frequency and intensity of training programmes designed to enhance a pilot's tolerance to applied +Gz acceleration remain to be comprehensively determined (Balldin, 1984; Banta and Grissett, 1985; Newman et al., 1999). However, based on what is currently known, some important generalisations can be made.

What is clear is that the pilot of a modern high-performance aircraft needs to be anaerobically strong in order to better tolerate the dynamic high +Gz environment, whether in civilian aerobatic competition or military air combat. Such types of flying are fatiguing in the extreme. An ACM sortie or aerobatic sequence is a dynamic, strength-related activity (Newman et al., 1999). The AGSM is a muscular endeavour. It stands to reason that an anaerobically fit pilot with well-developed muscle strength will be able to tolerate the AGSM for longer periods before becoming fatigued. This will allow him to avoid the danger of G-LOC for longer and to thus concentrate on the actual mission itself.

However, a moderate degree of aerobic fitness is also important for the high +Gz pilot, not necessarily in terms of +Gz tolerance but rather in terms of fatigue and mission tolerance. A level of aerobic fitness will help them withstand the generally fatiguing effects of high +Gz flight for longer (particularly with repetitive exposure to +Gz) and allow them to sustain a high in-flight workload for longer periods. It also seems reasonable to suggest that a degree of aerobic fitness will provide the high +Gz pilot with the ability to recover quickly from repeated strenuous ACM or aerobatic sorties. However, as seen above an excessive level of aerobic conditioning may actually reduce a pilot's +Gz tolerance.

Physical fitness makes an important contribution to the general health and well-being of a pilot. Based on the weight of current evidence, it seems that pilots exposed to the high +Gz environment should perform a balanced combination of physical conditioning activities, involving anaerobic training for +Gz tolerance and aerobic training for general cardiovascular health, as well as for quicker recovery times between flights. The ideal physical training regime that caters for all aspects of the pilot's demanding environment and optimises the proportions of aerobic and anaerobic training has not yet been developed. Should such a programme be developed, it will no doubt give the fast jet pilot even more of an edge in an air combat engagement, and the aerobatic pilot an edge in the competition environment. Indeed, when the high +Gz environment of the future is considered, the outcome of an air combat engagement may well be decided on the relative fitness of the pilots.

Miscellaneous Factors

Various other factors have been linked with G tolerance. A low blood sugar (hypoglycaemia), an empty stomach, infections and various nutritional supplements and medications (such as antihypertensive drugs) have all been reported to reduce G tolerance to varying degrees (Burton and Whinnery, 1999; Green, 2006b). A 50 per cent reduction in blood sugar has been linked to a reduction in the threshold for black-out of around 0.6 Gz (Howard, 1965). Interestingly, the physiological reaction to such a precipitous fall in blood sugar (catecholamine release, and so on) ultimately raises +Gz tolerance in the short term by around 0.5 Gz. An empty stomach allows the heart to descend more under high +Gz, thus effectively increasing the hydrostatic differential between the heart and brain. A full stomach helps splint the diaphragm and maintain the heart-to-brain distance. Distending the stomach by the consumption of 1.5 litres of water has been seen to increase the threshold for blackout by around 1 Gz (Green, 2006a).

Infections may raise body temperature, but also may adversely affect BP control mechanisms. Antihypertensive beta-blocking drugs such as propanolol have been shown to blunt the cardiovascular response to +Gz, particularly in terms of reducing the normal elevation in HR (Burton and Whinnery, 1996).

Caution is usually recommended in terms of the use of such drugs in pilots exposed to the high +Gz environment. In a recent case report, a US Navy F/A-18E pilot experienced a reduction in +Gz tolerance during BFM, manifested by visual loss (including complete black-out). This reduction in +Gz tolerance was attributed (in the absence of other likely explanations) to the pilot's recent consumption of a nutritional supplement (Barker, 2011). The supplement contained coenzyme Q10 and niacin, both of which have known haemodynamic effects that can potentially adversely affect +Gz tolerance. These include cutaneous vasodilation and reductions in BP. Significantly, after discontinuing the supplement the pilot's +Gz tolerance subsequently returned to normal.

Flight-Related Factors Affecting G Tolerance

There are a number of factors related to the actual flight environment at the time that can affect subsequent G tolerance. These include the nature of the flight manoeuvre (intensity, duration, rate of onset and offset, and so on), the frequency of exposure to the high G environment, G transition effects, and centrifuge training, among others. All of these flight-related factors will now be examined.

Seat-Back Angle

Increasing the seat-back angle (by reclining the seat back) has the effect of reducing the vertical distance between the heart and the brain and thereby reducing the hydrostatic differential between them. This should theoretically improve tolerance to any applied +Gz load (Burns, 1988; Burton and Whinnery, 1996; Burton and Shaffstall, 1980; Cohen, 1983; Dorman and Lawton, 1956; Green, 2006b; Logan et al., 1983; Nelson, 1987; Tong et al., 1994).

The HP differential between the heart and the brain and its relationship to seat-back angle is given by the following expression (Newman and Callister, 1999);

$HP = \rho.g.(h.cos\alpha)$
Where: HP = effective hydrostatic pressure differential.
                    ρ = fluid density.
                    g = acceleration due to gravity.
                    h = heart-brain distance.
                    α = seat-back angle.

Altering the seat-back angle to achieve an increase in +Gz tolerance is not new. Indeed, the Germans flight-tested some reclining seats in the 1930s, but did not operationally deploy them (Burton and Whinnery, 1996). In most fighter aircraft, the seat-back angle is around 13°, with the pilot effectively sitting upright. In the Swedish JAS-39 Gripen aircraft, the seat-back angle is 28° (Gronkvist et al., 2008) while in the F-16 it is 30° (Burton and Whinnery, 1996). In one centrifuge study, SACM tolerance times increased with greater seat-back angles: 170 ± 17 seconds at 13° seat-back angle and 541 ± 48 seconds at 65° (Burton and Shaffstall, 1980).

While a greater seat-back angle is theoretically advantageous in terms of G tolerance, it has some practical limitations. The seat is typically an ejection seat, so a greater recline can increase the chance of an ejection-related injury to the spine. A greater reclination angle will hamper the pilot's ability to turn their head to the rear of the aircraft in order to visually track an opponent during ACM. To offset this limitation, pilots might sit upright to maximise their visual scanning, but at the expense of any G tolerance enhancement produced by a reclining seat. The practical limitations tend to win out, such that the seat-back angle as a means of improving G tolerance is only of minor significance.

The Flight Manoeuvre

Being unprepared for the +Gz exposure is also a tolerance-reducing factor. The flying pilot, by virtue of awareness of what manoeuvre they are about to execute, coupled with the physical manipulation of the controls, tends to have a better tolerance of the subsequent +Gz load than another occupant of the aircraft who is unprepared and unaware of what is about to happen. This surprise effect can reduce their tolerance to the +Gz.

The rate of onset and offset of high +Gz has been discussed at length previously. In modern fast jet aircraft engaged in ACM, and civilian aerobatic aircraft engaged in competition, Gz onset rates can often be at the design limits of the aircraft, resulting in onset rates as high as +15 Gs^{-1}. At lower rates the visual symptoms can be used as an early warning or premonitory sign of approaching G-LOC. In practical terms, however, this does not often occur, for the pilot often needs to manoeuvre the aircraft quickly and forcefully, resulting in high G onset rates with consequently no visual warning signs.

Frequency of Exposure

Frequent, regular exposure to the high +Gz environment improves overall tolerance, via a process of cardiovascular adaptation. Most pilots of high-performance aerobatic and military fast jet aircraft have been aware of this for a long time. In recent years a body of scientific evidence has appeared in support of the anecdotal experience of pilots that they adapt to regular +Gz exposure over time (Convertino, 1998; Convertino et al., 1998; Morgan et al., 1994; Newman and Callister, 2008, 2009; Newman et al., 1998, 2000; Schlegel et al., 2003). This issue is explored in more detail in Chapter 9.

Aircrew with the highest number of flight hours have been found to have the highest tolerance to applied +Gz (Whinnery, 1979). Increased flying experience is closely linked with increased age, which in turn is often linked with increased weight (Whinnery, 1979). In a study that examined the link between flying experience and cardiovascular responses to orthostatic stress, it was found that a more favourable MAP response to acceleration was not achieved until approximately 800 hours of high +Gz flying experience, with the effect becoming greater as experience increases further (Newman and Callister, 2009). The authors argued that that the physiological mechanism underlying +Gz adaptation might not become apparent until a certain level of exposure to the high +Gz environment (in the region of 1,000 hours) has been experienced.

The Push–Pull Effect

The examination of G tolerance has so far only considered +Gz and –Gz separately, in isolation. Aerobatic flight as seen in Chapter 2 is highly dynamic, so it is important to consider the implications of so-called G transition effects, where +Gz and –Gz are seen in combination. The –Gz to +Gz transition effect has also become more popularly known as the 'push–pull effect' (PPE). The term refers to the actions of the pilot with respect to the control column – pushing forward for –Gz and then pulling back for +Gz (see Figure 8.4). In simple terms, the PPE refers to the transition between the –Gz state (or less than the usual +1 Gz state) to a high +Gz state. This might be achieved through unloading of the aircraft from a high +Gz to improve manoeuvring and roll rate before application of high +Gz again, which might result in an intervening exposure to less than +1 Gz or even a –Gz exposure. In a USAF study, such –Gz to +Gz transitions were observed to occur relatively frequently during air combat training missions, particularly those that involved ACM activities (Michaud et al., 1998). The PPE has been shown to reduce the pilot's tolerance to the subsequent high +Gz exposure (Banks and Gray, 1994; Banks et al., 1994, 1995; Bloodwell and Whinnery, 1982; Cheung and Bateman, 2001; Goodman and LeSage, 2002; Goodman et al., 2000, 2006; Liu et al., 2009, 2012; Mikuliszyn et al., 2005; Scott et al., 2007; Zhang et al., 2001). This might produce a G-LOC event at an earlier than predicted +Gz level.

Physiologically the PPE is a result of baroreflex activity. During the –Gz (or less than +1 Gz) component of the manoeuvre, the baroreflexes are attempting to deal with a perceived vascular over-filling issue. Just as they start to influence this situation, the high +Gz component is initiated. The cardiovascular system thus faces the high +Gz challenge in a far more hydrostatically unfavourable state, with a slow HR, poor cardiac contractility and a worsening peripheral vasodilatation. Tolerance to the high +Gz component is thus compromised by the out-of-phase baroreflex activity.

HR has been seen to change rapidly during high rate ±Gz transitions in civilian aerobatic aircraft, from 175 bpm to 40 bpm within a five-second period (Bloodwell and Whinnery, 1982). The PPE has also been seen to delay baroreflex-mediated peripheral vascular control at subsequent high +Gz levels, which leads to delayed head-level BP and consequent reduced +Gz tolerance (Goodman and LeSage, 2002).

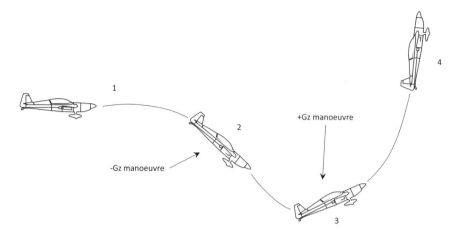

Figure 8.4   A manoeuvre resulting in the push–pull effect (PPE)

Centrifuge Training

While most air forces now make use of human centrifuges, they are also increasingly being used for training of commercial spaceflight participants (Blue et al., 2012; Jing et al., 2011). The modern centrifuge is an extremely sophisticated and capable device that can combine flight simulation with a high +Gz environment to produce a highly realistic flight experience for the pilot (Lau and Steinleitner, 1994; Newman, 2014). This latter situation is often termed Dynamic Flight Simulation (DFS).

The centrifuge can generate a level of +Gz acceleration equivalent to a fighter aircraft, albeit in a safe and reliable manner. The development of sophisticated human-in-the-loop active control systems now allows the pilot in the centrifuge to 'fly' the device, generating Gz loads via control column inputs as they would in the actual aircraft. Coupled with a simulated out-the-window view, accurate aircraft flight model, and comprehensive terrain and navigational databases, the centrifuge can essentially reproduce the aircraft flight envelope on the ground.

Centrifuges are used for various reasons, including research and development, training and even mission rehearsal. In some countries the centrifuge is used for qualification purposes, where (for example) pilots must be able to successfully tolerate +9 Gz for 20 to 30 seconds before being sent for F-16 training. The centrifuge can be used with either pre-programmed profiles or full active control profiles. Typical passive profiles include the GOR, where the centrifuge is taken to a peak of +9 Gz at an onset rate of +0.1 Gz per second, and the ROR, where the centrifuge is taken to a high +Gz level (usually +7 to +9) at an onset rate of +6 Gz per second. Either or both of these runs can be used for qualification purposes, where the peak +Gz must be tolerated for a given time interval. The accepted standard used by most air forces (in accordance with NATO Standardisation Agreement (STANAG) 3827) is successful tolerance of +7 Gz for 15 seconds on a ROR profile, while wearing an anti-G suit and performing an AGSM (Gillingham, 1987). For aircraft capable of sustaining +9 Gz, this value is used as the standard.

The main emphasis in centrifuge training is to improve an individual's G tolerance. There is little doubt that a comprehensive programme of centrifuge training can reduce the adverse consequences of exposure to the high G environment, and reduce the incidence of G-LOC. Consider the following examples. In the period 1982–84 the USAF G-LOC rate was four events per million flight hours. After implementing a centrifuge training programme in 1985, the G-LOC rate fell to only 1.3 G-LOC events per million flight hours in the period 1985–1990. The G-LOC rate reduction was directly attributed to the introduction of the centrifuge training programme (Lyons et al., 1992, 2004). After it introduced centrifuge training, the Turkish Air Force's G-LOC rate fell from 10 per cent in 1992 to 6 per cent in 1996 (Yilmaz et al., 1999). The rate reduction was attributed to improved AGSM instruction and technique over time through the centrifuge training programme. Some researchers have even argued that experiencing G-LOC (either inadvertently or deliberately) in a centrifuge could in itself improve G tolerance (Burton, 1991; Whinnery and Burton, 1987).

Conclusion

Tolerance to G is thus the end result of the influence of many factors. Addressing all of the individual factors before the flight, and understanding the impact of flight-related factors, will help maximise a given pilot's tolerance of their high G environment. The role of variation, both between and within individuals, must also be recognised. However, given the high G capabilities of modern aerobatic and military fast jet aircraft, these individual tolerance factors are generally not sufficient to ensure protection from G-LOC on a reliable basis. While regular and frequent exposure can lead to adaptation to G, as discussed in the next chapter, more specific countermeasures are required. These are considered in the final part of this book.

Chapter 9
Cardiovascular Adaptation to Acceleration

There is anecdotal evidence from the tactical fighter community which suggests that fighter pilots do experience a degree of adaptation arising from frequent exposure to high +Gz. The more they fly to high +Gz levels, the more they feel able to tolerate it. Is this increase in their tolerance due to adaptation of their cardiovascular system and/or baroreflexes to the high +Gz environment? Repetitive and frequent exposure to the high +Gz environment could act as a training or conditioning stimulus. If adaptation does occur in fighter pilots, it should be reflected in enhanced function, that is, the opposite of the situation that occurs with zero or microgravity exposure. This chapter examines the current literature dealing with cardiovascular adaptation in general and to high +Gz in particular.

Is Adaptation an Advantage?

Surprisingly, perhaps, the notion that individual pilots might physiologically adapt as a result of their frequent occupational exposure to high +Gz forces has not been the subject of much research. While the consequences of acute exposure are well understood (Burton and Whinnery, 1996; Gillingham and Crump, 1976; Houghton et al., 1985; Howard, 1965; Parkhurst et al., 1972; Whinnery, 1988; Whinnery et al., 1987), little has been known about the effects of chronic exposure to the high +Gz environment until relatively recently.

Any such adaptation to chronic +Gz exposure is theoretically advantageous in the tactical aviation environment, as it would tend to protect the pilot against G-LOC. In terms of Stoll's +Gz-time tolerance curve (discussed in Chapter 8), cardiovascular adaptation to +Gz would alter the shape of this curve. Enhanced baroreflex activity due to +Gz adaptation would be reflected in a change in the shape and/or position of the lower edge of the visual symptom band. The maximum activity of the baroreflexes might be reached in less than the usual 10 seconds or so. Furthermore, the trough representing minimum G tolerance in the Stoll curve (due to the temporal intersection of the metabolic energy reserve curve and that of the baroreceptors) might also be altered, reflecting a greater +Gz tolerance as a result of chronic +Gz exposure. These possible outcomes of enhanced cardiovascular function in the +Gz-adapted pilot are shown in Figure 9.1.

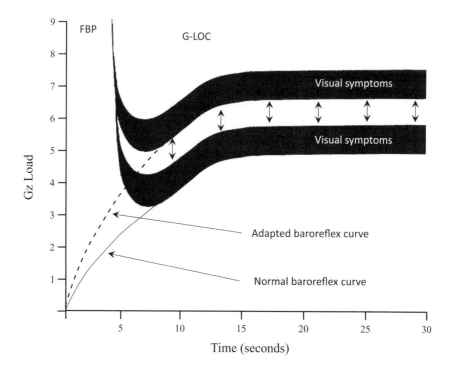

Figure 9.1   The effect of cardiovascular adaptation on the G-time tolerance curve

Such enhancement of cardiovascular function would clearly be beneficial, as it would allow the fighter pilot to more safely operate in the high +Gz environment with less danger and risk of inadequate cerebral perfusion. G-LOC is an important cause of pilot and aircraft losses. Any improvement in our understanding of the physiological effects of high +Gz exposure may well lead us to better ways of protecting the pilot from the potentially harmful effects of such exposure. Knowledge of the adaptation process would enable a safe and structured programme to be developed for pilots returning to flying fighter aircraft after long lay-off periods. Such a programme would allow them to return to the high +Gz environment as quickly and as safely as possible, maximising their +Gz tolerance and reducing their risk of G-LOC.

The practical benefits of protecting the pilots of high performance fighter aircraft from G-LOC are considerable, given the enormous cost in human and equipment terms of the loss of even one modern fighter aircraft. The benefits from an operational and tactical viewpoint of ensuring a fully conscious pilot throughout the entire flight envelope of the aircraft are equally as important.

The fully +Gz-adapted fighter pilot would have a significant physiological advantage, which would greatly improve their chances of survival.

Adaptation to Microgravity

Over the course of evolution, humans have successfully adapted to an upright existence in a +1 Gz terrestrial environment. In recent decades, humans have operated at both ends of the gravitational spectrum, that is, under conditions of zero or microgravity during spaceflight, and at high +Gz levels in fighter and aerobatic aircraft. Evidence of cardiovascular adaptation to altered gravitational states has been largely derived through human experience of the weightlessness of spaceflight and the microgravity of Earth orbit. The physiological effects of weightlessness have been well documented from analysis of the extensive biomedical results of the American, Russian and European manned space programmes from the late 1960s to the present time. The human experience of microgravity and weightlessness due to long-duration spaceflight has provided evidence of cardiovascular adaptation to the absence of gravity. This evidence now warrants a brief review.

Exposure to a microgravity environment results in several characteristic changes in the cardiovascular system. In the absence of the normal hydrostatic force, there is a central redistribution of blood volume, involving the cephalad translocation of some 1.5–2 litres from the legs and an unknown amount from the pelvic area (Buckey et al., 1996a, 1996b; Convertino, 1990; Montgomery, 1987, 1993; Moore and Thornton, 1987).

This volume shift results in facial puffiness, sinus congestion, periorbital swelling, engorged neck veins, a decrease in leg size and activation of the cardiopulmonary baroreceptors (Churchill and Bungo, 1997; Evans et al., 2013; Thornton et al., 1987, 1992). Enhanced renal filtration leads to a reduction in blood volume over time. Erythropoiesis is inhibited, leading to a generalised decrease in red cell mass. HR and BP remain normal or increase slightly during one-to-two weeks of spaceflight (Bungo, 1989). The cephalad fluid shift leads to increases in left ventricular end diastolic volume (LVEDV), SV and CO on initial exposure to microgravity (the first day typically). These parameters all then decrease with continued exposure beyond day one, with SV falling to approximately 15 per cent below baseline values (Bungo, 1989).

The important consequence of this altered cardiovascular state is that orthostatic intolerance becomes quite marked on return to the normal gravitational field of Earth. The orthostatic intolerance occurring as a result of constant exposure to a microgravity environment has been well documented, and is a feature common to astronauts from all space programs (Blamick et al., 1988; Blomqvist and Stone, 1983; Bungo, 1989; Bungo et al., 1985; Bungo and Johnson, 1983; Caiozzo et al., 2004; Convertino, 1990; Convertino et al., 1989; Evans et al., 2013; Fritsch-Yelle et al., 1994; Ten Harkel et al., 1992; Tomaselli et al., 1990). Astronauts undergoing post-flight tilt testing by and large demonstrate exaggerated cardiovascular responses. The symptoms reported range from a simple increase in HR to spontaneous syncope (Bungo and Johnson, 1983), but are generally manifested in the post-spaceflight period by a combination of increased HR, decreased MAP, systolic pressure and PP, and a variable change (often a decrease) in diastolic BP.

These changes all reflect a reduction in vascular filling. Human experience in the microgravity environment of Earth orbit and space has revealed that a decrease in orthostatic tolerance can occur after only nine hours exposure to the microgravity environment (Churchill and Bungo, 1997). These cardiovascular deconditioning (CD) effects have also been reproduced in ground-based microgravity-analogue studies (Convertino et al., 1990; Miller et al., 1964).

Bungo et al. (1983, 1985, 1989) carried out a series of experiments on returning Space Shuttle astronauts to investigate post-flight orthostatic intolerance. By comparing pre- and post-flight values for each individual, they were able to demonstrate the degree of CD in each subject, based on the results of a simple orthostatic challenge (five-minute stand test). This allowed them to develop a Cardiovascular Index of Deconditioning (CID), defined as the change in HR standing post-flight compared with pre-flight plus the difference between the changes in SP and DP. Although acknowledged as a somewhat simplistic interpretation of a complex issue, the authors found it to be a useful approximation with valid operational applications.

After CD occurred during spaceflight, the orthostatic challenge necessarily involved in a return to the +1 Gz environment of Earth universally resulted in HR increases in the astronauts. However, the BP responses to orthostasis fell into two groups. The first group experienced falls in both systolic and diastolic BP, reacting as if their circulations were encased in 'rigid pipes' (Bungo and Johnson, 1983). The second group, which Bungo and Johnson (1983) referred to as 'vascular hyper-responders', reacted with increases in DP, sometimes to hypertensive extents. After variable lengths of time post-flight, the orthostatic tolerance of astronauts generally returned to normal pre-flight levels. It can take up to several weeks for an astronaut's cardiovascular parameters to return to pre-flight levels. This return to pre-flight baseline values is essentially a function of the length of time in microgravity, and also reflects the individual astronaut's degree of cardiovascular adaptation to the microgravity environment.

Orthostatic intolerance can be explained physiologically by a shift in the position of the hydrostatic indifference point. In a manner similar to general dehydration and heat stress, exposure to microgravity with its resultant reduction in blood volume leads to a downward (footward) shift in the position of the HIP upon re-exposure to a +1 Gz environment. As has already been seen, under +1 Gz conditions the circulatory system is not completely filled, due to the distensible, compliant nature of the capacitance vessels. The reduction in circulating blood volume and the CD inherent in exposure to microgravity exacerbate the state of inadequate circulatory filling, thus shifting the HIP in a footward direction and increasing the susceptibility to orthostatic intolerance.

The precise mechanisms responsible for the evolution of orthostatic intolerance occurring after prolonged exposure to an actual or simulated microgravity environment remain unclear. However, it would appear from the results of several studies that such orthostatic intolerance is a multi-factorial phenomenon. It may well be due to the combined effects of several variables, chief among which seem to be reduced circulating blood volume and impaired arterial baroreflex function. These in turn are a result of the absence of the normal gravitational gradient that exists in the cardiovascular system under the +1 Gz conditions on Earth. It has been concluded by several researchers that the cardiovascular system adapts to the microgravity environment by means of fluid redistribution and the subsequent resetting of various control mechanisms such as the baroreflexes (Convertino et al., 1989, 1990; Thompson et al., 1990).

As has already been seen, the arterial baroreflex system is crucial for the effective control of BP. Given the degree of change that occurs in BP and other cardiovascular parameters as a result of exposure to altered gravitational field strengths, the role of the arterial baroreflex system in any consequent cardiovascular adaptation process becomes an important question.

Investigative Techniques

One of the fundamental techniques in physiological research involving investigation of a chronic change or adaptation in a given system is the use of a dynamic challenge to perturb that system. Understanding how the system responds to a range of normal and abnormal stimuli is integral to furthering an overall understanding of the operating mechanisms of the system.

In this chapter, the cardiovascular system's ability to adapt to repetitive +Gz exposure is the main focus. Given that the physiological consequences of exposure to the high +Gz environment are accentuations of the normal response to upright posture, a dynamic challenge is necessary for research purposes. Such a challenge must produce a HP differential in the longitudinal axis of the body. In doing so, the cardiovascular compensatory mechanisms such as the baroreflexes would be activated by the footward shift of fluid. Furthermore, the challenge should as closely as possible approximate the physiological consequences of exposure to high +Gz loads, with as few extraneous variables as possible. Based on these requirements, there are several options available, including (HUT), lower body negative pressure (LBNP) and orthostatic challenges such as active standing and the SST. These now warrant a brief consideration, in order to put the research findings that use these techniques to examine cardiovascular adaptation to +Gz into proper context.

Head-Up Tilt (HUT)

HUT is a commonly used technique for providing a dynamic orthostatic stimulus to the cardiovascular system, in order to determine its performance and functional integrity (Armstrong et al., 2010; Berry and Newman, 2007; Cooke et al., 1999; Deklunder et al., 1993; Evans et al., 2004; Gelinas et al., 2012; Gisolf et al., 2004; Graybiel and McFarland, 1941; Hyatt et al., 1975; Matzen et al., 1991; Vogt, 1966; Yamazaki et al., 2003). It has been proven to be a useful technique for the study of reflex control of the circulation (Mancia and Mark, 1983; Vogt, 1966). HUT has been used by several researchers to investigate the cardiovascular responses to postural and orthostatic challenges, and has found extensive applications in aerospace medicine research (Berry et al., 2003, 2006a, 2006b; Butler et al., 1990; Culbertson et al., 1951; Deklunder et al., 1993; Dikshit et al., 1986; El-Sayed and Hainsworth, 1995; Fulco et al., 1985; Gelinas et al., 2012; Graybiel and McFarland, 1941; Harrison et al., 1986; Hyatt et al., 1975; Jellema et al., 1996; Klein et al., 1969; Manen et al., 2011; Newman et al., 1998, 2000; Newman and Callister, 2008, 2009; Rickards and Newman, 2002; Self et al., 1996; Shvartz and Meyerstein, 1970, 1972; Smith et al., 1974; Spodick and Lance, 1977; Ten Harkel et al., 1992; Tuckman and Shillingford, 1966; Vogt, 1966). It is a simple, reliable, reproducible stimulus that closely mirrors the physiological effects of +Gz exposure. Due to its extensive use in both normal and clinicopathological populations there is an extensive literature dealing with the cardiovascular responses to HUT in these groups.

The physiological consequences of HUT are due to the imposition of a hydrostatic force on the closed-loop cardiovascular system and the system's responses to that force. These consequences have been discussed in Chapter 3. HUT involves a subject, resting on a table in a relaxed state (usually supine), being rotated about their centre of gravity while instrumented for recording of various cardiovascular parameters. The sine of the angle of tilt (relative to the horizontal plane) is directly proportional to the degree of hydrostatic force introduced, and as such determines the magnitude of the cardiovascular response. 30° of tilt produces 50 per cent of the hydrostatic effect of upright posture (that is, +0.5 Gz), while 75° produces 97 per cent.

The normal response to HUT is a decrease in CO, SV, PP and systolic pressure, while HR, DP and peripheral resistance increase (Fiorica and Kem, 1985; Fulco et al., 1985; Tanaka et al., 1996). MAP generally remains constant. These changes reflect the application of hydrostatic force and the concomitant activation of cardiovascular compensatory mechanisms (Gauer and Thron, 1965; Mancia and Mark, 1983; Pickering et al., 1971; Rowell, 1986, 1993; Tanaka et al., 1996; Tuckman and Shillingford, 1966). Renal blood flow decreases by as much as 32 per cent with 60° HUT, while 75° HUT leads to a 45 per cent increase in splanchnic vascular resistance (Culbertson et al., 1951). The physiological effects of HUT are comparable to those seen with upright posture. This is to be expected, given that the causative agent (hydrostatic force) is the same in both cases.

The time course of tilt varies considerably between studies, with typical times involving approximately 15–30 minutes of HUT or until the subject experiences syncope (Bartok et al., 1968; Fulco et al., 1985; Klein et al., 1969; Musgrave et al., 1969, 1971; Graybiel and McFarland, 1941; Shvartz and Meyerstein, 1970, 1972; Tanaka et al., 1996). As has been discussed previously, +Gz loads in high-performance aircraft are generally of rapid onset. Musgrave et al. (1969, 1971) and Tanaka et al. (1996) argue that passive HUT is the most appropriate and physiologically relevant ground-based analogue of acute +Gz exposure (other than a human centrifuge).

Lower-Body Negative Pressure

The effects of HUT have been compared with those of lower-body negative pressure (LBNP), which has been used extensively in the manned spaceflight program. HUT is unsuitable for space-based applications, as it takes up too much valuable and expensive space, as well as being dependent on Gz-mediated fluid shifts which are not possible in weightless or microgravity conditions. With LBNP, the negative pressure created around the lower body acts to draw blood into the lower extremities, thus causing a pressure gradient in the longitudinal axis (Frey et al., 1987; Hachiya et al., 2012; Hyatt et al., 1975; Sather et al., 1986). As such, LBNP has been evaluated for use as an in-flight countermeasure to the development of orthostatic intolerance in astronauts. Musgrave et al. (1969) found that 40 mmHg of LBNP produced similar fluid redistribution (total leg volume increases of 500–600ml) to both upright posture and 70° HUT. A follow-up study found that a greater level of LBNP (50 mmHg) was required to generate the same HR and arterial pressure changes as 70° HUT (Musgrave et al., 1971). Similar findings were reported by Bartok (1968). Musgrave et al. (1971) attributed their findings to the fact that with HUT the arterial baroreceptors are positioned above the heart, which does not occur with LBNP. Thus, as an investigative tool LBNP is not directly comparable to the effects of +Gz exposure.

Standing

There are some important differences between HUT and standing. HUT is typically a passive procedure, in that the subject is relaxed and does not use the lower limb muscles to assume the upright position. On the other hand, standing is clearly an active process. The lower limb muscles are used in both anti-gravity stabilisation and VR augmentation modes. In comparing the two, Tanaka et al. (1996) found that active standing caused a considerable rise in intra-abdominal pressure (43±22 mmHg) that was not observed in passive HUT. They attributed this pressure rise to the muscular contractions involved in assuming the upright posture. This increase in muscle tone is not present in a passive HUT (Rowell, 1993).

Related to this, they also found that active standing caused a transient but greater reduction in BP in the initial phases of standing (Tanaka et al., 1996). They attributed this to the effects of a rapid shift of blood from the splanchnic circulation due to the rise in intra-abdominal pressure, as well as from the contracting peripheral musculature. This shift of blood then activates the cardiopulmonary baroreceptors, leading to a transient systemic vasodilatation and reduction in BP. Once this initial effect was completed, there were no significant haemodynamic changes between active standing and passive HUT. Pickering et al. (1971) found no significant differences in the cardiovascular responses to either standing or sitting in the upright position.

The Squat–Stand Test

The SST is an active orthostatic challenge. A standard protocol for the SST has not been formally defined, but a commonly used version involves the subject squatting deeply and unassisted for a period of four minutes before standing upright as quickly as possible for a further two minutes (Berry et al., 2006a; Convertino et al., 1998; Rickards and Newman, 2003; Rossberg and Penaz, 1988).

The SST has been used in a variety of physiological and clinical contexts to examine cardiovascular reflex function (Claasen et al., 2009; Hanson et al., 1995; Lipsitz et al., 2000; Marfella et al., 1994; Van Lieshout et al., 1992; Zhang et al., 2009). In terms of cardiovascular adaptation to repetitive +Gz, it has also been used by several researchers (Berry et al., 2006a; Convertino et al., 1998; Rickards and Newman, 2003). These findings are discussed later.

The evidence suggests that the SST is a more exaggerated cardiovascular challenge for the baroreflexes to deal with than HUT (Rickards and Newman, 2003). This appears to be largely due to the consequences of the squat-induced 'tourniquet effect' on the lower limbs (Convertino et al., 1998; Rickards and Newman, 2003). Sudden standing then leads to large drops in arterial pressure due to reactive hyperaemia and vasodilatation in the lower limbs. Cardiopulmonary baroreceptor activation (due to the increased intra-abdominal pressure caused by standing) also tends to force BP down in the initial stages (Borst et al., 1982; Hainsworth, 1991; Sprangers et al., 1991; Tanaka et al., 1996). As such, SST tends to create a more pronounced challenge for the baroreflexes to deal with on standing, more so than the HUT (Rickards and Newman, 2003).

Adaptation of the Baroreflexes

It is clear from an analysis of the published evidence that the baroreflexes are capable of undergoing adaptation when required (Bungo and Johnson, 1983; Convertino, 1998; Convertino et al., 1990; Kasting et al., 1987; Newman et al., 1998, 2000; Newman and Callister, 2008, 2009; Mack et al., 1991; Schlegel et al., 2003; Smith et al., 1994). In this section, the evidence in support of baroreflex adaptation to various parameters is examined.

Convertino et al. (1990) showed that 6° bed-rest (a standard microgravity analogue) results in impaired baroreflex function, which appears to be independent of the fluid volume changes that are generally observed in microgravity. This impaired baroreflex function leads to increased orthostatic susceptibility, and as such reduces the affected individual's ability to tolerate transient changes in BP. The reduced pressure buffering capability of the cardiovascular system is thought to be an important contributing factor to post-spaceflight orthostatic intolerance.

Several investigators have examined baroreflex function in the setting of microgravity-induced alterations in central blood volume. Mack et al. (1991) found that an increase in central blood volume effectively attenuated the function of the low-pressure cardiopulmonary baroreceptors. Bungo's 'vascular hyper-responder' group of astronauts was considered to have had their 'cardiovascular controlling mechanisms', that is, the arterial baroreflexes, reset during the exposure to microgravity (Bungo and Johnson, 1983). Resetting of the carotid baroreceptor-cardiac reflex has been demonstrated by several investigators. Fritsch et al. (1989) found that drug-induced arterial pressure changes led to a chronic resetting of the threshold level for the carotid baroreflex, while Kasting et al. (1987) showed the continuous resetting ability of this reflex.

Other studies have confirmed these findings. During chronic severe hypertension, the baroreceptors continue to function and buffer acute arterial pressure changes by operating at a higher average set point (Downing, 1983; Krieger, 1970). While they are unable to counter the chronic elevation in pressure they do accurately buffer this new set point against acute, transient changes in arterial pressure. The system gradually resets (adapts) to a new high-pressure operating range, although evidence suggests that some reflex efficiency is lost in the process. The baroreceptors thus contribute to sustaining the hypertension induced by other mechanisms, once the new set point has been established (Downing, 1983). Baroreceptor resetting has been confirmed in dog and spontaneously hypertensive rat (SHR) models (Downing, 1983). In SHR studies, the threshold for hypotension-inducing baroreflex activity was found to be in the range of 120–140mmHg, which contrasts with the threshold values of 60–100mmHg in normotensive control rats. Conversely, a lower average set point is established during chronic hypotensive states (Downing, 1983; Krieger, 1970).

In renal hypertensive rabbits, changes in baroreceptor sensitivity (defined as the change in medullary input for a given pressure change) to arterial pressure fluctuations have been determined. In the hypertensive group, sensitivities were measured at an average of 0.64 impulse/s.mmHg^{-1}, compared with an average of 1.19 impulse/s.mmHg^{-1} in the control group. Reduced baroreceptor sensitivity has been demonstrated in several hypertensive animal models and also in hypertensive human subjects (Downing, 1983).

Billman et al. (1981) showed that carotid baroreceptor function in monkeys was attenuated by an increased central blood volume created by a rapid saline infusion.

Thompson et al. (1990) examined baroreceptor function in different volume states in humans. They found that acute changes in vascular volumes altered the function of the cardiopulmonary baroreceptors, but not that of the carotid baroreceptors. The disagreement with Billman's findings was attributed to relative differences in the degree of volume expansion achieved in the two studies.

Thompson's study supports the notion expressed by Convertino et al. that impaired carotid baroreceptor function contributes to orthostatic intolerance independent of reduced blood volume (Convertino et al., 1989; Thompson et al., 1990). Thompson et al. interpreted the results of their study as showing that volume expansion prior to return to Earth could return cardiopulmonary baroreceptor function to a more normal state, in order to protect against subsequent orthostatic intolerance (1990). In addition, they commented that microgravity-induced impaired carotid baroreceptor function would therefore require a specific countermeasure other than simple volume expansion to offset the increased orthostatic susceptibility (Thompson et al., 1990).

The Influence of Exercise on Baroreflex Function

Physical conditioning has been shown to induce a degree of cardiovascular adaptation, which may affect the physiological response to altered gravitational states (Forster and Whinnery, 1990; Mack et al., 1987). The question of physical conditioning and its effect on tolerance to applied +Gz acceleration is considered in detail in Chapter 8. However, here it is worth examining the influence of exercise on the function of the baroreflexes, in terms of their ability to adapt to change.

Aerobic or endurance training results in a number of well-documented changes in several cardiovascular variables (Wilmore and Costill, 1994). Resting HR slows down, due to increased parasympathetic (vagal) tone, and in highly conditioned athletes resting HRs of 30 to 40 beats per minute have been observed (Wilmore and Costill, 1994). SV increases, due to the combination of increases in LVEDV and cardiac contractility. These changes also tend to increase the cardiac ejection fraction. End-systolic volumes thus tend to be reduced. Venous compliance also tends to decrease, due to increased venous tone (Wilmore and Costill, 1994).

An important effect of endurance training is an increase in circulating blood volume, which is proportional to the degree of training (Mack et al., 1987; Wilmore and Costill, 1994). This increase is due to increases in blood plasma volume, due in turn to increased release of aldosterone and ADH. A relative decrease in haematocrit occurs, even though red cell mass actually increases. This is due to plasma volume increasing more than the red cell mass (Wilmore and Costill, 1994).

High levels of aerobic fitness appear to have a modifying influence on baroreflex function. In a study comparing endurance-trained athletes with non-athletes, Stegemann et al. (1974) found that the athletes had significantly smaller baroreflex gain factors than the non-athletes. They concluded that aerobic training can reduce the effectiveness of the baroreflexes as BP controlling mechanisms. Based on these findings, astronauts have been advised to limit pre-flight aerobic training in order to prevent significant orthostatic intolerance from occurring post-spaceflight (Klein et al., 1969).

The attenuation of the baroreflexes by aerobic training, while advantageous for dynamic exercise, may result in inadequate maintenance of cerebral perfusion under applied +Gz loads (Klein et al., 1969). According to Whinnery and Parnell, some aerobically-trained individuals are particularly sensitive to applied +Gz acceleration (1987). The high levels of vagal tone achieved by some individuals have been linked to the occurrence of various cardiac dysrhythmias under +Gz stress, such as sino-atrial block and atrioventricular dissociation (Gillingham, 1988; Whinnery et al., 1990). The issue remains the subject of debate.

Cardiovascular Adaptation to G

Exposure to high levels of applied +Gz represents an extreme orthostatic challenge, which can overcome the compensatory ability of cardiovascular countermeasures, such as the baroreflexes. The role of the baroreflexes in combating the deleterious effects of high +Gz exposure is easily understood when one considers G-LOC to be the ultimate consequence of failure of the cardiovascular system to tolerate an applied acceleration. Adaptation to the high +Gz environment would represent an advantageous and protective state for a pilot regularly exposed to it.

Cardiovascular adaptation to repetitive exposure to an altered gravitational field has been examined by several authors over many years, albeit in quite differing contexts. While the majority of this work has been done in relation to the microgravity of orbital spaceflight (Bungo, 1989; Bungo et al., 1985; Bungo and Johnson, 1983; Convertino et al., 1989, 1990; Fritsch et al., 1989; Fritsch-Yelle et al., 1994), there is an emerging body of evidence supporting the notion that repetitive +Gz exposure also leads to a degree of adaptation, reflected in enhanced cardiovascular performance in the face of an applied +Gz load.

Animal Studies

Several animal +Gz training studies have been conducted which indicate that cardiovascular adaptation to repetitive +Gz exposure does occur. Burton and Smith used a test population of adult male chickens using survival as the +Gz tolerance end-point to examine stress and adaptation responses to repetitive acceleration (1972). Their protocol involved a 162-day programme of daily exposure to either +2 or +3 Gz for different daily durations, ranging from 1–24 hours. After the intermittent daily exposure programme, the surviving birds were then chronically centrifuged at either +2 or +3 Gz for a further 111 days. They found that intermittent training exposures of +2 Gz produced a level of adaptation in the chickens, which was proportional to the duration of their daily training exposure. In contrast, intermittent training to +3 Gz greater than eight hours in duration produced physiological deterioration in that subject group. Burton and

Smith concluded that adaptation to an environmental stressor such as acceleration was a function of both duration and intensity of the stimulus.

Other animal studies have used changes in cardiovascular performance as a measure of adaptation. Duling (1967) centrifuged male Simonsen rats to +3 Gz continuously over a four-week period. The cardiovascular responses of the centrifuged rats were then compared with a control group of non-centrifuged rats. The centrifuged group demonstrated significantly greater increases in peripheral resistance when arterial pressures were altered pharmacologically than control rats. He concluded that centrifugation alters cardiovascular and baroreflex function.

Similarly, a French study involving repetitive exposure of rabbits to high +Gz levels (in the order of +8 to +9 Gz) found significant elevations in diastolic and systolic arterial pressures, as well as in the maximum rate of rise of left ventricular pressure (Borredon et al., 1985). They speculated that repeated exposure to high +Gz loads might cause '... persisting alterations to the functional state of the cardiovascular system'.

A Russian study by Vartbaronov et al. used canines as the experimental subjects in a programme of regular +Gz exposure over some two-to five months (1986). The end-point for the +Gz exposure was the onset of cardiac arrhythmia. Overall the animals increased their tolerance to high +Gz (longer time to onset of arrhythmia) by 20 to 30 per cent. In concert with this increase in tolerance was an observed steady decrease in HR during the experimental protocol. This was presumed to reflect accommodation or adaptation to the +Gz stressor (Vartbaronov et al., 1986).

Britton et al. (1946) exposed nine dogs to +6.3 Gz for up to 90 seconds per day, six days a week. After nine weeks, the dogs showed reductions in the tachycardia associated with subsequent centrifuge exposure. These HR effects were also presumed to reflect a lower degree of physiological stress response to +Gz exposures.

+Gz Training Studies in Humans

Training studies examining cardiovascular adaptation to repetitive +Gz stress in human subjects are much less common. The majority of these studies have used non-cardiovascular parameters as indices of tolerance to +Gz, such as the peak +Gz level reached or time to subject fatigue. Increases in both of these have been used as indicators of adaptation to +Gz.

Several authors have commented that subjects who were regularly exposed to high +Gz levels in human centrifuges appeared to tolerate the +Gz loads better with more experience of this environment (Epperson et al., 1982, 1985; Gillingham, 1988). The definition of tolerance used in each study was different, with peak +Gz level reached, time to exhaustion and time above +2 Gz being used. In one study the +Gz tolerance metric was not defined. According to Gillingham, the frequency of exposure seems to have an influence on the resultant level of +Gz tolerance (1988). He reported that centrifuge subjects and fighter pilots have a greater +Gz tolerance if exposed to +Gz three times per week than if exposed only once per week.

The overall role of flying experience has been investigated by several authors. Whinnery found that +Gz tolerance was correlated with flying experience (1979). Kobayashi et al. (2002) found that pilots with more flying experience were able to maintain a higher cerebral oxygen level at the same +Gz level than less experienced pilots. In a more recent study, a significant correlation was found between flying experience in the high +Gz environment and the cardiovascular response to an accelerative stress such as HUT (Newman and Callister, 2009).

Whinnery (1982a) reported that pilots who underwent a centrifuge training programme were able to increase their +Gz tolerance by at least an additional +2 Gz with regular exposure. Similar conclusions were also reached by other authors (Epperson et al., 1982, 1985; Frazier et al., 1982). Morgan et al. (1994) found that trained centrifuge subjects had less tolerance to a SACM profile after a 30-day lay-off.

The subjects used in the experiments discussed above were largely operational pilots or experienced centrifuge test subjects. They generally performed an AGSM, and in some of the studies also wore an anti-G suit. No cardiovascular data were presented in these studies, especially that related to acute responses of cardiovascular variables to the +Gz exposure. The performance of an AGSM masks any change in the cardiovascular system's response to +Gz due to repetitive exposure, making comparison with other experimental data a little problematic (Newman et al., 1998, 2000; Newman and Callister, 2008, 2009). In the absence of objective data on the acute cardiovascular response, the authors attributed the increased tolerance to +Gz of the subjects to improvement in their ability to perform the AGSM (Gillingham, 1988; Whinnery, 1982). Gillingham (1988), however, did speculate that an altered baroreflex sensitivity might provide a 'tempting' explanation for this phenomenon.

Only a few +Gz training studies have measured cardiovascular responses to +Gz exposures. In looking at the effect of 'lay-off' or time away from +Gz exposure, Toth et al. (1980) found that the HR response to +Gz exposure was greater after a period of non-exposure. HR was used as a measure of increased physiological workload, although not in terms of an acute response to +Gz. A study by Frazier et al. (1982), which examined tracking performance changes under conditions of combined Gz/Gy stress, used HR opportunistically as a gross measure of physiologic adaptation (after Toth et al., 1980). The time frame for the experiment was only short (seven days), and the HR data used was mean daily HR, and as such not a reflection of acute response to onset of +Gz. The change in HR was not statistically significant, but showed a trend to decrease over the week of experiments.

Lightfoot et al. (1989) used presyncopal symptom-limited LBNP to induce central hypovolaemia, and found that after only five LBNP exposures tolerance was increased by 47 per cent, with significant increases in maximum HR being observed after the third exposure. In addition, the rate–pressure product was significantly higher after the seventh exposure. Although the data was limited, they concluded that either the baroreflex mechanisms become more effective, or are reset to a different operating threshold.

In two studies, cardiovascular function after a period of high +Gz training was evaluated using the SST. Convertino et al. (1998) compared cardiovascular data from the final 10 heart beats of squatting with that of the initial 10 beats of standing. They documented significant changes in baroreflex function (manifested by higher SV and CO) due to repeated exposure to high +Gz forces. Kovitaya et al. investigated the cerebral haemodynamic response to repeated +Gz exposure in acceleration test panel subjects (1997). Their hypothesis was that if cardiovascular function is enhanced with repeated +Gz exposures, then cerebral haemodynamics should also be enhanced. They also used the SST, and measured middle cerebral artery blood flow velocity via transcranial Doppler sonography. The results of their study did not reveal any significant adaptations in cerebral blood flow velocities after three days of +Gz exposure. They attributed their lack of meaningful results to a potentially different form of adaptation in cerebrovascular function than that of the cardiovascular system, as well as the acknowledged limited overall +Gz exposure (approximately five minutes above +1 Gz) and wide individual variation in the subjects.

There is now an emerging body of scientific evidence supporting the +Gz adaptation notion (Berry et al., 2006a, 2006b; Convertino, 1998; Jouanin et al., 2005; Newman et al., 1998, 2000; Newman and Callister, 2008, 2009; Schlegel et al., 2003; Scott et al., 2013; Stevenson et al., 2014). Recent research examining the cardiovascular responses of fighter pilots suggests that they do indeed develop a degree of cardiovascular adaptation to the high +Gz environment in which they operate (Newman et al., 1998, 2000; Newman and Callister, 2008, 2009). These findings provide a physiological basis to the anecdotal experience of pilots of high-performance fighter aircraft that they adapt with regular and repetitive occupational exposure to high +Gz loads. Regular high +Gz exposure leads to the compensatory baroreflex system becoming more effective and efficient at dealing with the dynamic +Gz-induced BP changes (Newman et al., 1998, 2000; Newman and Callister, 2008).

A cross-sectional study comparing the cardiovascular responses to HUT between a group of actively flying fighter pilots and a matched group of non-pilots demonstrated a clear and fundamental difference in the cardiovascular responses of fighter pilots to HUT (Newman et al., 1998, 2000). This difference was attributed to the pilots' frequent and repetitive occupational exposure to the high +Gz environment, given that both groups were well matched in all other respects.

The pilot response to HUT was essentially an exaggerated or modified version of the normal response to tilt, as seen in Figure 9.2. This suggests that the fighter pilot's cardiovascular system has become much more effective at dealing with a sudden orthostatic challenge, such as HUT or applied +Gz loads. The fighter pilot is able to generate a significantly greater rise in MAP than that seen in the NP group. It does this by experiencing a smaller reduction in SV in the face of the HUT-mediated hydrostatic force, coupled with sustained increases in HR and more marked elevations in TPR (Newman et al., 1998, 2000).

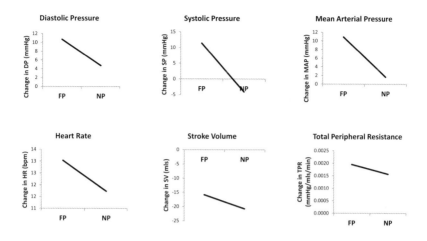

Figure 9.2   Cardiovascular responses to head-up tilt (HUT), G-adapted pilots vs non-pilots

The arterial baroreflex system appears to develop an increased sensitivity to changes in arterial pressure. The adapted baroreflex is able to generate an augmented dynamic cardiovascular response to an orthostatic challenge, reflected by better overall performance in the three determining variables of MAP, namely HR, SV and TPR (Newman et al., 1998, 2000).

A longitudinal study compared the cardiovascular response to HUT of fighter pilots before and after a period of high +Gz exposure (Newman and Callister, 2008). The pilots appeared to have developed an expanded circulating blood volume in the interval between HUT tests, with a higher resting MAP level. An increase in effective circulating blood volume results in a greater vasoactive reserve, with less vasoconstriction being required for a given orthostatic challenge (Convertino, 1998; Thompson et al., 1990). The pilots also developed a greater HR response with the second HUT test, which was significantly greater than that of their first test, as seen in Figure 9.3. This suggests an enhanced baroreflex sensitivity in the fighter pilots after they had returned to high +Gz flying, a finding that is consistent with earlier studies (Newman et al., 1998, 2000).

There are a number of published studies, particularly in the exercise physiology literature, that support the idea that blood volume expansion can occur as a chronic adaptation (Astrand and Rodahl, 1970; Convertino, 1998; Epperson et al., 1982; Holmgren et al., 1960; Oscai et al., 1968). An increase in total circulating blood volume after a centrifuge training programme has also been shown (Convertino, 1998). Furthermore, a reduction in blood volume has been seen following exposure to microgravity conditions (Bungo, 1989; Bungo et al., 1985; Bungo and Johnson, 1983; Convertino, 1990; Fritsch et al., 1989; Fritsch-Yelle et al., 1994; Thompson et al., 1990; Thornton et al., 1987; Tomaselli et al., 1990).

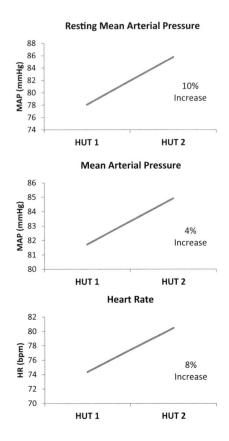

Figure 9.3   Longitudinal training effect of +Gz exposure on cardiovascular responses to head-up tilt (HUT)

It would seem reasonable from a theoretical viewpoint for blood volume expansion to occur under macrogravity conditions. This would be an advantageous phenomenon, both physiologically and hydrostatically. The vascular container in humans has been described as being chronically underfilled, due to the compliant nature of the venous side of the circulation (Rowell, 1986). If the vascular container was more completely filled (that is, more rigid) it should cope far better with +Gz-mediated hydrostatic challenges.

The underlying mechanisms for such blood volume expansion remain unclear. The reduction in circulating blood volume observed with exposure to microgravity has been the subject of much interest and speculation. Attention has focused on the renin-angiotensin-aldosterone system, since microgravity leads to central fluid shifts. Increased levels of plasma rennin and plasma aldosterone have been seen in some studies following exposure to microgravity (Convertino et al., 1996;

Haruna et al., 1997). Increased renal excretion of sodium ions under microgravity conditions may be due to a natriuretic mechanism rather than a previously hypothesised reduction in renal responsiveness to aldosterone (Convertino et al., 2000). The roles of atrial natriuretic peptide, angiotensin II and vasopressin in this mechanism remain undetermined. Endurance training has been found to increase the levels of ADH, aldosterone and plasma proteins, resulting in an overall increase in plasma volume. Red blood cell volume has also been shown to increase in some studies (Wilmore and Costill, 1994).

The mechanisms responsible for blood volume expansion under high +Gz conditions remain undetermined, and are the subject of emerging research. An increase in red blood cell content in subjects exposed to high +Gz has been documented, compared with the decrease that is seen in microgravity exposure (Blomqvist and Stone, 1983; Convertino, 1988). A +Gz-induced increase in circulating blood volume may well be mediated (at least in part) by changes in the activity of the renin-angiotensin-aldosterone system, due to chronic and repetitive exposure to +Gz acceleration. The baroreceptors (both cardiopulmonary and arterial) appear to have a role in signalling changes in blood volume, to which the renin-angiotensin-aldosterone system responds (Bishop and Sanderford, 2000; Colombari et al., 2000; Hasser et al., 2000; Thrasher, 1994). Baroreceptor function may in turn be modulated by humoral agents such as angiotensin II and arginine vasopressin (Bishop and Sanderford, 2000; Hasser et al., 2000; Sasaki and Dampney, 1990). An increase in the cellular component of the blood would appear to be a factor as well. More research is clearly needed to establish the basis for this protective +Gz adaptation.

A study by Schlegel et al. (2003) examined the effect of a single bout of prolonged +Gz exposure (to +3 Gz for up to 30 minutes) on cardiovascular function and tolerance to an orthostatic challenge (HUT). Their study showed that the prolonged +Gz exposure positively altered the subsequent tolerance to HUT, and there was also evidence that baroreflex responsiveness had been enhanced (Schlegel et al., 2003). These findings are consistent with those of earlier studies suggesting baroreflex adaptation due to chronic and repetitive +Gz exposure (Newman et al., 1998, 2000). More recent studies have also shown evidence of altered cardiovascular function as a result of chronic and repetitive +Gz exposure (Scott et al., 2013; Stevenson et al., 2014). Improved HUT tolerance after +Gz exposure appears to be a consistent finding (Newman et al., 1998, 2000; Scott et al., 2013).

During repetitive and chronic exposure to the high +Gz environment, as in ACM or aerobatic flight, the baroreflexes of the pilot are frequently exposed to what could be argued is a repetitive training stimulus. This is analogous to the concept of interval training documented in the exercise physiology literature (Fox et al., 1973, 1975), which involves frequent high-intensity short-duration periods of activity to induce persistent physiological adaptation. The nature of the training stimulus in the high +Gz environment is one of frequent, short-duration excursions to +Gz levels greater than the normal terrestrial value of +1 Gz.

The weight of experimental evidence thus suggests that a +Gz-induced hypervolaemic state coupled with enhanced baroreflex sensitivity (as shown by a significantly increased HR response) and a greater vasoactive reserve appear to be more than adequate to keep MAP at the required level and prevent orthostatic intolerance in the face of a HUT challenge (Newman et al., 1998, 2000; Newman and Callister, 2008, 2009). Such a state of cardiovascular conditioning would serve to protect the fighter pilot against severe orthostatic challenges such as applied high +Gz loads. Based on these studies, fighter pilots appear to develop a more advantageous cardiovascular state with repetitive +Gz exposure (Newman et al., 1998, 2000; Newman and Callister, 2008, 2009).

MAP and its three determining variables are influenced by both low- and high-pressure baroreflexes, and quite probably by the vestibular system. It seems logical that regulation of arterial pressure would be achieved via the neural integration of all available information concerning postural or +Gz-induced challenges with their attendant hydrostatic penalties. Such integrated information would include that provided by the arterial and cardiopulmonary baroreflexes, as well as the vestibular system. This would give a far more complete and accurate representation of the dynamic state of the circulation than that provided by one system alone. The integrated information would then form the basis for any corrective action that might need to be taken. Since tolerance to +Gz is a multi-factorial phenomenon, it seems logical that adaptation to +Gz will also be multi-factorial, involving improved performance of all reflex arcs concerned with cardiovascular control.

Future Research Directions

More research is clearly needed. Only in this way can a better understanding be achieved of the complex and intricate mechanisms responsible for regulation of the cardiovascular system in extreme environments such as high +Gz acceleration.

The current body of evidence points the way to further research into the phenomenon of cardiovascular adaptation to high +Gz. There are several lines of potential investigation to follow up. The use of a human centrifuge would allow a greater level of cardiovascular challenge to be given to the subjects, which would stress the cardiovascular system far more. Training studies involving larger numbers of pilots than were used in this study need to be done, in order to more fully document the +Gz training effect. A properly constructed study involving a sufficiently large number of completely untrained individuals subjected to a controlled +Gz exposure protocol in a human centrifuge is more likely to provide significant evidence of this effect. The time taken to lose any adaptation due to a lay-off from high +Gz flight also needs to be examined. The role of circulating blood volume expansion in chronic +Gz exposure needs to be addressed. Similarly, the roles of the VSR in the regulation of the cardiovascular system in general and in the response to applied +Gz in particular also warrant further investigation.

Finally, the emerging evidence that supports the notion of cardiovascular adaptation to high +Gz could provide the basis for development of safe and structured programmes for pilots returning to flying fighter aircraft after long lay-off periods. Such a programme would allow them to return to the high +Gz environment as quickly and as safely as possible, maximising their +Gz tolerance and reducing their risk of G-LOC. In addition, adaptation programmes could also be developed in order to maximise the +Gz tolerance of fighter pilots, with obvious tactical and operational advantages. This research has the potential to reduce the loss of pilots and aircraft due to the hazards of high +Gz flight.

Conclusion

There is now a body of scientific evidence that seems to confirm the anecdotal experience of fighter pilots that they adapt to the physiological demands of the high +Gz environment. The cardiovascular systems of fighter pilots who are regularly and repetitively exposed to the high +Gz environment develop a degree of functional adaptation, which is likely to be multi-factorial and not mediated by a single physiological system. Enhanced sensitivity of the arterial and cardiopulmonary baroreflexes, and an increase in effective circulating blood volume appear to be the underlying mechanisms of this functional adaptation. In addition, vestibular inputs into the regulation of the cardiovascular system under orthostatic or postural challenges may also be involved. Such cardiovascular adaptation would serve to protect the fighter pilot from the well-known hazards of operating in the high +Gz environment, such as G-LOC.

PART IV
Countermeasures

Chapter 10
The Anti-G Straining Manoeuvre

As the next chapters will show, there are several forms of anti-G protection available to pilots. These are in addition to the management of the various factors that determine tolerance to applied +Gz, as discussed in the previous chapters. One of the earliest forms of anti-G protection is the anti-G straining manoeuvre (AGSM). While there are several variations of AGSM, they all effectively share common elements. The beauty of the AGSM (in whatever manifestation) is that it requires no technology or equipment. It is a human-centred +Gz protective countermeasure. It requires adequate training in how to perform the manoeuvre, as well as practice to optimise its usefulness.

This chapter will explore the physiological basis of the AGSM, the different types of AGSM and its advantages and disadvantages. What will become clear is that if the AGSM is performed correctly it can provide a significant level of +Gz protection to the pilot of a civilian competition aerobatic aircraft or military fast jet.

The Physiological Basis of the Anti-G Straining Manoeuvre (AGSM)

The AGSM is a high-intensity, dynamic muscular activity, consisting of near-maximal isometric muscular contractions of nearly every major skeletal muscle group in the body, particularly the chest, abdominal wall and legs, combined with a repetitive short-duration forced expiratory strain against a closed glottis (Bain et al., 1994; Blomqvist and Stone, 1983; Buick et al., 1992; Burton et al., 1974; Burton and Whinnery, 1996; Chen et al., 2004; Eliasz et al., 2004; Gillingham and Fosdick, 1988; Green, 2006b; Kobayashi et al., 2012; Newman, 2014; Newman et al., 1999; Parkhurst et al., 1972; Scott et al., 2007; Weigman et al., 1995; Whitley, 1997; Yang et al., 2007). The fundamental physiological effect of this manoeuvre is to maintain head-level BP in the high +Gz environment (Bain et al., 1994; Blomqvist and Stone, 1983; Buick et al., 1992; Burton et al., 1974; Burton and Whinnery, 1996; Cooke et al., 2003; Green, 2006b; Newman, 2014; Newman et al., 1999; Williams et al., 1988; Yang et al., 2007). The ability to tolerate high +Gz loads is dependent, among other things, on the ability of the pilot to carry out the AGSM effectively and for protracted periods of time on a repetitive basis (Blomqvist and Stone, 1983; Burton, 1986a; Burton and Whinnery, 1996; Cornwall et al., 1994; Newman et al., 1999).

Muscle Tensing

As seen above, the AGSM consists of two elements – general isometric contraction of skeletal muscle groups, and an expiratory strain. Muscle tensing has been recognised as an important high +Gz countermeasure for many decades. Such tensing is able to generate up to +2 Gz worth of protection (Green, 2006b). Centrifuge testing has shown that subjects are able to generate significant force (up to 3150 N) on the rudder pedals as part of the leg muscle tensing element of the AGSM (Eliasz et al., 2004). Even teeth clenching has been found to produce a cardiovascular response in rats that maintained cerebral perfusion in a high +Gz setting (Takahata et al., 2011). In general, the greater the strength of the contracting muscles, the greater is the increase in arterial pressure, and as a result the greater the level of protection of cerebral perfusion (Oksa et al., 2003).

   The physiological mechanism responsible for this +Gz protection effect is an increase in applied pressure to arterioles and veins, increasing peripheral vascular resistance. This then tends to reduce peripheral pooling and subsequently increase VR to the heart. Additionally, abdominal muscle tensing helps to splint the diaphragm and reduce the +Gz-induced descent of the heart. This limits the increase in the HP differential between the heart and brain due to the application of high +Gz.

Expiratory Strain

The expiratory strain is effectively a repetitive, short-term Valsalva manoeuvre (Blomqvist and Stone, 1983; Burton and Whinnery, 1996; Green, 2006b; Shubrooks and Leverett, 1973). The Valsalva manoeuvre is well recognised in terms of its ability to develop high levels of intrathoracic pressure, in the order of 100 mmHg, aided by the marked reduction in chest wall compliance due to contraction of the muscles of the thoracic cage (Buick et al., 1992, Burton and Whinnery, 1996; Whitley, 1997; Williams et al., 1988). The physiological mechanism for the +Gz protective benefits of the Valsalva-like forced expiratory strain is that the increased intrathoracic pressure is transmitted directly to the heart and great vessels within the chest cavity, almost on a 1:1 basis, promoting blood flow to the brain (Buick et al., 1992; Burton and Whinnery, 1996; Green, 2006b; Hamilton et al., 1944; Newman, 2014; Williams et al., 1988).

   The transmission of intrathoracic pressure to the vascular system is the crucial +Gz-protective element, in that it helps maintain perfusion of the brain in the face of the significant +Gz challenge, thus ensuring the pilot remains conscious due to the continued supply of oxygen. At the same time, the pressure is also transmitted to the venous side of the circulation, which helps maintain the arterio-venous pressure gradient, thus allowing for the normal flow of blood to and from the brain. In a centrifuge study using near-infrared spectroscopy (NIRS) to measure oxygenation of the cerebral cortex during +Gz exposure, subjects who performed the AGSM correctly were not only able to tolerate the applied +Gz but were also able to maintain cerebral oxygen levels (Kobayashi et al., 2012).

Maintaining head-level BP is clearly the key to tolerating high levels of applied +Gz. However, the benefit of the expiratory strain is quickly lost if the manoeuvre is prolonged. The high level of intrathoracic pressure will restrict VR to the heart, thereby reducing CO and, ultimately, cerebral perfusion. In one study, the peak arterial pressure achieved with the L-1 type of AGSM (see below) occurred very early in the strain, but then started to decrease as VR began to suffer as a result of the persistent elevation in intrathoracic pressure (Williams et al., 1988). In the short term, then, the expiratory strain can boost head-level pressure, but in the long term it will lead to a reduced head-level pressure and increase the likelihood of G-LOC.

Timing of the Breathing Cycle

For these reasons, the expiratory strain component of the AGSM is not prolonged – it is effectively an interrupted or repeated short-term Valsalva manoeuvre. Ideally, the straining cycle should be in the order of three seconds (Gillingham and Fosdick, 1988; Lyons et al., 1997). This three-second cycle is important. If the increased intrathoracic pressure is maintained for more than this time, VR from the lower limbs is significantly affected as described above, and the AGSM becomes a counterproductive exercise. If the cycle is less than three seconds, the subject is in danger of hyperventilating, which carries the risk of unconsciousness in its own right. Timing the breathing cycle correctly is thus of paramount importance in terms of maximising the effectiveness of the AGSM as a high +Gz countermeasure.

From a respiratory point of view (and excluding for the moment the G protective nature of the skeletal muscle contraction), it must be remembered that in the high +Gz environment, only the straining component of the AGSM is protective. However, the pilot must also breathe in order to facilitate gas exchange and uptake of oxygen. The essential inspiration and expiration components of breathing must be completed as quickly as possible, for during this time interval the head-level BP will fall dramatically and the pilot is unprotected from the adverse effects of high +Gz. Once the strain is re-established, head-level BP is once again sustained and the pilot is protected (as seen in Figure 10.1). The inspiration–expiration component thus represents the nadir of protection during the AGSM, and so it is imperative that these essential actions be performed and the strain established as quickly as possible.

Helpfully, during the rapid inhalation phase, the relative negative intrathoracic pressure generated as a result tends to encourage VR from the lower legs. This is a beneficial side-effect, as it were, of the inhalation phase, as it means that cardiac filling will be optimised. Once the expiratory strain is initiated, chest wall compliance is reduced through contraction of the thoracic musculature, and the effect on head-level BP will be correspondingly maximised.

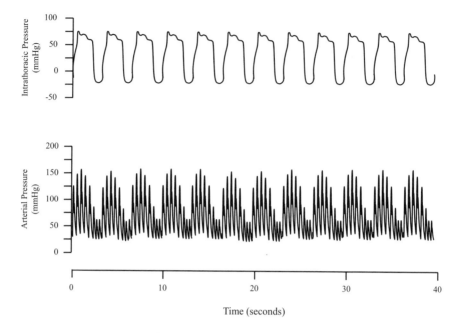

Figure 10.1   Anti-G straining manoeuvre (AGSM) effect on arterial blood pressure (BP)

The nature of the breathing component of the AGSM means that the respiratory demands of the pilot performing the AGSM increase quite dramatically. Inspiratory flow rates during a vigorous AGSM can be in the region of 5 litres per second (Buick et al., 1992; Whitley, 1997). In one centrifuge study, the maximum peak inhalatory flow was 274 litres per minute and the maximum peak exhalatory flow was 308 litres per minute (Whitley, 1997). The peak inspiratory flow values were seen to reduce with increasing applied +Gz level, which reflects the greater work of breathing (due to increased chest wall weight, and so on) under high +Gz and the effect of G-suit inflation (Whitley, 1997). Peak expiratory flow values also decreased with increasing +Gz level, but to a lesser extent. Clearly the breathing system installed in the aircraft must be capable of meeting such significant respiratory demands, or the G protection afforded by the AGSM will be negated by subsequent breathing difficulties.

The physiological effects of the Valsalva manoeuvre were used to develop a greater understanding of the relationship between pressure and volume in the lungs (Rahn et al., 1946). The intrathoracic pressure developed by the AGSM is a function of the pre-strain thoracic volume. When lung volume is at maximum vital capacity, a maximum effort AGSM can produce an intrathoracic pressure of over 170 mmHg (Buick et al., 1992). Due to the gas compression effect of the strain, the volume of the lungs will reduce over time, limiting the maximal intrathoracic pressure generated. The resultant intrathoracic pressure generated by the AGSM will thus reflect the interaction between the starting lung volume and the strain-induced reduction in lung volume. Based on these important facts, it can be seen that the most effective AGSM will involve as deep an inspiration as possible (approaching maximum lung volume), in order for the strain to develop the highest intrathoracic pressures possible.

Types of AGSM

There are basically three variations of AGSM, all of which are very similar. They are known as the M-1, the L-1 and the Hook manoeuvres (Burton and Murray, 1990; Burton and Whinnery, 1996; Clark, 1992; Green, 2006b; Williams et al., 1988; Zhang et al., 1994). The generic term AGSM is now used by convention to refer to any one of these three variations. The three-second repetitive cycles of expiratory straining effort that are integral to the AGSM can either be made against either a partially (M-1) or completely (L-1) closed glottis. When the straining is made against a partially closed glottis, the AGSM is known as the M-1 manoeuvre. When made against a closed glottis, it is known as the L-1 manoeuvre.

The L-1 manoeuvre was originally developed by the USAF, and named after Dr Sidney Leverett, who devised it. This manoeuvre is still the most widely recommended AGSM variant, very familiar to most of the world's fast jet aircrew.

The M-1 manoeuvre was developed by a team of researchers at the Biodynamics Research Unit of the Mayo Clinic in Rochester, including Dr Edward J. Baldes and Dr Earl H. Wood, based on earlier work in the 1930s in the UK by Steinforth (Burton and Whinnery, 1996; Clark, 1992). It is widely held that the M in the name M-1 refers to Mayo, but in a memoir by David M. Clark (1992) he cites that in describing the correct straining technique the researchers referred to their preferred manoeuvre as 'Manoeuvre 1', which was subsequently shortened to just M-1 when deployed as an operational countermeasure. The true derivation of the M term may well be lost to history, but it is an interesting item of G-related trivia nonetheless.

The Hook manoeuvre is a slight variation on the L-1 manoeuvre, developed and extensively used by the US Navy for its tactical fast jet aviators (Buick et al., 1992; Burton and Whinnery, 1996; Whinnery and Murray, 1990). It is somewhat difficult to put this manoeuvre into words that accurately describe how the pilot says the word 'Hook' that gives the manoeuvre its name. The pilot will effectively say the word 'Hook' as the strain is produced, held and then released. As the strain is developed and intrathoracic pressure is raised, the pilot will say 'Hook' (more accurately the pilot will say a clipped version of 'hook', without fully pronouncing the 'k') and then hold the strain for the usual three seconds (effectively straining against the held-back 'k' of the word 'Hook'). At the three-second mark, the pilot will release the intrathoracic air quickly as they pronounce the 'k' in an exaggerated fashion (as the syllable 'kah'), which facilitates the forced exhalation of air. So, put another way, the pilot will strain as they say 'Hook', hold this for three seconds, then say 'Kah' as they forcibly exhale the intrathoracic air and release the strain. Some might describe this manoeuvre more aptly as the 'Hook-Kah' manoeuvre, but in common usage it is known as the 'Hook'.

There are some other less well-recognised and less widely used forms of AGSM. The Qigong (Q-G) manoeuvre has been described by Chinese researchers, and is based on elements of traditional Chinese medicine (Guo et al., 1988, 1991; Zhang et al., 1991, 1992). This form of AGSM is worth mentioning here for the sake of completeness. While the Q-G manoeuvre is also a combination of breathing and muscle tensing, it is quite different mechanistically from the L-1, M-1 or Hook manoeuvres. The lower limb, abdominal, neck and respiratory muscles are preferentially designated for contraction.

The breathing component is markedly different from the other AGSM versions. It involves a rapid and shallow breathing cycle in which the inspiratory and expiratory phases are almost equal, in an ideal ratio of 0.85 (Guo et al., 1988, 1991; Zhang et al., 1991, 1992). In combination with the sequential muscle tensing, the Q-G manoeuvre apparently produces a pressure gradient between the abdominal cavity and the intrathoracic region, helping to facilitate VR (Zhang et al., 1991, 1992). In a centrifuge study, the maintenance of a thoraco-abdominal pressure gradient was observed up to +Gz levels of +7.5, with little fluctuation between abdominal and thoracic pressures during respiration (Zhang et al., 1992).

The breathing pattern therefore effectively uses the diaphragm as a form of vascular pump (Zhang et al., 1991, 1992, 1994). The Q-G manoeuvre thus does not seem to rely on high intrathoracic pressures to maintain head-level pressure under high +Gz, but instead relies on the resultant thoraco-abdominal pressure gradient to achieve +Gz protection. According to its proponents, one of the advantages of this manoeuvre is that the absence of an L-1 or M-1 style forced expiratory strain reduces the rapid BP drop during the subsequent inspiratory phase (Zhang et al., 1991, 1992).

The Q-G manoeuvre has not been extensively validated by researchers other than its proponents. In their centrifuge evaluation, Guo et al. (1988) reported that tolerance to a ROR profile increased by an average of almost +3 Gz when the Q-G manoeuvre was used. Such +Gz tolerance improvements have been confirmed in subsequent centrifuge studies, where ear-lobe pulse oximetry was also found to be maintained, reflecting good head-level oxygen delivery under high +Gz (Zhang et al., 1991). The same research team also reported that the Q-G manoeuvre was compatible with positive pressure breathing (a countermeasure discussed in more detail in Chapter 12), which they reported added to the protective effects of the Q-G manoeuvre (Zhang et al., 1994). The Q-G manoeuvre has not been adopted by Western countries, who almost universally prefer either the L-1 or Hook versions of the AGSM.

Advantages

The principal advantage of the AGSM (as the name suggests) is +Gz protection. If performed properly, the AGSM will give up to +3 to +4 Gz protection (Chen et al., 2004; Green, 2006b; Newman, 2014; Parkhurst et al., 1972; Yang et al., 2007). Failure to perform an AGSM correctly in the face of a high applied +Gz load will put the pilot at an increased risk of G-LOC. Several studies have documented that one of the more common reasons for G-LOC to occur is as a result of an incorrectly performed AGSM (Rayman, 1973a, 1973b; Whinnery, 1986). Seventy-two per cent of G-LOC events reported in a surveyed population of fighter pilots were attributed to a poor AGSM technique (Sevilla and Gardner, 2005). In the USAF in the 1980s, trained centrifuge panel subjects were found to have better, more effective AGSMs than current operational fighter pilots, suggesting an obvious training pathway to prevent G-related problems and maximise +Gz tolerance (Whinnery, 1982a). In a US Navy study, 53 per cent of surveyed pilots that reported A-LOC symptoms were not performing an AGSM at all (Morrissette and McGowan, 2000). The importance of the AGSM in promoting +Gz tolerance has been clearly established by many researchers (Chen et al., 2004; Lyons et al., 1992, 1997, 2004; Newman, 2014; Parkhurst et al., 1972; Shubrooks and Leverett, 1973; Webb et al., 1991; Whinnery, 1982a, 1986).

As discussed in Chapter 5, the AGSM also plays a role in prevention of acceleration atelectasis (Tacker et al., 1987). The increased intrathoracic pressure developed by the forced expiratory strain helps maintain inflation of the airways in the face of high +Gz exposure, use of 100 per cent oxygen and the action of the abdominal bladder of the G-suit.

From an operational perspective, the role of adaptation to the high +Gz environment (as discussed in Chapter 9) is important (Convertino, 1998; Convertino et al., 1988, 2003; Morgan et al., 1994; Newman et al., 1998, 2000; Newman and Callister, 2008, 2009). This cardiovascular adaptation to +Gz has an important effect in terms of how pilots perform the AGSM. As their baroreflexes become more effective at responding to applied +Gz loads, as a function of cardiovascular adaptation to +Gz based on repetitive exposure, pilots no longer necessarily need to perform a maximal AGSM. Indeed, they are able to titrate the AGSM to the level of protective effect required. As a result of this titration effect, the potentially limiting fatigue penalty (discussed below) can be mitigated. The pilots only need to develop sufficient strain to prevent grey-out and other G-related symptomatology. In the author's experience, fighter pilots who regularly operate in the high +Gz environment tend to do sub-maximal AGSMs. This reflects their increased cardiovascular performance due to +Gz adaptation allowing them to achieve the same level of +Gz tolerance with a reduced effort AGSM.

Interestingly, there is some evidence that repeated Valsalva manoeuvres can provide a short-term increase in baroreflex function, reflected in an elevated HR response to applied +Gz (Convertino et al., 2003). Experience in the high +Gz environment also allows pilots to perform less muscle tensing as part of their AGSM. In one study, subjects who were not pilots generated significant levels of footplate pressure that were far greater than required to cope with their +Gz exposure, and the authors suggested that this reflected their lack of skill in matching the degree of muscle tensing required to the +Gz profile (onset rate and peak) being experienced (Eliasz et al., 2004). In another centrifuge study using NIRS, it was found that pilots with more fighter flying hours were able to maintain a higher level of cerebral oxygenation at the same level of +Gz than fighter pilots with less flying time (Kobayashi et al., 2002).

Many questions remain to be answered about cardiovascular adaptation to +Gz, however, not least of which is how much G exposure (in terms of +Gz level, frequency of exposure, and so on) produces sufficient adaptation to the point where pilots can titrate their AGSM at will. Such questions require more research.

Disadvantages

While performing an AGSM correctly maximises the level of +Gz protection developed, it also produces a significant fatigue penalty in the pilot (Bain et al., 1995, 1997; Balldin et al., 1994; Buick et al., 1992; Burns and Balldin, 1988; Burton et al., 1987; Cornwall et al., 1994; Oksa et al., 1996, 1999; Epperson et al., 1982; Lyons et al., 1997; Newman, 2014; Whitley, 1997; Yang et al., 2007). In a study involving the SACM centrifuge profile and the use of electromyography (EMG) to examine muscle activity, it was found that as subjects neared the end of their tolerance time the work of inspiration had increased and the pressure generated during maximal AGSM had undergone a corresponding reduction. The authors suggested that it was this evident fatigue of the respiratory muscles (working to produce high intrathoracic pressures against a closed glottis) that was the cause of the subjects terminating the SACM profile (Bain et al., 1997).

In another study, a six-week programme of respiratory muscle training produced a measurable increase in respiratory muscle strength, but this did not translate into any significant cardiovascular benefit during performance of a simulated AGSM at +1 Gz (Yang et al., 2007). The authors suggest that respiratory muscle training might be helpful in improving tolerance of a high respiratory workload, and that further investigation at higher +Gz loads was needed.

The M-1 tends to not produce quite as much intrathoracic pressure as the L-1, due to the glottis only partially being closed (Buick et al., 1992). The lower level of intrathoracic pressure generated thus tends to reduce the overall +Gz protective benefit. This is a clear disadvantage of the M-1 manoeuvre, as it also comes with a similar fatigue penalty to the other AGSM variants. The M-1, by its nature, also tends to interfere with communications and has been linked with the development of irritated vocal cords (Gillingham and Fosdick, 1988). Based on these issues, the M-1 manoeuvre is less commonly used than the L-1 or Hook variants of the AGSM.

The AGSM is designed to increase G intensity tolerance, by allowing the individual to reach and sustain cerebral perfusion at a higher G level than would otherwise be possible. However, it must be remembered that tolerance to applied +G can be described in several ways (as discussed in Chapter 8). While increased G intensity might be desirable, some operational scenarios might require G duration tolerance to be a more important priority. This might occur during ACM against a similarly equipped adversary with similar aircraft performance, which might produce an engagement where a given G level might be experienced for an extended period of time. In such circumstances, tolerating a given G load for a longer period of time than the adversary might be the key ingredient to success. Given the muscular effort and concentration required to achieve a good AGSM, it is perhaps not surprising that the fatigue penalty created by the AGSM can actually detract from G duration tolerance at a certain point.

Body position has been seen to influence the cardiac responses to the Valsalva manoeuvre, and has also been examined in relation to the AGSM (Olschewski and Bruck, 1990; Williams et al., 1988). One study found that the ability to generate high arterial pressures with the AGSM was not significantly different across a range of body positions (Williams et al., 1988). It has been found that in some aircraft the required seating position forces the pilot to flex forward, which can affect the ability to generate the required force through muscle tensing when exposed to high +Gz (Oksa et al., 2003). The use of a simple lumbar support was found to alter the spinal position enough that the effectiveness of the AGSM was enhanced (Oksa et al., 2003).

The high intrathoracic and intra-abdominal pressures generated by the AGSM have caused some theoretical concern in terms of promoting urinary incontinence in female pilots operating in the high +Gz environment. Research done to date suggests that the AGSM by itself does not lead to a greater incidence of urinary incontinence (Benjamin and Hearon, 2000).

Conclusion

The AGSM is a critical technique for pilots of civilian aerobatic aircraft and military fast jets to master in order to protect themselves from the adverse effects of high +Gz loads. Failure to perform this technique correctly will significantly increase the risk of G-LOC. While there are some disadvantages such as fatigue, the level of +Gz protection afforded by a properly executed AGSM make it an essential tool of survival for the pilot operating in a high +Gz environment.

Chapter 11
The G-Suit

The G-suit has become a standard item of flight equipment for the pilot of a high-performance fast jet aircraft operating in the high +Gz environment. The G-suit has a relatively long history, and while there are newer forms of suit being developed and deployed operationally, the G-suit in common use around the world today has not significantly changed from the design dating back to the 1940s and 1950s.

This chapter will examine the G-suit as an important anti-G countermeasure. While it is a standard form of G protection for military fast jet pilots, the G-suit has found a role in protecting astronauts from the orthostatic intolerance inherent in return to Earth after prolonged spaceflight (Bungo and Johnson, 1983; Lee et al., 2011; Nicogossian, 1989; Perez et al., 2003; Platts et al., 2009). In civilian aerobatic competition, the G environment involves much shorter duration +Gz exposures (although the peak +Gz might be very high), and as such most pilots in this domain do not use G-suits.

History of the G-Suit

The G-suit has had a long history of development. The earliest G-suit design can be traced back to the beginning of the twentieth century, more or less to the time of the Wright brothers' first powered flight in 1903. An American surgeon named George Crile discovered that compression of the abdomen and extremities of experimental animals raised their BP. He used this discovery to develop a suit for human use containing a number of rubber bags which were inflated with air to compress the abdomen and limbs (Crile, 1905). While successful in maintaining BP in patients with shock, the suit was somewhat cumbersome and ultimately was replaced by the now conventional use of intravenous fluid and blood transfusions.

As discussed in Chapter 4, by the late 1920s and early 1930s G-LOC events were being experienced due to the increasing agility of aircraft at that time. Several efforts were made by various researchers to develop an effective countermeasure for this emerging G-LOC problem. In 1932 a USN researcher, Lieutenant Commander Poppen, designed a pneumatic abdominal belt which was inflated by the pilot with a hand bulb prior to +Gz exposure (Wood et al., 1946). This belt underwent several years of development, and was noted to give some degree of +Gz protection.

During the Second World War, a major advance in G-suit design was made. In 1940, Professor Frank Cotton, working at Sydney University in Australia, successfully designed a pneumatic G-suit that covered the abdomen as well as the lower limbs (Brook, 1990; Cotton, 1945; Green, 2006b). The suit's internal rubber sacs inflated in proportion to the level of +Gz force experienced, and compression of the abdomen and lower limbs was assisted by the non-distensible nature of the suit's outer layer. The Cotton G-suit was initially tested in 1941 on a small centrifuge at Sydney University, and then flight-tested in a variety of high-performance aircraft including the Spitfire. The suit was found to confer around +2 Gz worth of protection.

In the United States, other forms of pneumatic suit were under development. These included so-called graded pressure suits, in which the applied pressure was highest at the distal end of the lower limbs, and then reduced gradually towards the thorax, so as to produce a driving pressure gradient that could help propel blood to the heart (Green, 2006b). Capstan suits were also developed, which used +Gz-induced inflation of a small external tube to increase the tension of the fabric covering the lower limbs (Burton et al., 1973; Green, 2006b). Ultimately these variations of Cotton's pneumatic G-suit did not prove as successful.

It is worth mentioning here the water-filled G-suit developed by the Canadians at much the same time as Cotton developed his pneumatic suit (Brook, 1990; Green, 2006b). The idea of a water-filled suit had been in existence for some years, and had been proposed by the Germans in 1934 (Green, 2006b). The Franks suit, named after its Canadian originator, Dr Wilbur Franks, worked in much the same way as the pneumatic suit, with the exception being that the rubber sacs were filled with water before flight. This arrangement gave apparently very good +Gz protection, but this was largely offset by the increased weight of the suit, which made it bulky, cumbersome and difficult to move with (Brook, 1990; Burton and Whinnery, 1996; Green, 2006b). Furthermore, comparisons with the pneumatic suit failed to show that the water-filled suit offered enough of a +Gz protective advantage in the face of its inherent disadvantages (Green, 2006b). As a result, the water-filled suit was not widely adopted. The modern G-suit as used today is thus based on the principle of gas-inflatable bladders, and by and large is much the same as the pneumatic suit first developed in the Second World War.

Mode of Operation

The G-suit in use today will be familiar to anyone who has flown in a high-performance military aircraft. In most Western nations, the CSU-13B/P G-suit (originally developed for the USAF) is a popular choice. Other suits are effectively locally produced variations of this widely used suit. The G-suit is worn as a pair of trousers, in effect, over the flight suit. The abdominal belt has a zipper on one side, and the legs have zippers on each inside length. Once these zippers are fastened, a series of laces at the rear of the abdominal component and each leg can be used to tighten the suit against the pilot's body. If done correctly, this will ensure a tight fit every time the pilot dons the G-suit. This lacing is generally done once to ensure a good fit, with the zippers then being used for routine donning and doffing. On each outer thigh there is an additional zip, which can be closed once the G-suit is donned to create a higher level of tension in the fabric cover and to ensure an even tighter fit.

Internally, the G-suit consists of five interconnecting pneumatic bladders, one of which compresses the lower abdomen and the remaining four compress both thighs and both calves. The bladders are contained within a non-distensible fabric cover (usually made of flame-resistant material such as Nomex®) and are non-circumferential, providing somewhere in the region of 30 per cent coverage of the lower body. Inflation of the G-suit bladder system is achieved via a source of bleed air from the compressor stage of the jet engine. This air is delivered to the bladders through an integrated hose connected to an anti-G valve (AGV) installed in the aircraft (Burton, 1988a; Burton and Shaffstall, 1980; Green, 2006b). The hose connects to the AGV via a relatively simple push-in/pull-out mechanism.

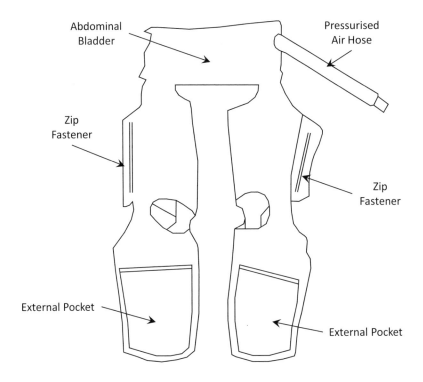

Figure 11.1   Standard G-suit

As the suit inflates in proportion to the +Gz load, the calves, thighs and lower abdomen of the pilot are compressed. This forces blood back to the heart, prevents dilatation of the capacitance vessels of the lower limbs, reduces the increase in mean transit time (peripheral pooling) in peripheral blood vessels seen with +Gz, and the abdominal bladder acts to splint the diaphragm and prevent the downward displacement of the heart. The abdominal bladder also increases vascular resistance in the splanchnic region, directing considerable abdominal blood volume back to the heart. In overall terms, TPR is thus increased by the G-suit, which delays the filling of the capacitance vessels.

This is an important point. It takes some seconds for TPR to increase in the face of an orthostatic challenge such as +Gz exposure. Experimental evidence in fighter pilots undergoing HUT suggests that in the +Gz-adapted state only the magnitude of response appears to change, with no change occurring in terms of the time course of the response of TPR to HUT (Newman and Callister, 2008). This finding supports the continued use of G-suits by fast jet pilots. The action of the G-suit in providing external compression and increased vascular resistance helps to minimise the potentially adverse problems associated with the time lag between the +Gz stimulus and the resultant baroreflex-mediated change in peripheral vascular resistance (Newman and Callister, 2008).

As was discussed in Chapter 3, the principal problem faced by the cardiovascular system when exposed to high +Gz loads is the HP effect, driving blood away from the heart and limiting its return from the lower limbs. In the giraffe, the sheer height of the animal and the distance of the heart from the lower limbs means that HP has a large impact on its circulatory system. To counteract this adverse hydrostatic effect, one of the countermeasures that the giraffe employs is the fact that the skin over the limbs is essentially non-distensible in nature. The hide of the giraffe's legs thus acts as a natural form of G-suit (Schmidt-Neilsen, 1991; Warren, 1974). Humans, however, with their relatively elastic and loose skin over the lower legs, do not have this inbuilt anti-hydrostatic mechanism, and must instead rely on an applied technological supplement, that is, the G-suit.

The standard AGV fitted to most high performance +Gz-capable aircraft is a mechanically-operated device which controls the pressure and rate of inflation of the G-suit bladders. Inflation is generally delayed until a level of +1.75 to +2 Gz is reached (Burton and Whinnery, 1996; Green, 2006b). Inflation of the suit is achieved via a linear pressure schedule, which matches inflation pressure to +Gz level. In the United Kingdom, the G-suit pressure schedule is an inflation pressure of 1.25 lb/square inch (8.6 kPa) per G, whereas in the United States a slightly different schedule is used, with an inflation pressure of 1.5 lb/square inch (10.3 kPa) per G (Burton and Whinnery, 1996; Green, 2006b). The maximum pressure generally attained with full suit inflation is around 10 lb/square inch, or 70 kPa (Balldin et al., 2008; Burton and Whinnery, 1996). Once the applied +Gz load has decreased, the high pressure in the G-suit opens up the AGV and the suit pressure is dumped.

Advantages

The principal advantage and the whole point of the G-suit is to increase tolerance to applied +Gz (Burton, 1992; Burton and Whinnery, 1996; Green, 2006b; Peterson et al., 1977). The standard G-suit provides up to +2 Gz worth of protection under ideal conditions. In practical terms, the generally accepted level of protection is in the order of about +1–1.5 Gz when the suit is properly fitted. Simply donning a correctly fitted G-suit results in around +0.5 Gz worth of protection (Burton and Whinnery, 1996). The reminder of the available +Gz protection is split between the abdominal bladder and the lower limb bladders in an 80:20 ratio (Burton and Whinnery, 1996). A well-trained and +Gz-experienced pilot who wears a G-suit and properly executes the AGSM (discussed in Chapter 10) can operate at +Gz levels of up to +9 Gz (although this is particularly fatiguing). This is of course subject to some individual variation and represents an optimal situation.

Several authors have examined cardiovascular performance under high applied +Gz loads in the absence of G-suits. In a study using trans-cranial Doppler to measure cerebral blood flow velocity, a French study found that average velocity fell by 10 per cent for each additional +Gz. With an inflated standard G-suit, however, the reduction in blood flow velocity was only 6 per cent per +Gz (Njemanze et al., 1993). Another study found a 49 per cent reduction in middle cerebral artery blood flow in participants subjected to +4 Gz without an inflated G-suit (Ossard et al., 1994). Tripp et al. (1994) found that the normal +Gz-induced falls in cardiac EDV and SV were reduced by the inflation of a G-suit. The results of these studies ably demonstrate the significant contribution that the G-suit can make in protecting the cardiovascular system from the well-recognised adverse consequences of exposure to the high +Gz environment.

The importance of the G-suit in providing a greater level of +Gz tolerance is keenly demonstrated when it is no longer available, such as might occur if it were to fail during flight. Failure of the G-suit during manoeuvring flight is not common, but the removal of its +Gz protective effects will lead to greatly reduced +Gz tolerance (Eiken and Gronkvist, 2013; Stevenson and Scott, 2014). In a survey of F-16 and F-15 pilots, G-suit malfunction was the cause of 19 per cent of G-LOC events (Sevilla and Gardner, 2005).

The G-suit also provides a vital function in supporting VR from the lower limbs to the heart when positive pressure breathing systems are being used for high +Gz protection. It helps to maintain the pressure gradient between the lower limbs and the thorax, such that the driving pressure is towards the heart, which therefore maximises VR. G-suit failure is of particular significance during the use of positive pressure breathing in the high +Gz setting. The absence of an operational G-suit can increase the risk of pressure syncope due to inability to maintain adequate VR from the lower limbs against the high level of intrathoracic pressure. Furthermore, there is some evidence that the abdominal bladder provides airway counterpressure during positive pressure breathing, which helps maximise transmission of pressure from the airways to the thorax, which is beneficial for +Gz protection (Eiken et al., 2011). In some cases the abdominal bladder pressure may be directly transmitted to the heart (Eiken et al., 2011). The issue of pressure breathing for +Gz protection and the role of the G-suit are covered in more detail in Chapter 12.

There is also some evidence that use of the G-suit may increase the responsiveness of the cardiovascular system to activation of the carotid baroreflex, which would be protective in the high +Gz environment through limitation of blood pooling in the lower limbs (Convertino and Reister, 2000). The significance of this in terms of the overall ability of the cardiovascular system to adapt to repetitive and frequent +Gz exposure (as discussed in Chapter 9) remains to be determined.

The orthostatic intolerance seen in astronauts on return to Earth after prolonged spaceflight has led to the use of G-suits as a countermeasure (Buckey et al., 1996b; Bungo, 1989; Bungo et al., 1985; Bungo and Johnson, 1983; Churchill and Bungo, 1997; Convertino et al., 1989, 1990; Fritsch-Yelle et al., 1994; Lee et al., 2011; Perez et al., 2003; Platts et al., 2009). The suit worn by NASA astronauts is known as an inflatable anti-gravity suit (AGS), and for all intents and purposes is similar to the standard five-bladder military pilot G-suit (Platts et al., 2009). The AGS can be inflated to pressures up to 2.5 psi. According to NASA standard operating procedures, astronauts must inflate the AGS to at least 1 psi during re-entry after spaceflights with a duration likely to cause orthostatic intolerance, in order to maintain arterial pressure during re-exposure to Earth's +1 Gz environment (Perez et al., 2003; Platts et al., 2009).

Russian cosmonauts use a different system: their suit is known as the Kentavr, which is an elastic, non-inflatable garment that provides constant compression. Similar to the G-suit, there are laces that allow for a customised individual fit (Platts et al., 2009; Vil-Viliams et al., 1998). The Kentavr suit provides a nominal pressure of around 0.6 ± 0.1 psi (Vil-Viliams et al., 1998). The effectiveness of the AGS and the Kentavr suit in protecting the wearer from orthostatic tolerance during re-entry and landing has been well documented in a number of studies (Kotovskaya et al., 2003; Krutz et al., 1994; Perez et al., 2003; Vil-Viliams et al., 1998).

The ability of the G-suit to effectively support the cardiovascular system against the adverse hydrostatic effects of high +Gz has seen the G-suit adapted for other purposes. It has been successfully used to treat postural hypotension including in patients with Shy–Drager syndrome (Brook, 1994; Burton, 1975; Stanford, 1961). It has also been used in emergency and critical care settings to support the circulatory system and maintain the BP of patients who have suffered life-threatening hypovolaemic events. In these settings, the suit is not known as a G-suit but as a pneumatic anti shock garment, or PASG (Garvin et al., 2014). The PASG (also known as a MAST suit, for Military Anti Shock Trousers) is able to increase VR to the heart and increase peripheral vascular resistance in exactly the same way as the G-suit. Rather than an AGV and bleed air from the engine of the aircraft, the G-suit in PASG form needs an integral inflation device, which is often a small compressed air source or a simple foot pump.

Disadvantages

The standard G-suit does have some limitations. It is reasonably uncomfortable by its very nature, especially the abdominal bladder which can produce a significant degree of discomfort at high +Gz levels. This has led to some pilots opting to not plug their G-suits in, preferring to accept a lower +Gz tolerance rather than experience the attendant discomfort (Alvim, 1995; Johanson and Pheeny, 1988). There is also potential for the G-suit to increase the thermal burden on the wearer, offsetting the increased +Gz protection provided by the suit (Green, 2006b; Perez et al., 2003).

The G-suit's effectiveness is limited by the rate at which it can inflate. Any delays in inflating to maximum pressure will create a potentially large enough time interval that G-LOC can occur before the G-suit can be fully operational. The standard AGV fitted to most fast jet aircraft is designed to inflate in no more than 2–3 seconds, in order to give maximum protection (Burton, 1988b, 1992; Burton and Whinnery, 1996; Green, 2006b). The AGV thus limits the G-suit's ability to deal with rapid onset rates of +Gz. If a level of +5 Gz is reached almost immediately (as is common in ACM), the pilot may have reached the stage of G-LOC before the G-suit is optimally inflated. The AGSM thus begins to assume greater importance. The difficulty with this situation is that the pilot's principal focus of attention may well be the tactical situation they are faced with rather than on the need to properly perform the AGSM as they manoeuvres the aircraft under high G loads. With the current mechanical AGV, the fast jet pilot may well negate the protective effect of the +1.5 Gz suit if the G-onset rate is too high.

Advanced G-Suit Designs

While the standard G-suit has largely remained unchanged since the 1940s, in recent years efforts have been made to develop more advanced G-suits. These recent advances in G-suit technology essentially represent variations on a theme. Many countries are working on such new generation G-suits. While they have some inherent design differences, all of these new advanced technology G-suits have one thing in common: they all rely on extended bladder coverage. As such, they represent a design evolution of the standard G-suit to meet the demands of more G-capable advanced tactical fighter aircraft.

Several of these extended coverage G-suits (ECGS) are in service with several air forces, and are said to provide a higher level of +Gz protection than that of the standard G-suit (around +2 to +2.5 Gz worth of protection compared with the standard suit's +1 to +1.5 Gz).

While standard G-suits such as the CSU-13B/P (or the CSU-15 A/P suit used by the US Navy) cover somewhere in the region of 30 per cent of the lower body, the various ECGS provide coverage of around 80–90 per cent (Buick, 1992; Goodman et al., 1993; Green, 2006b; Morgan et al., 1993; Ossard et al., 1995;

Paul, 1996; Paul and Ackles, 1993). They are thus a more complete lower-body garment than existing G-suits. The bladder system is circumferential, wrapping almost completely around the thighs and calves, and in some cases there is also a larger, augmented abdominal bladder.

There are several of these ECGS systems in either use or development. The United States has several versions of an ECGS. The USAF has its Advanced Technology Anti-G Suit (ATAGS) which is part of a wider integrated life support system known as COMBAT EDGE (Combined Advanced Technology Enhanced Design Anti-G Ensemble). The ATAGS suit is a significant innovation, combining extended bladder coverage with optional pressure socks (Morgan et al., 1993). The US Navy has its own version of this suit, known as the Eagle G-suit.

The RAF has developed an ECGS, known as the Full Coverage Anti-G Trouser, FCAGT (Stevenson et al., 2013). This suit is in service in the Eurofighter Typhoon aircraft. The Swedish Air Force's ECGS is in operational use in the JAS-39 Gripen fighter aircraft, as part of the Gripen's AGE-39 integrated life support system (Eiken et al., 2002; Montmerle and Linnarsson, 2005). The Finnish Air Force has been using an ECGS (combined with PBG) in its F/A-18 tactical fighter force since 1996 (Siitonen et al., 2003). The French Air Force uses an ECGS known as the ARZ 830 G-suit (Ossard et al., 1995). STING is the name for the advanced technology G protective system developed by the Canadian Armed Forces, and consists of an ECGS and a positive pressure breathing system (similar to COMBAT EDGE). The use of pressure socks has also been investigated by the Canadians (Paul and Ackles, 1993).

Each of these advanced designs has been extensively evaluated both in the centrifuge and in some cases in high-performance aircraft in operational fighter squadrons. The results of these evaluations warrant further attention. The USAF ATAGS suit has been extensively evaluated in the centrifuge, and flight-tested in both F-15 and F-16 fighter aircraft (Morgan et al., 1993). Pilots using the ATAGS suit consistently reported an increased G tolerance when compared with the standard G-suit. Ten out of 11 pilots expressed a preference to use the ATAGS suit for every high G flight. Each participating pilot reported that with ATAGS it was easier to sustain a high G loading. Ten out of 11 pilots preferred the foot pressurisation option with ATAGS. Nine out of 11 pilots reported improved tactical performance while using the ATAGS suit (Morgan et al., 1993).

A Canadian study demonstrated that an ECGS with pressure socks provided a higher level of G tolerance ($+10.6$ Gz$\pm$ 0.4) than the same suit without pressure socks ($+10.1$ Gz$\pm$ 0.4), and both of these combinations provided more G tolerance than the standard G-suit alone ($+9.4$ Gz$\pm$ 0.5). These results were with subjects performing an AGSM. Relaxed G tolerances were reported as $+5.54$ Gz$\pm$ 0.37 with the ECGS, and $+4.66$ Gz$\pm$ 0.19 with the standard G-suit. These centrifuge-derived results indicate a marked improvement in G tolerance with the new generation G-suits (Paul and Ackles, 1993).

There is also some evidence that ECGS provide greater support to VR during positive pressure breathing, allowing higher levels of breathing pressure to theoretically be used (Goodman et al., 1993). This support of VR is also adequate at lower rates of G-suit inflation (Goodman et al., 1995). The Finnish Air Force used single photon emission computed tomography (SPECT) to examine cerebral blood flow under high –in-flight +Gz with the aircrew wearing the standard Finnish ECGS. The results of this study showed that ECGS and PBG as a combination were able to maintain cerebral blood flow at +6 Gz without the need for the pilots to perform an AGSM (Siitonen et al., 2003).

As might have been predicted, these new suits are not without their own limitations. The increased size of the suits can create problems with mobility, especially when the larger bladders are inflated. There is also an increased potential for thermal stress in pilots wearing these suits, which can of itself reduce any +Gz protective benefit of the ECGS (Balldin et al., 2008; Green, 2006b). The increased bulk of these G-suits requires careful assessment of any adverse interaction with other life support equipment or cockpit structures. Several authors have noted the imperative to ensure correct fit to maximise +Gz protection (Green, 2006b; Stevenson et al., 2013).

In recent years a new version of an old idea has appeared. A new water-filled suit has been developed, which uses fluid-filled columns in a tight-fitting suit (Eiken et al., 2002; Green, 2006b). This suit has the obvious advantage of not requiring a direct connection with the aircraft. In theory, it provides instantaneous +Gz protection, as the hydrostatic force developed by the +Gz manoeuvre is applied equally and instantaneously to the fluid in the suit. This then creates an external compression on the lower body, supporting VR in the same way as a traditional pneumatic suit (Eiken et al., 2002). This suit has found a role in some forms of civilian aerobatic competition, largely because it requires no modification of the aircraft and can theoretically provide instantaneous protection at high +Gz onset rates.

Past experience with the Franks suit has shown the inherent difficulties with a water-filled suit. Water immersion per se can provide good +Gz protection, up to +2 Gz when the body is immersed up to the ribcage (Burns, 2005; Green, 2006b). Integrating this immersion protection capability into a suit to be worn by a pilot is not without its challenges. This new suit is a refinement on an old idea.

A centrifuge-based evaluation of this new water-filled suit demonstrated that it was not capable of providing an adequate level of +Gz protection in a +9 Gz aircraft (Eiken et al., 2002). G intensity tolerance was +9 Gz while using the AGE-39 ECGS system for the Gripen fighter, but was only +6.3 Gz while using the new water-filled suit. From an operational perspective, the finding that only one subject was able to complete a SACM profile while using the water-filled suit is of some significance (Eiken et al., 2002).

A novel approach to +Gz protection could involve electrical stimulation of lower limb muscles. A recent interesting study showed that a lower body suit with inbuilt muscle stimulating electrodes produced an equivalent level of arterial BP at +1 Gz as a standard G-suit and the AGSM (Balldin et al., 2008). Whether this finding could result in a new approach to G-suit design remains unknown, but the authors noted the potential for further exploration.

Anti-G Valve (AGV) Developments

The AGV in an aircraft is an essential part of the overall anti-G system, as it is this which allows the G-suit to operate. As discussed previously, the current mechanical AGV may not be fast enough to ensure optimal inflation of the G-suit under very high G onset rates (Burton, 1988b, 1992; Burton and Whinnery, 1996; Gillingham and Winter, 1976; Green, 2006b). While a lot of attention has been directed at improving the G-suit itself, some research attention has also been focused on improving the performance of the AGV.

The French ARZ 830 ECGS is associated with an electronically controlled AGV. This valve is capable of very rapid inflation rates, in the order of 100hPa per G. Experimental studies in the centrifuge suggest an optimal inflation rate of only 70hPa/G which can still afford improved +Gz protection. The ARZ 830 system with its electronic AGV is designed as standard life support equipment for the Dassault Rafale advanced tactical fighter (Ossard et al., 1995).

The USAF has also been developing an improved AGV, which also relies on sophisticated electronics. The Rate Sensitive Anti-G Valve (RSAGV) is electronically controlled and is very responsive to both high absolute levels of G and high onset rates. During centrifuge testing it demonstrated a +0.5 Gz increase in protection over the current AGV. It has also been extensively tested in-flight (Wanstall, 1990). Work in the United States has involved matching digital electronics to the valves in order to produce variable inflation rates that correlate with the G-onset profile of the aircraft. Microprocessor-controlled systems have also been designed to 'pulse' the G-suit pressure, to produce, in effect, a VR pump (Van Patten, 1988).

There is little doubt that the high-performance fighter pilot of tomorrow will require more in the way of anti-G protection than is presently available. The optimum anti-G protective system has so far not been developed, but the various advanced technology G-suits employing extended bladder coverage seem to provide a higher level of G protection than the standard G-suit used today. It seems likely that whatever G-suit system ultimately becomes standard in the next century it will consist not just of an ECGS but will also involve the incorporation of an electronic rate-sensitive AGV. Only in this way will maximum G protection be afforded to the fighter pilot.

Conclusion

The G-suit has been an integral part of the military fast jet pilot's flight clothing for many decades. In recent years it has undergone something of a design revolution, extending its coverage in an attempt to provide greater G protection in aircraft with significantly enhanced operational G environments. The introduction of super-agile aircraft has helped drive this revolution. However, at the extreme end of the high +Gz environment, more must be done to protect the pilot. The next chapter looks at what that involves.

Chapter 12
Positive Pressure Breathing for G Protection

Perhaps the most recent development in terms of countermeasures for high +Gz exposure is positive pressure breathing. Positive pressure breathing for G protection (PBG) involves breathing air which is progressively pressurised as the applied +Gz load increases. Pressure breathing is not like normal breathing, and is effectively a reversal of the usual breathing cycle. As a result, PBG requires pilots to undergo appropriate ground-based training in its use so that they are familiar with it and are equipped with the skills to cope with it. While PBG has some significant G protection advantages, it also has some inherent problems which have been well documented in the scientific literature in recent years. These problems are important in that they can limit the utility of PBG in an operational environment.

There are various PBG systems in use around the world. Most current fourth generation fighter aircraft in operation around the world make use of some form of PBG system, often in combination with an enhanced coverage G-suit such as the USAF ATAGS suit or the UK's full coverage anti-G suit (FCAGT). Examples of PBG systems in use include the USAF's Combined Advanced Technology Enhanced Designed G-Ensemble (COMBAT EDGE) system, as well as the AGE 39 system used in the Swedish JAS 39 Gripen fighter aircraft and the Eurofighter aircrew equipment assembly (AEA) used in the Typhoon aircraft.

Physiology of Positive Pressure Breathing for G Protection (PBG)

In Chapter 10, the AGSM was considered in detail. One of the issues with the AGSM is the muscular fatigue penalty it brings to each pilot, which can limit the G duration tolerance of the pilot. This can clearly be an operational limitation for a fast jet pilot. In an effort to address this issue, PBG was developed. The central underlying idea with PBG is effectively one of converting the usual AGSM into an automatic process requiring little conscious effort on the part of the pilot while achieving a similar +Gz tolerance outcome. A conventional PBG countermeasure suite involves a pressure delivery regulator operating in accordance with a given pre-determined pressure schedule, a G-suit and a chest counterpressure garment (CCPG). When a counterpressure garment is used this is referred to as assisted PBG, whereas PBG without a counterpressure garment is referred to as unassisted PBG. Modifications to the flight helmet and oxygen mask are also required to cope with the additional delivered breathing pressure.

PBG exploits the physiological consequences of delivering breathing air under pressure to the lungs. As seen in Chapter 10, the increased pressure of the air in the lungs is essentially transmitted to the vascular system on an almost 1:1 basis (Buick et al., 1992; Green, 2006b; Hamilton et al., 1944; Newman, 2014). Normally with an AGSM the forced expiratory straining activities of the pilot generate an elevated intra-thoracic pressure, which is transmitted to the blood vessels and heart. With PBG, however, the same effect is achieved via the delivered high-pressure air, without the need to actively strain on the part of the pilot (Ackles et al., 1978; Burns, 1988; Burns and Balldin, 1988; Clere et al., 1993; Domaszuk, 1983; Fernandes et al., 2003; Harding and Bomar, 1990; Krock et al., 1994, 1997; Lauritzsen and Pfitzner, 2003; Lu et al., 2007; Njemanze et al., 1993; Pecaric and Buick, 1992; Shaffstall and Burton, 1979; Shubrooks, 1973; Travis and Morgan, 1994).

The high level of pressure in the thoracic cavity due to PBG has several physiological consequences. Firstly, of course, is the transmission of intrathoracic pressure to the vascular system. As was seen in Chapter 10 with the AGSM, this raised intrathoracic pressure helps promote CO and cerebral perfusion, keeping the pilot conscious in the face of a high +Gz load. As with the AGSM, the raised pressure is also transmitted to the venous part of the circulation, thus maintaining the arterio-venous pressure gradient and the normal flow of blood to and from the brain. Indeed, some studies have shown that PBG prevents the collapse of the internal jugular vein that is normally seen with +Gz exposure, thus helping maintain cerebral blood flow (Cirovic et al., 2003).

Secondly, the efficiency of the pressure transmission from the airways to the vascular system is somewhat compromised by the PBG-induced intrathoracic pressure increase. This pressure increase will cause the lungs to distend and the chest wall to elevate and expand (opposite to what happens during a forced expiratory strain with the AGSM). This chest wall elevation and expansion will tend to reduce how much of the pressure increase is transmitted to the vascular system, thus limiting the protective component of the PBG. This adverse effect is offset to an extent by the increased effective weight of the chest wall due to the high level of applied +Gz being experienced. This is even more pronounced when the seat-back angle of the pilot is progressively reclined. This G-induced weight increase limits the degree of chest wall expansion and therefore the reduction in pressure transmission efficiency. It also helps limit the associated increase in the work of breathing caused by the increased intrathoracic pressure. This chest wall counterpressure effect is considered in more detail later in this chapter.

Thirdly, the increased intrathoracic pressure leads to distension of the lungs, which can potentially lead to parenchymal disruption if the pressure exceeds the structural integrity limits of the lungs. PBG thus is associated with a theoretical increased risk for spontaneous pneumothorax, particularly in the apical regions, and especially if the individual has a pre-existing pulmonary condition such as an apical bulla (Balldin et al., 2005).

Pressure Schedule

Positive pressure is delivered according to a pre-defined pressure schedule. A study by Pecaric et al. (1992) determined experimentally that a pressure schedule that introduced pressure into the mask cavity at +4.85 Gz and then linearly increased by 41.55 mmHg per +Gz would result in a maximum pressure of 73 mmHg being generated. This PBG schedule would protect all subjects to at least +6.6 Gz without the need to perform an anti-G strain. Using this schedule, the average increase in relaxed +Gz tolerance would be in the order of +2.2 Gz. They then modified this schedule to take into account individual variation, +Gz onset rate and visual criteria. Their modified schedule was to begin PBG at +3.3 Gz, with a linear increase of 42 mmHg per +Gz to at least 73 mmHg.

With most PBG systems in current use, positive pressure starts feeding into the breathing gas supplied to the pilot at around +4 to +5 Gz, and increases in a linear fashion with increasing +Gz load, reaching a level of 60 mmHg positive pressure at +9 Gz (Pecaric and Buick, 1992; Travis and Morgan, 1994).

A generic PBG schedule is shown at Figure 12.1.

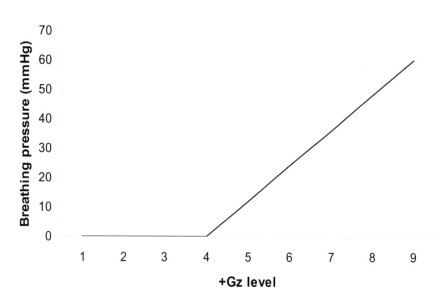

**Figure 12.1 Positive pressure breathing for G protection (PBG)
pressure schedule**

The Role of the G-Suit

The G-suit is an essential component of a PBG system. There are two fundamental physiological reasons as to why this is so: the prevention of pressure syncope and the efficient transmission of pressure.

Pressure Syncope

There are some adverse characteristics of PBG as a result of the way the normal human cardiovascular system responds to the increased intra-thoracic pressure. To an extent, this is a consequence of human anatomy and the fact that in the upright posture the heart is a long way from the ground and at the upper end of what is effectively a closed-loop column of blood.

The increased intra-thoracic pressure due to PBG tends to prevent the return of blood from the areas of the body below the heart. This blood has to travel upwards to the heart against the HP generated by high +Gz. While non-return valves in the leg veins and other control mechanisms such as the baroreflexes attempt to return blood to the heart, they can be overwhelmed by the addition of PBG-generated elevated intra-thoracic pressures. Blood is thus trapped in the lower body, and VR and SV are both reduced. As a consequence, CO is reduced, restricting cerebral perfusion and the delivery of oxygen to the brain. This will ultimately result in what is known as pressure syncope, where consciousness in the pilot is lost due to insufficient VR from the lower body as a result of elevated intrathoracic pressure.

To prevent this adverse cardiovascular outcome, VR to the heart from the rest of the body must be supported via the simultaneous use of an anti-G suit. Crucially, the pressure in the suit must always be higher than that supplied to the chest, in order to sustain a pressure gradient from the lower body to the heart that facilitates blood flow towards the heart (Ackles et al., 1978; Green, 2006b; Krock et al., 1997). No matter what pressure is delivered to the chest, a higher G-suit pressure will result in the ongoing flow of blood to the heart, and thence to the brain via the lungs. The blood volume delivered to the upper body and heart is thus optimised while blood pooling in the legs and abdomen is correspondingly reduced. Failure of the G-suit to maintain this pressure gradient (via non-use or inadvertent disconnection) will result in sudden onset pressure syncope.

Efficient Pressure Transmission

As discussed earlier, the intra-thoracic pressure generated by the AGSM or PBG is not completely transmitted to the vascular system, due to the elastic nature of the lung parenchyma and the expansion of the chest wall. The elastic properties of the lung and chest wall thus tend to limit the efficiency of pressure transmission from the airways to the vascular system. The G-suit performs an important role in helping to reduce this transmission loss. Eiken et al. (2011) found that during PBG, the abdominal bladder of the G-suit not only limits the well recognised caudal displacement of the heart and blood volume but also applies pressure to the lower part of the thorax. They found that the pressure transmission is almost unaffected when the G-suit abdominal bladder is pressurised, and that the performance of the AGSM was easier when wearing a G-suit than when not wearing one (Eiken et al., 2011). This helps produce a higher level of +Gz protection at a given PBG level.

The abdominal bladder of the G-suit seems to counteract the elastic recoil of the lung and chest wall, thereby improving the efficiency of pressure transmission. For such reasons, it is readily apparent that a G-suit is an essential component of a PBG system. Without a G-suit, the pressure generated by PBG is not efficiently used. This does come with a price, however. Acceleration atelectasis is a potential risk with such countermeasures, and this is discussed in more detail later in this chapter.

PBG and AGSM in Combination

Theoretically, the addition of PBG to the anti-G countermeasure suite should remove the need for pilots to manually perform an AGSM. It has been shown that in general PBG replaces the need for a straining manoeuvre rather than adding to it (Buick et al., 1992; Eiken et al., 2003, 2007). Eiken et al. (2003) found no evidence that PBG increases the maximal +Gz tolerance attained by an individual. They did note, however, that at a level of +9 Gz, subjects in their centrifuge study needed to also perform an AGSM on top of the PBG being used. The use of PBG thus seems to reduce the magnitude of the AGSM performed, which will reduce the subjective fatigue felt by the pilot over time.

Eiken et al. (2007) found that PBG plus a G-suit provided a combined level of G protection of +4.6 Gz. Interestingly, they found that the G-suit contributed +3 Gz of this protection, and approximately a third of the G-suit's protection was due to the abdominal bladder component of the suit.

Burton (2000a, 2000b) predicted that the protection afforded by the AGSM and PBG would be additive when used in combination. However, Buick et al. (1992) and Eiken et al. (2003) both found that this is in fact not the case. The combination of PBG and AGSM does not produce the same increase in intrathoracic pressure that would be predicted by simply adding their individual effects together. The reasons for this are the inadequate counterpressure provided by the G-suit and the inherent elastic properties of the thoracic cage.

Buick et al. (1992) commented that PBG's inflationary effect on the lungs without the need to achieve expiratory muscle activation places those muscles at a subsequent advantage in terms of being able to generate additional pressure on top of that developed by PBG. Indeed, centrifuge subjects report that the ability to perform an AGSM is enhanced by the presence of PBG, with or without a counterpressure vest, due to the slight effort required to exhale (Balldin et al., 2005).

The consensus view, therefore, appears to be that the levels of +Gz intensity protection obtained separately from PBG and the AGSM are not simply additive. The physiological interaction of these two protective measures appears to be far more complex than that.

The Role of Chest Counterpressure

The lungs are relatively delicate structures, and will suffer damage (with potentially severe consequences for the pilot) if certain pressures are exceeded. The delicate nature of the lung architecture is worth bearing in mind when considering the physiological implications of using PBG. In a relaxed subject, full distension of the lungs is achieved at a breathing pressure of 20 mmHg. If the chest wall is not supported the lungs will rupture when the breathing pressure exceeds 40–50 mmHg.

Support of the chest wall can be achieved through simple contraction of the muscles of the thoracic cage, an expiratory strain (such as occurs when performing an AGSM) or use of a chest counterpressure system. Such chest wall support can allow a breathing pressure of up to 80 mmHg to be tolerated safely with no risk to the structural integrity of the lungs. In addition, the lungs can sustain very short-term peak pressures in the region of 200–300 mmHg (as occurs during sneezing or coughing) and up to 120 mmHg (16 kPa) if the forced expiratory strain is held for a few seconds (as in an AGSM). However, if the straining pressure or muscular contractions are suddenly released the lungs are no longer supported and may then experience traumatic damage due to the high level of distending breathing pressure.

Given all of this, it is important that at high levels of positive pressure (as occurs at high levels of +Gz) the chest wall must be supported. As seen in Figure 12.1, the pressure delivered to the lungs at +9 Gz is in the order of 60 mmHg. Without chest wall support from the CCPG, rupture of the lungs could potentially be expected at this pressure level.

The conventional way of supporting the chest wall during PBG is via a chest counterpressure garment (CCPG). This is generally a sleeveless vest worn as an integral component of a PBG system. The CCPG is usually constructed with an outer layer of flame-resistant material such as Nomex® and an internal inflatable bladder applied to the frontal aspect of the chest, with a hose connecting this internal bladder to the pressurised air system of the aircraft (via the anti-G valve).

The vest inflates with pressurised air supplied by the anti-G valve system. It inflates to the same pressure as that supplied to the lungs via the PBG system. This prevents over-distension of the lungs and ensures an equal balance of pressures across the lung wall. This is an important point – the pressure delivered into the chest must be the same as that supplied to the counterpressure garment. Any differential in pressure between the inside of the chest and the outside of the chest will be translated into difficulty and discomfort with the normal breathing cycle. To a pilot this will mean difficulty breathing out (when chest pressure exceeds CCPG pressure), and breathing in (when CCPG pressure exceeds chest pressure). By keeping the trans-chest pressure equal, the work of breathing is normalised and the pilot is able to breathe in an essentially normal manner, despite the potentially high breathing pressures.

The function of the CCPG can therefore be summarised in three main areas: facilitation of effective pressure transmission from the airways to the arterial system, assistance with expiration through reducing the work of breathing, and protection of the lung parenchyma from trauma associated with overdistension.

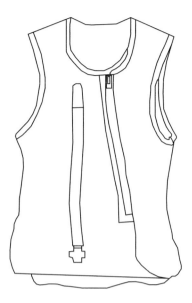

Figure 12.2   Chest counterpressure garment (CCPG)

It has been argued that increasing the size of the CCPG (in terms of the size and coverage of the internal inflatable bladders) might generate greater intrathoracic pressures and therefore greater G tolerance (Buick et al., 1992). However, this introduces a practical issue. The extent of protection must be balanced by an appropriate level of comfort. The pilot must still be able to fly the aircraft and manipulate the controls. Too much bladder coverage by a CCPG might adversely impinge on this ability, thus rendering the G countermeasure system impracticable and somewhat redundant.

Is Counterpressure Necessary?

In recent years the need to provide counterpressure via an externally worn garment has been questioned. There is some evidence that the increased weight of the chest wall under +Gz (a linear relationship between chest mass and applied G) may on its own compensate for the increased work of exhalation due to pressure in the chest when a CCPG is not worn (Balldin et al., 2005; Green, 2006b; Gronkvist et al., 2005). Indeed, some researchers have suggested that this natural G-induced counterpressure effect may be effective enough at moderate G levels such that a specific CCPG may not be needed, especially when the abdominal bladder of the G-suit is also providing compression of the lower thoracic region (Balldin et al., 2005; Gronkvist et al., 2005, 2008).

A Swedish study found that the CCPG did not appear to actually facilitate pressure transmission from the airways to the arterial system, as it was intended to do (Gronkvist et al., 2005). A follow-on study also showed that the work of breathing was unaffected by the addition of the CCPG to the PBG ensemble, although other studies have shown that the work of breathing is reduced by a CCPG (Gronkvist et al., 2003, 2008). Balldin et al. (2005) found that the +Gz tolerance achieved by the combination of PBG and the AGSM was not affected by the additional use of a CCPG. Subjects were still able to successfully achieve +9 Gz and complete a simulated air combat manoeuvring (SACM) centrifuge profile without the CCPG. However, four episodes of G-LOC were reported in this study, and all involved the use of PBG without a CCPG (Balldin et al., 2005).

While these G-LOC numbers are clearly too small to draw a definitive conclusion, it does support the argument that at high levels of +Gz it is beneficial to have a CCPG in place as an added +Gz protective measure. Most current operationally deployed PBG systems do tend to incorporate a CCPG as an integral component of the anti-G countermeasure system. The safety and operational utility of unassisted PBG remains to be comprehensively determined. However, there does appear to be a growing body of experimental evidence that suggests that the use of a CCPG is somewhat redundant, and some air forces reportedly no longer use counterpressure with their PBG systems (Green, 2006b).

The Pressure Regulator

In general, exposure to the high +Gz environment will see pilots experience a higher breathing rate and minute volume, as well as increases in peak expiratory flow. PBG will see pilots experience a higher respiratory frequency and a greater TV (the amount of air in each breathing cycle, normally about 500 mls). The volume of air expelled from the lungs per minute (minute volume) also increases with PBG, and is approximately 50 per cent above resting values (resting being roughly 500 mls per breath, with a breathing frequency of 12–14 breaths/min). Given this respiratory situation, oxygen equipment should be able to supply enough breathing gas to meet inspiratory peak flows of up to 200 litres per min, and a maximum rate of change of 20 litres per sec^2 at these peak flows.

As mentioned earlier, it is a key and vital distinction to make at this point that the pressure supplied via the regulator to the vest should be identical to the pressure supplied to the lungs via the face mask. In the design of most PBG systems, the pressure source for the external counterpressure vest and the mask is the same – the high-pressure air is simply delivered to two final destinations (vest and mask), from the same originating source. The reason for this is (as described above) that the pressures to the mask and the vest must be the same to allow for a normal pressure breathing cycle, particularly at high levels of PBG and high levels of applied +Gz.

Pressure Variations

Another area worthy of mention is the effect of any variations or oscillations of delivered pressure. If the pressure oscillations are mild, it is highly unlikely that under operational circumstances they will be noticed by the pilot during PBG. However, there are two crucial oscillation scenarios to avoid:

• where the pressures delivered to the chest and the CCPG are not equal;
• the G-suit pressure is not maintained at a higher level than supplied to the chest.

These two oscillations will potentially compromise the pilot's ability to remain conscious during the +Gz application and the PBG cycle. Unequal delivery pressures to the chest and CCPG will cause difficulties in breathing, as discussed earlier, such that the workload of the pilot under high +Gz will increase, with potentially adverse consequences for +Gz protection.

If the G-suit pressure is not maintained at a higher level than chest-supplied pressure, an adverse pressure gradient will be established along the long axis of the body (Green, 2006b). From a HP perspective, this will lead to potentially significant pooling of blood in the lower limbs, with a resultant fall in VR to the heart. This will then cause problems with reduced CO, and ultimately the volume of blood delivered to the brain will reduce. The end result of this sequence of events is an increase in the likelihood of +Gz-induced loss of consciousness.

The pressure breathing regulator developed for use with the PBG system should therefore be driven by signal inputs from the anti-G valve, according to the pressure schedule. The signal inputs should be constructed such that PBG cannot be initiated without anti-G suit inflation. This will prevent the onset of pressure syncope due to the loss of pressure gradient if the G-suit does not inflate to a higher pressure than the chest/CCPG combination.

In general, provided that any oscillations in the supplied pressure are equal for the chest and CCPG, are mild, and in the same direction as the preferred lower body-chest pressure gradient, the pressure oscillations will probably not be noticed.

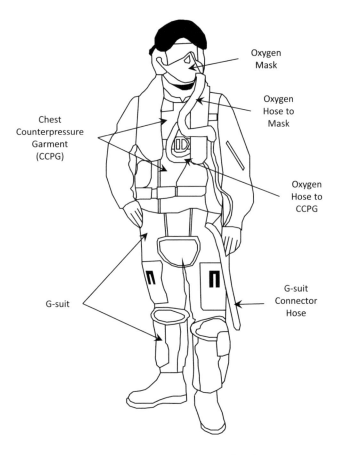

**Figure 12.3   Typical positive pressure breathing for G protection (PBG)
              ensemble as worn by a fast jet pilot**

Advantages of Positive Pressure Breathing for G Protection (PBG)

The two main advantages of PBG are the ability to tolerate a higher numerical
value for +Gz, and also the ability to tolerate operationally normal +Gz levels
for longer periods with a much reduced fatigue penalty (Ackles et al., 1978;
Burns, 1988; Burns and Balldin, 1988; Eiken et al., 2011; Fernandes et al., 2003;
Gronkvist et al., 2005, 2008; Lauritzsen and Pfitzner, 2003; Shaffstall and Burton,
1979; Shubrooks, 1973; Tong et al., 1998b). The pressure associated with PBG
not only boosts head-level BP but also helps take care of inspiration (making
it essentially passive rather than active). These features have the overall effect
of reducing the pilot's physiological workload while simultaneously improving
head-level BP and oxygen delivery to the brain (Ackles et al., 1978; Burns and

Balldin, 1988; Burns, 1988; Eiken et al., 2011; Fernandes et al., 2003; Green, 2006b; Gronkvist et al., 2005, 2008; Lauritzsen and Pfitzner, 2003; Shaffstall and Burton, 1979; Shubrooks, 1973; Tong et al., 1998b).

Increased +Gz Tolerance

The increase in +Gz tolerance associated with the use of PBG (either with or without CCPG) has been demonstrated in several studies (Ackles et al., 1978; Burns, 1988; Burns and Balldin, 1988; Fernandes et al., 2003; Gronkvist et al., 2005, 2008; Lauritzsen and Pfitzner, 2003; Shaffstall and Burton, 1979; Shubrooks, 1973; Sowood and O'Connor, 1994; Tong et al., 1998b). Shaffstall and Burton compared PBG and G-suit only in terms of +Gz tolerance (1979). They found that the use of PBG increased relaxed +Gz tolerance compared with the use of a G-suit only (+6.5 Gz compared with +3.6 Gz). They also found that time tolerance to a SACM centrifuge profile also increased with use of PBG compared with the G-suit only condition (138 seconds compared with 101 seconds for the G-suit condition). The increase in tolerance time to SACM centrifuge profiles has been confirmed in other studies, including one in which the tolerance time with PBG was twice that without PBG (Burns and Balldin, 1988). These studies have also commented on the fatigue-reducing ability of PBG (Balldin et al., 2003b; Burns and Balldin, 1988; Shaffstall and Burton, 1979; Shubrooks, 1973).

It is well accepted that one of the reasons contributing to episodes of G-LOC is breakdown in the AGSM performed by the pilot, which can be a function of fatigue arising from protracted ACM engagements. The use of a PBG system reduces the degree of +Gz-related fatigue experienced by the pilot, thus allowing him or her to continue the flight operations for longer and/ or to a higher level. While reducing the workload associated with high +Gz protection, PBG allows a pilot to therefore be adequately protected from the adverse characteristics of the high +Gz environment while at the same time allowing them to be more heavily focused on the mission they are required to perform.

Given this, PBG can be considered as a unique physiological force multiplier, since it helps promote mission effectiveness against a background high level of +Gz protection.

Reported Problems with Positive Pressure Breathing for G Protection (PBG)

As might be predicted from the nature of this technology, positive pressure breathing systems have had some disadvantages and problems reported with their introduction into service. For the most part, these issues are a side-effect of the pressures being generated by the breathing system.

Adverse Pressure Problems

The high-pressure air delivered to the face mask can cause a number of adverse effects. The high-pressure air can distend the upper respiratory passages and interfere with the ability to close the glottis (Buick et al., 1992; Ernsting, 1966). The pressurised air can enter the naso-lacrimal ducts and create a jet of air directed at the eye, particularly with breathing pressures in the order of 60 mmHg. This can lead to blepharospasm, discomfort and visual impairment. By the same process, the high-pressure air can enter the Eustachian tube and lead to middle ear pain and discomfort, again when breathing pressures are around 60 mmHg. The mechanism of this appears not to be a direct overpressure of the middle ear, but an occlusion of the pharyngeal end of the Eustachian tube (Howard, 1965). Tracheal stretching at high pressures (around 70 mmHg) and conjunctival suffusion at breathing pressures of 30 mmHg have also been described.

Mask Leakage

One practical problem is leakage of high-pressure air from around the face mask. While aviator-style masks tend to have a reflected edge seal to encourage good mask-face adhesion, the high pressures generated by positive pressure breathing (especially at high +Gz levels) can overcome the natural seal of the mask and produce a high-pressure air leak.

This can cause several problems. One of these is that not all of the high-pressure air is now being delivered into the lungs of the wearer. This creates an overall inefficient breathing system, with a consequent potential for significant reduction in +Gz protection. The escaping high-pressure air can also produce a high-pitched or squealing noise, which can be annoying to the wearer, a source of distraction in a critical phase of flight operations, and can also interfere with communications.

In an effort to overcome this problem, several positive pressure breathing systems have an inflatable bladder mounted at the back of the helmet, which will inflate as positive pressure is delivered, and thus help to ensure a tight-fitting seal on the face of the pilot (Burton and Whinnery, 1996; Green, 2006b). Additional mask tensioning systems (some of which are automatic) are also used. It is important to make sure that the helmet does not move relative to the head when pressure breathing is in operation, particularly when helmet-mounted sighting and display systems are in use.

Arm Pain

One of the major problems reported with positive pressure breathing for +Gz protection is the development of arm pain, usually in the forearm (Burton and Whinnery, 1996; Eiken and Kolegard, 2001; Green, 1997, 2006b; Green et al., 2007a, 2007b; Howard and Garrow, 1958; Linde and Balldin, 1998; Watkins et al., 1998). While pilots exposed to high +Gz have reported the development of arm pain during the +Gz exposure, such arm pain is more common and tends to occur at a lower +Gz level when positive pressure breathing for +Gz protection is used (Burton and Whinnery, 1996; Green, 2006b; Green et al., 2007a, 2007b; Whitley, 1992).

The main operational effect of this pain is that pilots who experience it will generally not fly the aircraft to the level of +Gz at which the pain occurs. That is, they will titrate their +Gz exposure to essentially avoid arm pain. In so doing, of course, they do not exploit the full capabilities of the aircraft, and therefore remain more vulnerable to the opposing aircraft in an air combat setting. As Chapter 2 demonstrated, the G environment of the civilian competition aerobatic aircraft is quite different from that of the military fast jet. From a G-time tolerance point of view, the civilian aerobatic aircraft operates at higher peak G levels but sustains the G level for much shorter periods of time than a military fast jet. As a result, PBG is a military fast jet-specific countermeasure, as it is predominantly aimed at improving pilot tolerance of high +Gz (in terms of tolerating a sustained G load for a longer period of time and reducing pilot fatigue). As such, G-related arm pain is usually only seen in military fast jet aircraft. The issue of G-related arm pain has thus received significant research attention over the recent past, mainly since the widespread introduction of PBG systems for enhancing G tolerance.

The underlying mechanism responsible for the development of this high +Gz-induced pain is still yet to be fully understood. It has not been conclusively established as to whether the pain originates in either the arteries or veins of the arms or in some combination. The experimental evidence does seem to suggest that the pain is of vascular origin, as denying blood flow to the arms via occlusion cuffs prevents the pain from developing under high +Gz (Green, 1997). What is known is that as forearm vascular pressure rises (which occurs during the use of PBG) the level of reported pain also increases (Green, 2006b). Early work in the 1950s showed that the general increase in sympathetic drive and catecholamine release (as discussed in Chapter 7) that causes widespread vasoconstriction leads to reduced blood flow in the forearm (Howard and Garrow, 1958).

However, more recent work (Eiken and Kolegard, 2001; Green, 1997; Green et al., 2007a, 2007b) suggests that the underlying problem appears to be overdistension of the forearm vasculature. Vasodilatation rather than vasoconstriction thus appears to be the underlying cause of the pain. In a centrifuge-based study, a reduction in forearm vascular resistance (FVR) when the arms were in a dependent position was seen at +6 Gz and beyond (Green et al., 2007b). The earlier work by Howard and Garrow (1958) was performed at +Gz levels up to +3 Gz with the arms in a non-dependent position. Green et al. (2007b) found that the addition of PBG seems to make the pain worse, but has no effect on forearm venous pressure (FVP), suggesting that venous distension is not the cause of the pain. The weight of evidence thus seems to indicate that at high Gz levels (+6 and beyond) the significant increase in vascular transmural pressure leads to a failure of vascular autoregulation, which in turn results in a dramatic fall in FVR and the subsequent development of distension-related arm pain.

An effective solution to the problem of arm pain in the high +Gz setting is still somewhat elusive. Beyond the decision of the pilot to avoid +Gz levels that induce pain, various other technological aspects have been considered in an effort to mitigate the pain. Suggested solutions have included such things as a fundamental re-design of the fast jet cockpit. This might involve raising the control stick and throttles to a position closer to the level of the heart such that the arms are not in as dependent a position as they usually are, thereby reducing the hydrostatic differential between the heart and the arms. Changing the control stick from the more conventional central floor-mounted position to a side-stick type of control can also reduce this hydrostatic differential. This does not seem to entirely eliminate the PBG-arm pain, however.

Arterial occlusion has been shown to prevent the development of PBG-induced pain (Green, 1997). This is clearly not a viable long-term solution to the problem, since the complete lack of blood flow to the arms causes other health and performance issues. Adding pressurised sleeves and even gloves to the CCPG has been examined as a potential solution (Green, 1997; Linde and Balldin, 1998; Self et al., 2000). Theoretically this would make sense to do, as these sleeves and gloves extend the pressure applied to the upper body by the CCPG and apply pressure directly to the arms. However, the results of pilot use of sleeves and gloves have so far been equivocal (Green, 1997; Linde and Balldin, 1998; Self et al., 2000). The work to resolve the issue of PBG-induced arm pain in fast jet aircrew remains ongoing.

Acceleration Atelectasis

The use of 100 per cent oxygen as a breathing gas for PBG (rather than normal air with 21 per cent oxygen content) poses some special risks for high +Gz pilots. As discussed in Chapter 5, the combination of 100 per cent oxygen, a G-suit with an abdominal bladder and a +Gz level greater than +3 can lead to acceleration atelectasis (Burton and Whinnery, 1996; Green, 2006a; Tacker et al., 1987). This involves collapse of the lower inch or two of the lung, due to the air spaces in that part of the lung being closed off by the dual action of the overlying G-suit (in particular the abdominal belt) and the applied +Gz, with the 100 per cent oxygen then being rapidly absorbed from the closed air sacs which then collapse. To a pilot this leads to some chest pain and discomfort, a sense of tightness in the chest, some shortness of breath and a dry, irritating cough.

As shown in Chapter 5, atelectasis produced by +Gz exposure can be progressively reduced with the addition of an inert gas (such as nitrogen) into the breathing mixture, by the use of unassisted positive pressure breathing and by use of the AGSM (Tacker et al., 1987). The 'problem' with PBG in this setting is that it tends to be supported by chest counterpressure, thus allowing atelectasis to potentially remain a problem. According to Tacker et al. (1987), assisted or supported PBG may not be as effective in preventing the development of acceleration atelectasis as unassisted PBG, since the action of chest counterpressure produces less overall increase in lung volumes.

Increased Thermal Burden

The use of PBG with its CCPG clearly adds another layer of equipment and clothing to the pilot. This can potentially create an additional thermal burden for the pilot, especially in combination with a high workload in air combat settings and hot ambient flight conditions (Balldin et al., 2002; Balldin and Siegborn, 1992; Nunneley et al., 1978, 1995; Nunneley and Stribley, 1979; Sowood and O'Connor, 1994). This thermal stress can lead to impaired performance and reduction in +Gz tolerance via dehydration, as discussed in Chapter 8.

While thermal stress is a potential issue with the use of a CCPG, most studies have not shown a significant difference in operational thermal load with the use of a CCPG. Balldin et al. (2002) found that subjects wearing a CCPG as part of the COMBAT EDGE PBG ensemble did not experience an increase in heat load compared with subjects wearing the standard flight clothing ensemble. Relaxed +Gz tolerance was much higher with the PBG ensemble during a GOR centrifuge exposure, and also led to a reduction in subjective stress scores.

In another study involving hot weather operations in F-16 pilots, core temperatures were not seen to be significantly different with or without the CCPG (Nunneley et al., 1995). A study by the RAF found that the use of a CCPG as part of the Eurofighter AEA in a warm climate led to an increase in thermal stress that was not regarded as unacceptable, while +Gz tolerance was improved (Sowood and O'Connor, 1994). There is some early evidence that when pilots are indeed thermally stressed the use of PBG does tend to increase their +Gz endurance (Balldin and Siegborn, 1992).

While the evidence seems to suggest that increased thermal stress is not a significant issue with use of the CCPG, it stands to reason that the only real way to maximise the avoidance of any thermal stress-related degradation in pilot performance with PBG systems is to ensure that the cockpit has a working and efficient environmental conditioning system. This will ensure that the subjective comfort of the pilot and the operational benefits of PBG are both maximised.

Conclusion

Positive pressure breathing for +Gz protection (PBG) is thus an effective means of protecting the fighter pilot from the potentially deleterious effects of high +Gz exposure. The principal benefit from PBG is a reduction in workload and fatigue associated with high +Gz exposure. This benefit is achieved with some penalties – namely arm pain and an increased thermal burden. In an increasingly sophisticated and complex operational environment, PBG offers the pilot of next-generation fighter aircraft an important means of ensuring survival.

References

Ackles, K.N., Porlier, J.A., Holness, D.E., Wright, G.R., Lambert, J.M. and McArthur, W.J. (1978). Protection against the physiological effects of positive pressure breathing. *Aviation Space & Environmental Medicine*, 49, pp. 753–8.

Adler, A., Ruskin, K.J. and Greer, D.M. (2013). Traumatic carotid artery dissection during acrobatic flight associated with $-G_z$ acceleration. *Aviation Space & Environmental Medicine*, 84, pp. 1201–4.

Aerospace Medical Association Commercial Spaceflight Working Group. (2011). Position paper: suborbital commercial spaceflight crewmember medical issues. *Aviation Space & Environmental Medicine*, 82, pp. 475–84.

AGARD Aerospace Medicine Panel Working Group 18. (1997). Echocardiographic findings in NATO pilots: do acceleration (+Gz) stresses damage the heart? *Aviation Space & Environmental Medicine*, 68, pp. 596–600.

Aghina, J.C. (1984). Othematoma associated with ill-fitting helmet and high G load: a case report. *Aviation Space & Environmental Medicine*, 55, pp. 143–4.

Albano, J.J. and Stanford, J.B. (1998). Prevention of minor neck injuries in F-16 pilots. *Aviation Space & Environmental Medicine*, 68, pp. 1193–9.

Albery, W.B. (1999). Echocardiographic evaluation of female centrifuge subjects for chronic changes in cardiac function. *Aviation Space & Environmental Medicine*, 70, pp. 561–4.

Albery, W.B. (2004). Acceleration in other axes affects +Gz tolerance: dynamic centrifuge simulation of agile flight. *Aviation Space & Environmental Medicine*, 75, pp. 1–6.

Alcorn, C.W., Croom, M.A., Francis, M.S. and Ross, H. (1996). The X-31 aircraft: advances in aircraft agility and performance. *Progress in Aerospace Sciences*, 32, pp. 377–413.

Allnutt, R.A., Chelette, T.L., Post, D.L. and Tripp, L.D. (1999). Disappearing colors at G and luminance [abstract]. *Aviation Space & Environmental Medicine*, 70, p. 85.

Allnutt, R.A. and Tripp, L.D. (1998). Color hue shift during gradual onset Gz acceleration. *Proceedings SAFE, 36th Annual Symposium*, pp. 446–53.

Alricsson, M., Harms-Ringdahl, K., Larsson, B., Linder, J. and Werner, S. (2004). Neck muscle strength and endurance in fighter pilots: effects of a supervised training program. *Aviation Space & Environmental Medicine*, 75, pp. 23–8.

Alricsson, M., Harms-Ringdahl, K., Schüldt, K., Ekholm, J. and Linder, J. (2001). Mobility, muscular strength and endurance in the cervical spine in Swedish Air Force pilots. *Aviation Space & Environmental Medicine*, 72, pp. 336–42.

Alvim, K. (1995). Greyout, blackout, and G-loss of consciousness in the Brazilian Air Force: a 1991–92 survey. *Aviation Space & Environmental Medicine*, 66, pp. 675–7.

Andersen, H.T. (1988). Neck injury sustained during exposure to high G forces in the F-16B. *Aviation Space & Environmental Medicine*, 59, pp. 356–8.

Äng, B., Linder, J. and Harms-Ringdahl, K. (2005). Neck strength and myoelectric fatigue in fighter and helicopter pilots with a history of neck pain. *Aviation Space & Environmental Medicine*, 76, pp. 375–80.

Äng, B.O. and Kristoffersson, M. (2013). Neck muscle activity in fighter pilots wearing night-vision equipment during simulated flight. *Aviation Space & Environmental Medicine*, 84, pp. 125–33.

Anton, D., Burton, R., Flageat, J., Leger, A. and Oosterveld, W.J. (1994). *The Musculoskeletal and Vestibular Effects of Long Term Repeated Exposure to Sustained High G*. Neuilly-sur-Seine, France: AGARD.

Armstrong H.G. and Heim J.W. (1938). The effect of acceleration on the living organism. *Journal of Aviation Medicine*, 9, pp. 199–215.

Armstrong, R.G., Seely, A.J., Kilby, D., Journeay, W.S. and Kenny, G.P. (2010). Cardiovascular and thermal responses to repeated head-up tilts following exercise-induced heat stress. *Aviation Space & Environmental Medicine*, 81, pp. 646–53.

Assa, A., Prokupetz, A., Wand, O., Harpaz, D. and Grossman, A. (2011). Echocardiographic evaluation and follow-up of cardiac and aortic indexes in aviators exposed to acceleration forces. *Journal of the American Society of Echocardiography*, 24, pp. 1163–7.

Astrand, P. and Rodahl, K. (1970). *Textbook of Work Physiology*. New York: McGraw-Hill.

Averty, C. and Green, N.D.C. (2005). Prevalence of high-G neck injury in fast jet flying instructors [abstract]. *Aviation Space & Environmental Medicine*, 76, p. 217.

Bain, B., Jacobs, I. and Buick, F. (1994). Electromyographic indices of muscle fatigue during simulated air combat maneuvering. *Aviation Space & Environmental Medicine*, 65, pp. 193–8.

Bain, B., Jacobs, I. and Buick, F. (1997). Respiratory muscle fatigue during simulated air combat maneuvering (SACM). *Aviation Space & Environmental Medicine*, 68, pp. 118–25.

Balldin, U.I. (1984). Physical training and +Gz tolerance. *Aviation Space & Environmental Medicine*, 55, pp. 991–2.

Balldin, U., Annicelli, L., Gibbons, J. and Kisner, J. (2008). An electrical muscle stimulation suit for increasing blood pressure. *Aviation Space & Environmental Medicine*, 79, pp. 914–18.

Balldin, U.I., Derefeldt, G., Eriksson, L., Werchan, P.M., Andersson, P. and Yates, J.T. (2003a). Color vision with rapid-onset acceleration. *Aviation Space & Environmental Medicine*, 74, pp. 29–36.

Balldin, U.I., Kuronen, P., Rusko, H. and Svensson, E. (1994). Perceived exertion during submaximal G exposures before and after physical training. *Aviation Space & Environmental Medicine*, 65, pp. 199–203.

Balldin, U.I., O'Connor, R.B., Isdahl, W.M. and Werchan, P.M. (2005). Pressure breathing without a counter-pressure vest does not impair acceleration tolerance up to 9 G. *Aviation Space & Environmental Medicine*, 76, pp. 56–62.

Balldin, U.I., O'Connor, R.B., Werchan, P.M., Isdahl, W.M., Demitry, P.F., Stork, R.L. and Morgan, T.R. (2002). Heat stress effects for USAF anti-G suits with and without a counter-pressure vest. *Aviation Space & Environmental Medicine*, 73, pp. 456–9.

Balldin, U.I. and Siegborn, J. (1992). G-endurance during heat stress and balanced pressure breathing. *Aviation Space & Environmental Medicine*, 63, pp. 177–80.

Balldin, U.I., Tong, A., Marshall, J.A. and Regna, M. (1999). Premature ventricular contractions during +Gz with and without pressure breathing and extended coverage anti-G suit. *Aviation Space & Environmental Medicine*, 70, pp. 209–12.

Balldin, U.I., Werchan, P.M., French, J. and Self, B. (2003b). Endurance and performance during multiple intense high +Gz exposures with effective anti-G protection. *Aviation Space & Environmental Medicine*, 74, pp. 303–8.

Banks, R.D. and Gray, G. (1994). 'Bunt bradycardia': two cases of slowing of heart rate inflight during negative Gz. *Aviation Space & Environmental Medicine*, 65, pp. 330–31.

Banks, R.D., Grissett, J.D., Saunders, P.L. and Mateczun, A.J. (1995). The effect of varying time at -Gz on subsequent +G_z physiological tolerance (push–pull effect). *Aviation Space & Environmental Medicine*, 66, pp. 723–7.

Banks, R.D., Grissett, J.D., Turnipseed, G.T., Saunders, P.L. and Rupert, A.H. (1994). The 'push–pull effect'. *Aviation Space & Environmental Medicine*, 65, pp. 699–704.

Banta, G.R. and Grissett, J.D. (1985). Relationship of cardiopulmonary fitness to flight performance in tactical Aviation. In: *Medical Selection and Physiological Training of Future Fighter Aircrew*.AGARD CP-396, December.

Barker, P.D. (2011). Reduced G tolerance associated with supplement use. *Aviation Space & Environmental Medicine*, 82, pp. 140–43.

Bartok, S.J., Carlson, L.D. and Walters, R.F. (1968). Cardiovascular changes during tilt and leg negative pressure tests. *Aerospace Medicine*, 39, pp. 1157–62.

Bartusiak, M. (2000). *Einstein's Unfinished Symphony: Listening to the Sounds of Space-Time*. Washington, DC: Joseph Henry Press.

Bateman, W.A., Jacobs, I. and Buick, F. (2006). Physical conditioning to enhance +Gz tolerance: issues and current understanding. *Aviation Space & Environmental Medicine*, 77, pp. 573–80.

Bayer, A., Yumuşak, E., Şahin, Ö.F. and Uysal, Y. (2004). Intraocular pressure measured at ground level and 10,000 feet. *Aviation Space & Environmental Medicine*, 75, pp. 543–5.

Beckman, E.L., Duane, T.D., Ziegler, J.E. and Hunter, H. (1954). Some observations on human tolerance to acceleration stress. Phase IV. Human tolerance to high positive G applied at a rate of 5 to 10 G per second. *Aviation Space & Environmental Medicine*, 25, pp. 50–66.

Benjamin, C.R. and Hearon, C.M. (2000). Urinary continence in women during centrifuge exposure to high+ Gz. *Aviation Space & Environmental Medicine*, 71, pp. 131–6.

Berry, N.M., Rickards, C.A. and Newman, D.G. (2003). The effect of caffeine on the cardiovascular responses to head-up tilt. *Aviation Space & Environmental Medicine*, 74, pp. 725–30.

Berry, N.M., Rickards, C.A. and Newman, D.G. (2006a). Squat-stand test response following ten consecutive episodes of head-up tilt. *Aviation Space & Environmental Medicine*, 77, pp. 1125–30.

Berry, N.M., Rickards, C.A. and Newman, D.G. (2006b). Acute cardiovascular adaptation to ten consecutive episodes of head-up tilt. *Aviation Space & Environmental Medicine*, 77, pp. 494–9.

Berry, N.M. and Newman, D.G. (2007). Head-up tilting – new applications for a dynamic cardiovascular challenge. *Aviation Space & Environmental Medicine*, 78, p.635.

Bevegard, S., Castenfors, J. and Lindblad, L.E. (1977). Effect of carotid sinus stimulation on cardiac output and peripheral vascular resistance during changes in blood volume distribution in man. *Acta Physiologica Scandinavica*, 101, pp. 50–57.

Beyer, R.W. and Daily, P.O. (2004). Renal artery dissection associated with Gz acceleration. *Aviation Space & Environmental Medicine*, 75, pp. 284–7.

Biernacki, M.P., Jankowski, K.S., Kowalczuk, K., Lewkowicz, R. and Dereń, M. (2012). +G$_z$ centrifugation and mood. *Aviation Space & Environmental Medicine*, 83, pp. 136–9.

Biernacki, M.P., Tarnowski, A., Lengsfeld, K., Lewkowicz, R., Kowalczuk, K. and Dereń, M. (2013). +G$_z$ load and executive functions. *Aviation Space & Environmental Medicine*, 84, pp. 511–15.

Billman, G.E., Dickey, D.T., Teoh, K.K. and Stone, H.L. (1981). Effects of central venous blood volume shifts on arterial baroreflex control of heart rate. *American Journal of Physiology*, 241(Heart Circ Physiol 10), pp. H571–H575.

Bishop, V.S. and Sanderford, M.G. (2000). Angiotensin II modulation of the arterial baroreflex: role of the area postrema. *Clinical and Experimental Pharmacology and Physiology*, 27, pp. 428–31.

Blamick, C.A., Goldwater, D.J. and Convertino, V.A. (1988). Leg vascular responsiveness during acute orthostasis following simulated weightlessness. *Aviation Space & Environmental Medicine*, 59, pp. 40–43.

Blomqvist, C.G. and Stone, H.L. (1983). Cardiovascular adjustments to gravitational stress. In: *Handbook of Physiology. The Cardiovascular System*, Sect. 2, Vol III, Ch. 28. Bethesda: American Physiological Society.

Bloodwell, R.D. and Whinnery, J.E. (1982). Acceleration exposure during competitive civilian aerobatics. *Preprint of Paper Presented at Meeting of the Aerospace Medical Association*. Florida: Bal Harbour, pp. 167–8.

Blue, R.S., Riccitello, J.M., Tizard, J., Hamilton, R.J. and Vanderploeg, J.M. (2012). Commercial spaceflight participant G-force tolerance during centrifuge-simulated suborbital flight. *Aviation Space & Environmental Medicine*, 83, pp. 929–34.

Blumberg, N., Arbel, R. and Dabby, D. (2002). Avulsion of the triceps tendon during acceleration stress. *Aviation Space & Environmental Medicine*, 73, pp. 931–3.

Borchart, C.J., Allnutt, R.A. and Tripp, L.D. (2000). Using the cyan to central (C2C) interval in training centrifuge subjects [abstract]. *Aviation Space & Environmental Medicine*, 71, p. 269.

Borredon, P., Paillard, F., Liscia, P. and Nogues, C. (1985). Hypertension induced by repeated exposure to high sustained +Gz (HS +Gz) stress. *Aviation Space & Environmental Medicine*, 56, pp. 328–32.

Borst, C., Wieling, W., Van Brederode, J.F.M., Hond, A., De Rijk, L.G. and Dunning, A.J. (1982). Mechanisms of initial heart rate response to postural change. *American Journal of Physiology*, 243, pp. H676–H681.

Bovim, G., Schrader, H. and Sand, T. (1994). Neck pain in the general population. *Spine*, 19, pp. 1307–9.

Boyum, K.E., Pachter, M. and Houpis, C.H. (1995). High angle of attack velocity vector rolls. *Control Engineering Practice*, 3, pp. 1087–93.

Braunstein, M.L. and White, W.J. (1962). Effects of acceleration on brightness discrimination. *Journal of the Optical Society of America*, 52, pp. 931–3.

Britton, S.W., Corey, E.L. and Stewart, G.A. (1946). Effects of high acceleration forces and their alleviation. *American Journal of Physiology*, 146, pp. 33–57.

Brook, W.H. (1990). The development of the Australian anti-G suit. *Aviation Space & Environmental Medicine*, 61, pp. 176–82.

Brook, W.H. (1994). Postural hypotension and the anti-gravity suit. *Australian Family Physician*, 23, p. 1945.

Buckey, J.C., Gaffney, F.A., Lane, L.D., Levine, B.D., Watenpaugh, D.E., Wright, S.J., Yancy, C.W., Meyer, D.M., Blomqvist, C.G. (1996a). Central venous pressure in space. *Journal of Applied Physiology*, 81, pp. 19–25.

Buckey, J.C., Lane, L.D., Levine, B.D., Watenpaugh, D.E., Wright, S.J., Moore, W.E., Gaffney, F.A. and Blomqvist, C.G. (1996b). Orthostatic intolerance after spaceflight. *Journal of Applied Physiology*, 81, pp. 7–18.

Buick, F. (1992). Advanced +Gz protection systems and their physiologic bases. *The Physiologist*, 35(1, Suppl.), pp. S158–61.

Buick, F., Hartley, J. and Pecaric, M. (1992). Maximum intra-thoracic pressure with anti-G straining maneuvers and positive pressure breathing during +Gz. *Aviation Space & Environmental Medicine*, 63, pp. 670–77.

Bulbulian, R., Crisman, R.P., Thomas, M.L. and Meyer, L.G. (1994). The effects of strength training and centrifuge exposure on +Gz tolerance. *Aviation Space & Environmental Medicine*, 65, pp. 1097–104.

Bungo, M.W. (1989). The cardiopulmonary system. In: Nicogossian, A.E., Huntoon, C.L. and Pool, S.L. (eds), *Space Physiology and Medicine*. Philadelphia: Lea and Febiger.

Bungo, M.W., Charles, J.B. and Johnson, P.C. (1985). Cardiovascular deconditioning during space flight and the use of saline as a countermeasure to orthostatic intolerance. *Aviation Space & Environmental Medicine*, 56, pp. 985–90.

Bungo, M.W. and Johnson, P.J. (1983). Cardiovascular examinations and observations of deconditioning during space shuttle orbital flight test program. *Aviation Space & Environmental Medicine*, 54, pp. 1001–4.

Burnett, A.F., Naumann, F.L. and Burton, E.J. (2004). Flight-training effect on the cervical muscle isometric strength of trainee pilots. *Aviation Space & Environmental Medicine*, 75, pp. 611–15.

Burns, J.W. (1988). Prevention of loss of consciousness with positive pressure breathing and supinating seat. *Aviation Space & Environmental Medicine*, 59, pp. 20–22.

Burns, J.W. (1992). High-G cardiovascular physiology. *The Physiologist*, 35(1 Suppl.), pp. S131–34.

Burns, J.W. (2005). Hemodynamics of graded water immersion in the baboon: +Gz protection potential. *Aviation Space & Environmental Medicine*, 76, pp. 430–34.

Burns, J.W. and Balldin, U.I. (1988). Assisted positive pressure breathing for augmentation of acceleration tolerance time. *Aviation Space & Environmental Medicine*, 59, pp. 225–33.

Burns, J.W., Ivan, D.J., Stern, C.H., Patterson, J.C., Johnson, P.C., Drew, W.E. and Yates, J.T. (2001). Protection to +12 Gz. *Aviation Space & Environmental Medicine*, 72, pp. 413–21.

Burns, J.W., Kruyer, W.B., Celio, P.V., Deering, J., Loecker, T.H., Richardson, L.A., Fanton, J.W., Davis, H. and Dick, E.J. Jr. (2008). Cardiac ischemia model for +G_z using miniature swine and baboons. *Aviation Space & Environmental Medicine*, 79, pp. 374–83.

Burns, J.W., Loecker, T.H., Fischer Jr, J.R. and Bauer, D.H. (1996). Prevalence and significance of spinal disc abnormalities in an asymptomatic acceleration subject panel. *Aviation Space & Environmental Medicine*, 67, pp. 849–53.

Burns, J.W., Werchan, P.M., Fanton, J.W. and Dollins, A.B. (1991). Performance recovery following +Gz-induced loss of consciousness. *Aviation Space & Environmental Medicine*, 62, pp. 615–17.

Burton, R.R. (1975). Clinical application of the anti-G suit. *Aviation Space & Environmental Medicine*, 46, p. 745.

Burton, R.R. (1986a). A conceptual model for predicting pilot group G tolerance for tactical fighter aircraft. *Aviation Space & Environmental Medicine*, 57, pp. 733–44.

Burton, R.R. (1986b). Simulated aerial combat manoeuvring tolerance and physical conditioning: current status. *Aviation Space & Environmental Medicine*, 57, pp. 712–14.

Burton, R.R. (1988a). G-induced loss of consciousness: definition, history, current status. *Aviation Space & Environmental Medicine*, 59, pp. 2–5.

Burton, R.R. (1988b). Anti-G suit inflation rate requirements. *Aviation Space & Environmental Medicine*, 59, pp. 601–5.

Burton, R.R. (1991). Panel on deliberate G-induced loss of consciousness: introduction. *Aviation Space & Environmental Medicine*, 62, pp. 609–11.

Burton, R.R. (1992). Protecting the pilot during high-G loading. *The Physiologist*, 35(1, Suppl.), pp. S155–7.

Burton, R.R. (2000a). Mathematical models for predicting G-level tolerances. *Aviation Space & Environmental Medicine*, 71, pp. 506–13.

Burton, R.R. (2000b). Mathematical models for predicting G-duration tolerances. *Aviation Space & Environmental Medicine*, 71, pp. 981–90.

Burton, R.R., Cohen, M.M. and Guedry, F.E. (1988). G-LOC panel: questions, answers and discussion. *Aviation Space & Environmental Medicine*, 59, pp. 36–9.

Burton, R.R. and Jaggars, J.L. (1974). Influence of ethyl alcohol ingestion on a target task during sustained +Gz centrifugation. *Aerospace Medicine*, 45, pp. 290–96.

Burton, R.R., Leverett, S.D. and Michaelson, E.D. (1974). Man at high sustained +Gz acceleration: a review. *Aerospace Medicine*, 45, pp. 1115–36.

Burton, R.R. and MacKenzie, W.F. (1975). Joint Committee on Aviation Pathology: II. Heart pathology associated with exposure to high sustained +Gz. *Aviation Space & Environmental Medicine*, 46, pp. 1251–3.

Burton, R.R., Parkhurst, M.J. and Leverett Jr, S.D. (1973). + Gz protection afforded by standard and preacceleration inflations of the bladder and capstan type G-suits. *Aerospace Medicine*, 44, pp. 488–94.

Burton, R.R. and Shaffstall, R.M. (1980). Human tolerance to aerial combat manoeuvres. *Aviation Space & Environmental Medicine*, 51, pp. 641–8.

Burton, R.R. and Smith, A.H. (1972). Stress and adaptation responses to repeated acute acceleration. *American Journal of Physiology*, 222, pp. 1505–10.

Burton, R.R. and Whinnery, J.E. (1985). Operational G-induced loss of consciousness: something old; something new. *Aviation Space & Environmental Medicine*, 56, pp. 812–17.

Burton, R.R. and Whinnery, J.E. (1996). Biodynamics: sustained acceleration. In: DeHart, R.L. (ed.), *Fundamentals of Aerospace Medicine*. Baltimore: Williams and Wilkins.

Burton, R.R., Whinnery, J.E. and Forster, E.M. (1987). Anaerobic energetics of the simulated aerial combat maneuver (SACM). *Aviation Space & Environmental Medicine*, 58, pp. 761–7.

Butler, G.C., Xing, H. and Hughson, R.L. (1990). Cardiovascular responses to 4 hours of 6° head-down tilt or 30° of head-up tilt bed rest. *Aviation Space & Environmental Medicine*, 61, pp. 240–46.

Caiozzo, V.J., Rose-Gottron, C., Baldwin, K.M., Cooper, D., Adams, G., Hicks, J. and Kreitenberg, A. (2004). Hemodynamic and metabolic responses to hypergravity on a human-powered centrifuge. *Aviation Space & Environmental Medicine*, 75, pp. 101–8.

Cammarota, J.P. (1991). Symptoms of +Gz induced incapacitation during simulated aerial combat. *Aviation Space & Environmental Medicine*, 62(5, Suppl.), p. A41.

Cammarota, J.P. (1994). A dynamic percolation model of the central nervous system under acceleration (+Gz) induced ischemic/hypoxic stress [PhD thesis]. Philadelphia, PA: Drexel University.

Cammarota, J.P. (1997a). The point of no return: G-LOC at low G induced by a +GZ pulse. [Abstract]. *Aviation Space & Environmental Medicine*, 68, p. 631.

Cammarota, J.P., Forster, E.M. and McGowan, D.G. (1997b). Alteration and loss of consciousness induced by a +Gz pulse [abstract]. *Aviation Space & Environmental Medicine*, 68, p. 631.

Campbell, M.R. and Garbino, A. (2011). History of suborbital spaceflight: medical and performance issues. *Aviation Space & Environmental Medicine*, 82, pp. 469–74.

Carminati, M.-V., Griffith, D. and Campbell, M.R. (2011). Sub-orbital commercial human spaceflight and informed consent. *Aviation Space & Environmental Medicine*, 82, pp. 144–6.

Carter, D., Pokroy, R., Azaria, B., Matetzky, S., Prokopetz, A., Barenboim E., Harpaz, D. and Goldstein, L. (2006). Effect of G-force on bicuspid aortic valve in aviators. *Cardiology*, 108, pp. 124–7.

Carter, D., Prokupetz, A., Harpaz, D. and Barenboim, E. (2010). Effects of repeated exposure to acceleration forces (+Gz) and anti-G manoeuvres on cardiac dimensions and performance. *Experimental & Clinical Cardiology*, 15, pp. e10–e12.

Chelette, T.L., Allnutt, R.D., Tripp, L.D. and Post, D.L. (1999). Do some colors disappear at high G? [abstract]. *Aviation Space & Environmental Medicine*, 70, p. 85.

Chen, H.-H., Wu, Y.-C. and Kuo, M.-D. (2004). An electromyographic assessment of the anti-G straining maneuver. *Aviation Space & Environmental Medicine*, 75, pp. 162–7.

Cheung, B. and Bateman, W.A. (2001).G-transition effects and their implications. *Aviation Space & Environmental Medicine*, 72, pp. 758–62.

Cheung, B. and Hofer, K. (1999). Degradation of visual pursuit during sustained +3 Gz acceleration. *Aviation Space & Environmental Medicine*, 70, pp. 451–8.

Cheung, B. and Hofer, K. (2003). Acceleration effects on pupil size with control of mental and environmental factors. *Aviation Space & Environmental Medicine*, 74, pp. 669–74.

Cheung, R. (2004). Nonvisual illusions in flight. In: Previc, F.H. and Ercoline, W.R. (eds), *Spatial Disorientation in Aviation – Progress in Astronautics and Aeronautics*. Reston: AIAA.

Chou, P.-I., Wen, T.-S., Wu, Y.-C., Horng, C.-T. and Liu, C.-C. (2003). Contrast sensitivity after +Gz acceleration. *Aviation Space & Environmental Medicine*, 74, pp. 1048–51.

Chung, K.Y. and Lee, S.J. (2001). Cardiac arrhythmias in F-16 pilots during aerial combat maneuvers (ACMS): a descriptive study focused on G-level acceleration. *Aviation Space & Environmental Medicine*, 72, pp. 534–8.

Churchill, S.E. and Bungo, M.W. (1997). Responses of the cardiovascular system to spaceflight. In: Churchill, S.E. (ed.), *Fundamentals of Space Life Sciences*, vol. 1. Malabar: Krieger.

Cirovic, S., Walsh, C. and Fraser, W.D. (2000). A mathematical model of cerebral perfusion subjected to Gz acceleration. *Aviation Space & Environmental Medicine*, 71, pp. 514–21.

Cirovic, S., Walsh, C., Fraser, W.D. and Gulino, A. (2003). The effect of posture and positive pressure breathing on the hemodynamics of the internal jugular vein. *Aviation Space & Environmental Medicine*, 74, pp. 125–31.

Claassen, J.A., Levine, B.D. and Zhang, R. (2009). Dynamic cerebral autoregulation during repeated squat-stand maneuvers. *Journal of Applied Physiology*, 106, pp. 153–60.

Clark, D.M. (1992). *The E.J Baldes I Knew*. Worcester: David Clark Company.

Clere, J.M., Ossard, G. and Melchior, F. (1993). Physiological considerations concerning positive pressure breathing (PBG) during +Gz. *Physiologist*, 36(1 Suppl), pp. S102–5.

Coakwell, M.R., Bloswick, D.S. and Moser, R. Jr. (2004). High-risk head and neck movements at high G and interventions to reduce associated neck injury. *Aviation Space & Environmental Medicine*, 75, pp. 68–80.

Coburn, K.R. (1970). Physiological endpoints in acceleration research. *Aerospace Medicine*, 41, pp. 5–11.

Cohen, M.M. (1970). Hand-eye coordination in altered gravitational fields. *Aerospace Medicine*, 41, pp. 647–9.

Cohen, M.M. (1983). Combining techniques to enhance protection against high sustained accelerative forces. *Aviation Space & Environmental Medicine*, 54, pp. 338–42.

Colombari, D.S.A., Colombari, E., Lopes, O.U. and Cravo, S.L. (2000). Afferent pathways in cardiovascular adjustments induced by volume expansion in anesthetized rats. *American Journal of Physiology*, 279, pp. R884–90.

Comens, P. (1998). Effect of 100% oxygen on EKG changes and serum myoglobin in fighter pilots. *Aviation Space & Environmental Medicine*, 69, pp. 149–53.

Comens, P., Reed, D. and Mette, M. (1987). Physiologic responses of pilots flying high-performance aircraft. *Aviation Space & Environmental Medicine*, 58, pp. 205–10.

Convertino, V.A. (1987). Aerobic fitness, endurance training and orthostatic intolerance. *Exercise and Sports Sciences Reviews*, 15, pp. 223–59.

Convertino, V.A. (1998). High sustained +Gz acceleration: physiological adaptation to high-G tolerance. *Journal of Gravitational Physiology*, 5, pp. P51–4.

Convertino, V.A. (1990). Physiological adaptations to weightlessness: effects on exercise and work performance. *Exercise and Sports Sciences Reviews*, 18, pp. 119–66.

Convertino, V.A., Doerr, D.F., Eckberg, D.L., Fritch, J.M. and Vernikos-Danellis, J. (1989). Carotid baroreflex response following 30 day to simulated microgravity. *Physiologist*, 32(Suppl.), pp. 67–8.

Convertino, V.A., Doerr, D.F., Eckberg, D.L., Fritch, J.M. and Vernikos-Danellis, J. (1990). Head-down bed rest impairs vagal baroreflex responses and provokes orthostatic hypotension. *Journal of Applied Physiology*, 68, pp. 1458–64.

Convertino, V.A., Engelke, K.A., Ludwig, D.A. and Doerr, D.F. (1996). Restoration of plasma volume after 16 days of head-down tilt induced by a single bout of maximal exercise. *American Journal of Physiology*, 270, pp. R3–10.

Convertino, V.A., Luetkemeier, M.J., Elliott, J.J., Ludwig, D.A. and Wade, C.E. (2000). Renal responsiveness to aldosterone during exposure to simulated microgravity. *Journal of Applied Physiology*, 89, pp. 1737–43.

Convertino, V.A., Ratliff, D.A., Doerr, D.F., Ludwig, D.A., Muniz, G.W., Benedetti, E., Chavarria, J., Koreen, S., Nguyen, C. and Wang, J. (2003). Effects of repeated Valsalva maneuver straining on cardiac and vasoconstrictive baroreflex responses. *Aviation Space & Environmental Medicine*, 74, pp. 212–19.

Convertino, V.A. and Reister, C.A. (2000). Effect of G-suit protection on carotid-cardiac baroreflex function. *Aviation Space & Environmental Medicine*, 71, pp. 31–6.

Convertino, V.A., Tripp, L.D., Ludwig, D.A., Duff, J. and Chelette, T.L. (1998). Female exposure to high G: chronic adaptations of cardiovascular functions. *Aviation Space & Environmental Medicine*, 69, pp. 875–82.

Cooke, W.H., Carter, J.R. and Kuusala, T.A. (2003). Muscle sympathetic nerve activation during the Valsalva maneuver: interpretive and analytical caveats. *Aviation Space & Environmental Medicine*, 74, pp. 731–7.

Cooke, W.H., Hoag, J.B., Crossman, A.A., Kuusela, T.A., Kari, U.O. and Eckberg, D.L. (1999). Human responses to upright tilt: a window on central autonomic integration. *Journal of Physiology*, 517, pp. 617–28.

Cooper, K.H. and Leverett, S.D. (1966). Physical conditioning versus +Gz tolerance. *Aerospace Medicine*, 37, pp. 462–5.

Cornwall, M.W., Krock, L.P. and Wagner, L.M. (1994). Muscular fatigue and recovery following alternating isometric contractions at different levels of force. *Aviation Space & Environmental Medicine*, 65, pp. 309–14.

Côté, P., Cassidy, J.D. and Carroll, L. (1998). The Saskatchewan Health and Back Pain Survey. The prevalence of neck pain and related disability in Saskatchewan adults. *Spine*, 23, pp. 1689–98.

Côté, P., Cassidy, J.D., Carroll, L.J. and Kristman, V. (2004). The annual incidence and course of neck pain in the general population: a population-based cohort study. *Pain*, 11, pp. 267–73.

Cotton, F.S. (1945). An aerodynamic suit for the protection of pilots against black-out. *The Australian Journal of Science*, 7, p. 161.

Crile, G.W. (1905). The resuscitation of the apparently dead and a demonstration of the pneumatic rubber suit as a means of controlling the blood pressure. *Transactions of the Southern Surgical & Gynecological Association*, 16, pp. 362–70.

Cui, L., Xu, X.-R., Chu, J.-G., Fu, Z.-J., Bi, Y.-M. and Wang, J.-C. (2012). A fighter pilot case of pulmonary sequestration. *Aviation Space & Environmental Medicine*, 83, pp. 1171–5.

Culbertson, J.W., Wilkins, R.W., Ingelfinger, F.J. and Bradley, S.E. (1951). The effect of the upright posture upon hepatic blood flow in normotensive and hypertensive subjects. *Journal of Clinical Investigation*, 30, pp. 305–11.

D'Andrea, A., Limongelli, G., Caso, P., Sarubbi, B., Della Pietra, A., Brancaccio, P., Cice, G., Scherillo, M., Limongelli, F., and Calabro, R. (2002). Association between left ventricular structure and cardiac performance during effort in two morphological forms of athlete's heart. *International Journal of Cardiology*, 86, pp. 177–84.

Dalecki, M., Bock, O. and Guardiera, S. (2010). Simulated flight path control of fighter pilots and novice subjects at +3 G$_z$ in a human centrifuge. *Aviation Space & Environmental Medicine*, 81, pp. 484–8.

Davis, C., Cammarota, J., Hamilton, R. and Whinnery, J. (1991). Case report: benign paroxysmal positional vertigo associated with centrifuge acceleration exposure [abstract]. *Aviation Space & Environmental Medicine*, 62, p. 474.

Deklunder, G., Lecroart, J.-L., Chammas, E., Goullard, L. and Houdas, Y. (1993). Intracardiac haemodynamics in man during short periods of head-down and head-up tilt. *Aviation Space & Environmental Medicine*, 64, pp. 43–9.

De Loose, V., Van den Oord, M., Burnotte, F., Van Tiggelen, D., Stevens, V., Cagnie, B., Danneels, L. and Witvrouw, E. (2009a). Functional assessment of the cervical spine in F-16 pilots with and without neck pain. *Aviation Space & Environmental Medicine*, 80, pp. 477–81.

De Loose, V., Van den Oord, M., Burnotte, F., Van Tiggelen, D., Stevens, V., Cagnie, B., Witvrouw, E. and Danneels, L. (2008). Individual, work-, and flight-related issues in F-16 pilots reporting neck pain. *Aviation Space & Environmental Medicine*, 79, pp. 779–83.

De Loose, V., Van den Oord, M., Keser, I., Burnotte, F., Van Tiggelen, D., Dumarey, A., Cagnie, B., Witvrouw, E. and Danneels, L. (2009b). MRI study of the morphometry of the cervical musculature in F-16 pilots. *Aviation Space & Environmental Medicine*, 80, pp. 727–31.

Derefeldt, G., Andersson, P.J. and Eriksson, L. (2000). Color identification and discrimination during moderately elevated +Gz-load [abstract]. *Aviation Space & Environmental Medicine*, 71, p. 269.

Dern, S., Vogt, T., Abeln, V., Strüder, H.K. and Schneider, S. (2014). Psychophysiological responses of artificial gravity exposure to humans. *European Journal of Applied Physiology*, pp. e1–11.

De Voogt, A.J. and van Doorn, R.R.A. (2009). Accidents associated with aerobatic maneuvers in U.S. aviation. *Aviation Space & Environmental Medicine*, 80, pp. 732–3.

Dikshit, M.B., Banerjee, P.K. and Rao, P.L.N. (1986). Orthostatic tolerance of normal Indians and those with suspected abnormal cardiovascular reflex status. *Aviation Space & Environmental Medicine*, 57, pp. 168–73.

Doba, N. and Reis, D.J. (1974). Role of the cerebellum and the vestibular apparatus in regulation of orthostatic reflexes in the cat. *Circulation Research*, 34, pp. 9–18.

Domaszuk, J. (1983). The application of positive pressure breathing for improving +Gz acceleration tolerance. *Aviation Space & Environmental Medicine*, 54, pp. 334–7.

Dooley, J.W., Hearon, C.M., Shaffstall, R.M. and Fischer, M.D. (2001). Accommodation of females in the high-G environment: the USAF Female Acceleration Tolerance Enhancement (FATE) Project. *Aviation Space & Environmental Medicine*, 72, pp. 739–46.

Dorf, R.C. (1989). *Modern Control Systems*. Reading: Addison-Wesley Publishing Company.

Dorman, P.J. and Lawton, R.W. (1956). Effect on G tolerance of partial supination combined with the anti-G suit. *Journal of Aviation Medicine*, 27, pp. 491–6.

Dowell, A.R., Shropshire, S. and McCally, M. (1968). Ventilation and pulmonary gas exchange during headward (+Gz) gradient acceleration. *Aerospace Medicine*, 39, pp. 926–34.

Dowell, R.T. (1983). Cardiac adaptations to exercise. *Exercise and Sports Sciences Reviews*, 11, pp. 99–117.

Downing, S.E. (1983). Baroreceptor regulation of the heart. In: *Handbook of Physiology. The Cardiovascular System*, Sect. 1, vol. III, Ch. 17. Bethesda: American Physiological Society.

Drew Sr, W.E. (2000). Spinal symptoms in aviators and their relationship to G-exposure and aircraft seating angle. *Aviation Space & Environmental Medicine*, 71, pp. 22–30.

Duling, B.R. (1967). Effects of chronic centrifugation at 3G's on cardiovascular reflexes of the rat. *American Journal of Physiology*, 213, pp. 466–72.

Dyson, F. (2013). Is a graviton detectable? *International Journal of Modern Physics*, 28(25), pp. 1–14.

Eckberg, D.L., Rea, R.F., Andersson, O.K., Hedner, T., Pernow, J., Lundberg, J.M. and Wallin, B.G. (1988). Baroreflex modulation of sympathetic activity and sympathetic neurotransmitters in humans. *Acta Physiologica Scandinavica*, 133, pp. 221–31.

Edelberg, R., Henry, J.P., Maciolek, J.A., Salzman, E.W. and Zuidema, G.D. (1956). Comparison of human tolerance to accelerations of slow and rapid onset. *Aviation Space & Environmental Medicine*, 27, pp. 482–9.

Eichler, W., Frank, I., Nehring, M., Welsch, H. and Klotz, K.-F.(2004). Hypergravity and dehydration-induced shifts of interstitial fluid in the skin monitored by ultrasound. *Aviation Space & Environmental Medicine*, 75, pp. 760–63.

Eiken, O., Bergsten, E. and Grönkvist, M. (2011). G-protection mechanisms afforded by the anti-G suit abdominal bladder with and without pressure breathing. *Aviation Space & Environmental Medicine*, 82, pp. 972–7.

Eiken, O. and Grönkvist, M. (2013). Signs and symptoms during supra-tolerance $+G_z$ exposures, with reference to G-garment failure. *Aviation Space & Environmental Medicine*, 84, pp. 196–205.

Eiken, O. and Kölegärd, R. (2001). Relationship between arm pain and distension of arteries and veins caused by elevation of transmural pressure in local vascular segments. *Aviation Space & Environmental Medicine*, 72, pp. 427–31.

Eiken, O., Kölegärd, R., Bergsten, E. and Grönkvist, M. (2007). G protection: interaction of straining maneuvers and positive pressure breathing. *Aviation Space & Environmental Medicine*, 78, pp. 392–8.

Eiken, O., Kölegärd, R., Lindborg, B., Aldman, M., Karlmar, K.E., Linder, J. and Kölegoård, R. (2002). A new hydrostatic anti-G suit vs. a pneumatic anti-G system: preliminary comparison. *Aviation Space & Environmental Medicine*, 73, pp. 703–8.

Eiken, O., Kölegärd, R., Lindborg, B., Mekjavic, I.B. and Linder, J. (2003). The effect of straining maneuvers on G-protection during assisted pressure breathing. *Aviation Space & Environmental Medicine*, 74, pp. 822–6.

Eiken, O., Mekjavic, I.B. and Kölegärd, R. (2012). Local intravascular pressure habituation in relation to G-induced arm pain. *Aviation Space & Environmental Medicine*, 83, pp. 667–72.

Eliasz, J., Mikuliszyn, R.S. and Dereń, M. (2004). Measurement of force exerted on footplates by centrifuge subjects. *Aviation Space & Environmental Medicine*, 75, pp. 551–3.

El-Sayed, H. and Hainsworth, R. (1995). Relationship between plasma volume, carotid baroreceptor sensitivity and orthostatic tolerance. *Clinical Science*, 88, pp. 463–70.

Epperson, W.L., Burton, R.R. and Bernauer, E.M. (1982).The influence of differential physical conditioning regimes on simulated aerial combat manoeuvring tolerance. *Aviation Space & Environmental Medicine*, 53, pp. 1091–7.

Epperson, W.L., Burton, R.R. and Bernauer, E.M. (1985). The effectiveness of specific weight training regimens on simulated aerial combat maneuvering G tolerance. *Aviation Space & Environmental Medicine*, 56, pp. 534–9.

Ericsson, L.E. (1995). Challenges in high-alpha vehicle dynamics. *Progress in Aerospace Sciences*, 31, pp. 291–334.

Ernsting, J. (1966). *Some Effects of Raised Intrapulmonary Pressure in Man.* London: McKay. AGARDograph 106.

Essandoh, L.K., Duprez, D.A. and Shepherd, J.T. (1988). Reflex constriction of human resistance vessels to head-down neck flexion. *Journal of Applied Physiology*, 64, pp. 767–70.

Evans, J.M., Mohney, L., Wang, S., Moore, R.K., Elayi, S.-C., Stenger, M.B., Moore, F.B. and Knapp, C.F. (2013). Cardiovascular regulation during body unweighting by lower body positive pressure. *Aviation Space & Environmental Medicine*, 84, pp. 1140–46.

Evans, J.M., Stenger, M.B., Moore, F.B., Hinghofer-Szalkay, H., Rössler, A., Patwardhan, A.R., Brown, D.R., Ziegler, M.G. and Knapp, C.F. (2004). Centrifuge training increases presyncopal orthostatic tolerance in ambulatory men. *Aviation Space & Environmental Medicine*, 75, pp. 850–58.

Fejer, R., Kyvik, K.O. and Hartvigsen, J. (2006). The prevalence of neck pain in the world population: a systematic critical review of the literature. *European Spine Journal*, 15, pp. 834–48.

Fernandes, L., Linder, J., Krock, L.P., Balldin, U.I. and Harms-Ringdahl, K. (2003).Muscle activity in pilots with and without pressure breathing during acceleration. *Aviation Space & Environmental Medicine*, 74, pp. 626–32.

Feynman, R.P. (1965). *The Character of Physical Law*. London: Penguin Books.

Feynman, R.P. (1985). *QED: The Strange Theory of Light and Matter*. London: Penguin Books.

Feynman, R.P. (1996). *Six Easy Pieces*. Reading: Addison-Wesley Publishing Company.

Fiorica, V. and Kem, D.C. (1985). Plasma norepinephrine, blood pressure and heart rate response to graded change in body position. *Aviation Space & Environmental Medicine*, 56, pp. 1166–71.

Florence, G., Riondet, L., Serra, A., Etienne, X., Huart, B., Van Beers, P., Bonneau, D., Gomez-Merino, D., Drogou, C. and Pradeau, P. (2005). Psychostimulants and G tolerance in rhesus monkeys: effects of oral modafinil and injected caffeine. *Aviation Space & Environmental Medicine*, 76, pp. 121–6.

Folkow, B., Heymans, C. and Neil, E. (1965). Integrated aspects of cardiovascular regulation. In: *Handbook of Physiology. Circulation*, Sect. 2, vol. III, Ch. 49. Bethesda: American Physiological Society.

Fong, K.L. and Fan, S.W. (1997). An overview of the physiological effects of sustained high +Gz forces on human being. *Annals of the Academy of Medicine Singapore*, 26, pp. 94–103.

Forster, E.M. and Cammarota, J.P. (1993). The effect of G-LOC on psychomotor performance and behaviour. *Aviation Space & Environmental Medicine*, 64, pp. 132–8.

Forster, E.M. and Whinnery, J.E. (1988). Recovery from +Gz-induced loss of consciousness: psychophysiologic considerations. *Aviation Space & Environmental Medicine*, 59, pp. 517–22.

Forster, E.M. and Whinnery, J.E. (1990). Dynamic cardiovascular response to +Gz stress in aerobically trained individuals. *Aviation Space & Environmental Medicine*, 61, pp. 303–6.

Fox, E.L., Bartels, R., Billings, C., Matthews, D., Bason, R. and Webb, W.M. (1973). Intensity and distance of interval training programs and changes in aerobic power. *Medicine and Science in Sports*, 5, pp. 18–22.

Fox, E.L., Bartels, R., Billings, C., O'Brien, R. and Bason, R. (1975). Frequency and duration of interval training programs and changes in aerobic power. *Journal of Applied Physiology*, 38, pp. 481–4.

Frankenhaeuser, M. (1958). Effects of prolonged gravitational stress on performance. *Acta Psychologica*, 14, pp. 92–108.

Frazier, J.W., Repperger, D.W., Toth, D.N. and Skowronski, V.D. (1982). Human tracking performance changes during combined +Gz and +Gy stress. *Aviation Space & Environmental Medicine*, 53, pp. 435–9.

Freedman, D.Z. and van Nieuwenhuizen, P. (1978). Supergravity and the unification of the laws of physics. *Scientific American*, Feb, pp. 126–43.

Frey, M.A.B., Mathes, K.L. and Hoffler, G.W. (1987). Aerobic fitness in women and responses to lower body negative pressure. *Aviation Space & Environmental Medicine*, 58, pp. 1149–52.

Fritsch, J.M., Rea, R.F. and Eckberg, D.L. (1989). Carotid baroreflex resetting during drug-induced arterial pressure changes in humans. *American Journal of Physiology (Regulatory Integrative Comparative Physiology)*, 256, pp. R549–53.

Fritsch, J.M., Smith, M.L., Simmons, D.T. and Eckberg, D.L. (1991). Differential baroreflex modulation of human vagal and sympathetic activity. *American Journal of Physiology*, 260, pp. R635–41.

Fritsch-Yelle, J.M., Charles, J.B., Jones, M.M., Beightol, L.A. and Eckberg, D.L. (1994). Spaceflight alters autonomic regulation of arterial pressure in humans. *Journal of Applied Physiology*, 77, pp. 1776–83.

Froom, P., Barzilay, J., Caine, Y., Margaliot, S., Forecast, D. and Gross, M. (1986). Low back pain in pilots. *Aviation Space & Environmental Medicine*, 57, pp. 694–5.

Fulco, C.S., Cymerman, A., Rock, P.B. and Farese, G. (1985). Hemodynamic responses to upright tilt at sea level and high altitude. *Aviation Space & Environmental Medicine*, 56, pp. 1172–6.

Gallo, E. and Marolf, D. (2009). Resource Letter BH-2: Black Holes. *American Journal of Physics*, 77, pp. 294–307.

Galvagno, S.M. Jr, Massa, T.V. and Price, S.C. (2004). Acceleration risk in student fighter pilots: preliminary analysis of a management program. *Aviation Space & Environmental Medicine*, 75, pp. 1077–80.

Gan, W.H., Lam, P.M., Chong, C.H., Tan, B.C.B., Fong, K.L. and Tan, H.Y.R. (2008). Pneumomediastinum diagnosed by chest radiography after centrifuge training. *Aviation Space & Environmental Medicine*, 79, pp. 424–8.

Ganse, B., Limper, U., Bühlmeier, J. and Rittweger, J. (2013). Petechiae: reproducible pattern of distribution and increased appearance after bed rest. *Aviation Space & Environmental Medicine*, 84, pp. 864–6.

Garvin, N.M., Levine, B.D., Raven, P.B. and Pawelczyk, J.A. (2014). Pneumatic antishock garment inflation activates the human sympathetic nervous system by abdominal compression. *Experimental Physiology*, 99, pp. 101–10.

Gauer, O.H. and Henry, J.P. (1964). Negative (–G) acceleration in relation to arterial oxygen saturation, subendocardial hemorrhage and venous pressure in the forehead. *Journal of Aviation Medicine*, 35, pp. 533–45.

Gauer, O.H. and Thron, H.L. (1965). Postural changes in the circulation. In: *Handbook of Physiology. Circulation*, Sect. 2, vol. III, Ch. 67. Bethesda: American Physiological Society.

Gelinas, J.C., Marsden, K.R., Tzeng, Y.C., Smirl, J.D., Smith, K.J., Willie, C.K., Lewis, N.C., Binsted, G., Bailey, D.M., Bakker, A., Day, T.A. and Ainslie, P.N. (2012). Influence of posture on the regulation of cerebral perfusion. *Aviation Space & Environmental Medicine*, 83, pp. 751–7.

Gerzer, R. (2009). Hypergravity and microgravity influence haemostasis. *Thrombosis & Haemostasis*, 101, p. 799.

Gillingham, K.K. (1987). G tolerance standards for aircrew training and selection. *Aviation Space & Environmental Medicine*, 58, pp. 1024–6.

Gillingham, K.K. (1988). High-G stress and orientational stress: physiologic effects of aerial maneuvering. *Aviation Space & Environmental Medicine*, 59(11,Suppl.), pp. A10–20.

Gillingham, K.K. and Crump, P.P. (1976). Changes in clinical cardiologic measurements associated with high +Gz stress. *Aviation Space & Environmental Medicine*, 47, pp. 726–33.

Gillingham, K.K. and Fosdick, J.P. (1988). High-G training for fighter aircrew. *Aviation Space & Environmental Medicine*, 59, pp. 12–19.

Gillingham, K.K., Freeman, J.J. and McNee, R.C. (1977). Transfer functions for eye-level blood pressure during +Gz stress. *Aviation Space & Environmental Medicine*, 48, pp. 1026–34.

Gillingham, K.K., Plentzas, S. and Lewis, N.L. (1985). G environments of F-4, F-5, F-15 and F-16 aircraft during F-15 tactics development and evaluation. Brooks AFB, TX: USAF, 1985; USAFSAM-TR-85–51.

Gillingham, K.K., Schade, C., Jackson, W. and Gilstrap, L. (1986). Women's G tolerance. *Aviation Space & Environmental Medicine*,57, pp. 745–53.

Gillingham, K.K. and Winter, W.R. (1976). Physiologic and anti-G suit performance data from YF-16 flight tests. *Aviation Space & Environmental Medicine*, 47, p. 672.

Girgenrath, M., Göbel, S., Bock, O. and Pongratz, H. (2005). Isometric force production in high Gz: mechanical effects, proprioception, and central motor commands. *Aviation Space & Environmental Medicine*, 76, pp. 339–43.

Gisolf, J., Akkerman, E.M., Schreurs, A.W., Strackee, J., Stok, W.J. and Karemaker, J.M. (2004). Tilt table design for rapid and sinusoidal posture change with minimal vestibular stimulation. *Aviation Space & Environmental Medicine*, 75, pp. 1086–91.

Glaister, D.H. (1970). Distribution of pulmonary blood flow and ventilation during forward (+Gx) acceleration. *Journal of Applied Physiology*, 29, pp. 432–9.

Göbel, S., Bock, O., Pongratz, H. and Krause, W. (2006). Practice ameliorates deficits of isometric force production in +3 Gz. *Aviation Space & Environmental Medicine*, 77, pp. 586–91.

Goodman, L.S., Banks, R.D., Grissett, J.D. and Saunders, P.L. (2000). Heart rate and blood pressure responses to +G$_z$ following varied-duration –Gz. *Aviation Space & Environmental Medicine*, 71, pp. 137–41.

Goodman, L.S., de Yang, L., Kelso, B. and Liu, P. (1995). Cardiovascular effects of varying G-suit pressure and coverage during +1 Gz positive pressure breathing. *Aviation Space & Environmental Medicine*, 66, pp. 829–36.

Goodman, L.S., Fraser, W.D., Ackles, K.N., Mohn, D. and Pecaric, M. (1993). Effect of extending G-suit coverage on cardiovascular responses to positive pressure breathing. *Aviation Space & Environmental Medicine*, 64, pp. 1101–7.

Goodman, L.S., Grosman-Rimon, L. and Mikuliszyn, R. (2006). Carotid sinus pressure changes during push-pull maneuvers. *Aviation Space & Environmental Medicine*, 77, pp. 921–8.

Goodman, L.S. and LeSage, S. (2002). Impairment of cardiovascular and vasomotor responses during tilt table simulation of 'push-pull' maneuvers. *Aviation Space & Environmental Medicine*, 73, pp. 971–9.

Goodstein, D.L. and Goodstein, J.R. (1997). *Feynman's Lost Lecture*. London: Vintage.

Graybiel, A. and McFarland, R.A. (1941). The use of the tilt-table test in aviation medicine. *Journal of Aviation Medicine*, 12, pp. 194–211.

Green, J. and Miller, M. (1973). A model describing the response of the circulatory system to acceleration stress. *Annals of Biomedical Engineering*, 1, pp. 455–67.

Green, N.D. (1997). Arm arterial occlusion cuffs as a means of alleviating high +Gz-associated arm pain. *Aviation Space & Environmental Medicine*, 68, pp. 715–21.

Green, N.D., Brown, M.D. and Coote, J.H. (2007a). Failure of vascular autoregulation in the upper limb with increased +Gz acceleration. *European Journal of Applied Physiology*, 100, pp. 621–6.

Green, N.D., Brown, M.D. and Coote, J.H. (2007b). Pain and changes in peripheral resistance at high vascular transmural pressure in the human forearm. *European Journal of Applied Physiology*, 100, pp. 627–35.

Green, N.D. and Ford, S.A. (2006). G-induced loss of consciousness: retrospective survey results from 2259 military aircrew. *Aviation Space & Environmental Medicine*, 77, pp. 619–23.

Green, N.D.C. (2003). Acute soft tissue neck injury from unexpected acceleration. *Aviation Space & Environmental Medicine*, 74, pp. 1085–90.

Green, N.D.C. (2006a). Effects of long-duration acceleration. In: Rainford, D.J. and Gradwell, D.P. (eds), *Ernsting's Aviation Medicine*. 4th edn. London: Hodder Arnold.

Green, N.D.C. (2006b). Protection against long-duration acceleration. In: Rainford, D.J. and Gradwell, D.P. (eds), *Ernsting's Aviation Medicine*. 4th edn. London: Hodder Arnold.

Green, N.D.C. and Brown, L. (2004). Head positioning and neck muscle activation during air combat. *Aviation Space & Environmental Medicine*, 75, pp. 676–80.

Grönkvist, M., Bergsten, E. and Eiken, O. (2008). Lung mechanics and transpulmonary pressures during unassisted pressure breathing at high G_z loads. *Aviation Space & Environmental Medicine*, 79, pp. 1041–6.

Grönkvist, M. and Bergsten, E. (2003). Is the counterpressure jerkin needed during positive pressure breathing at high+ Gz-loads [abstract]. *Aviation Space & Environmental Medicine*, 74, pp. 469–70.

Grönkvist, M., Bergsten, E., Kölegård, R., Linder, J. and Eiken, O. (2005). G tolerance and pulmonary effects of removing chest counterpressure during pressure breathing. *Aviation Space & Environmental Medicine*, 76, pp. 833–40.

Grossman, A., Wand, O., Harpaz, D., Prokupetz, A. and Assa, A. (2011). Acceleration forces and cardiac and aortic indexes in jet fighter pilots. *Aviation Space & Environmental Medicine*, 82, pp. 901–3.

Guardiera, S., Bock, O., Pongratz, H. and Krause, W. (2007a). Acceleration effects on manual performance with isometric and displacement joysticks. *Aviation Space & Environmental Medicine*, 78, pp. 990–94.

Guardiera, S., Bock, O., Pongratz, H. and Krause, W. (2007b). Isometric force production in experienced fighter pilots during +3G_z centrifuge acceleration. *Aviation Space & Environmental Medicine*, 78, pp. 1072–4.

Guardiera, S., Dalecki, M. and Bock, O. (2010). Stability of simulated flight path control at +3 G_z in a human centrifuge. *Aviation Space & Environmental Medicine*, 81, pp. 394–8.

Guardiera, S., Schneider, S., Noppe, A. and Strüder, H.K. (2008). Motor performance and motor learning in sustained +3 G_z acceleration. *Aviation Space & Environmental Medicine*, 79, pp. 852–9.

Guez, M., Hildingsson, C., Nilsson, M. and Toolanen, G. (2002). The prevalence of neck pain. *Acta Orthopaedica*, 73, pp. 455–9.

Guggisberg, C.A.W. (1969). *Giraffes*. London: Arthur Barker Ltd.

Guo, H.Z., Zhang, S.X. and Jing, B.S. (1991). The characteristics and theoretical basis of the Qigong maneuver. *Aviation Space & Environmental Medicine*, 62, pp. 1059–62.

Guo, H.Z., Zhang, S.X., Jing, B.S. and Zhang, L.M. (1988). A preliminary report on a new anti-G maneuver. *Aviation Space & Environmental Medicine*, 59, pp. 968–72.

Gustafsson, T., Kölegärd, R., Sundblad, P., Norman, B. and Eiken, O. (2013). Elevations of local intravascular pressures release vasoactive substances in humans. *Clinical Physiology & Functional Imaging*, 33, pp. 38–44.

Guyton, A.C. and Hall, J.E. (1996). *Textbook of Medical Physiology*. 9th edn. Philadelphia: W.B. Saunders.

Hachiya, T., Hashimoto, I., Saito, M. and Blaber, A.P. (2012). Peripheral vascular responses of men and women to LBNP. *Aviation Space & Environmental Medicine*, 83, pp. 118–24.

Hainsworth, R. (1991). Reflexes from the heart. *Physiological Reviews*, 71, pp. 617–58.

Hainsworth, R. and Al-Shamma, Y.M.H. (1988). Cardiovascular responses to stimulation of carotid baroreceptors in healthy subjects. *Clinical Science*, 75, pp. 159–65.

Hamalainen, O. (1993). Flight helmet weight, +Gz forces, and neck muscle strain. *Aviation Space & Environmental Medicine*, 64, pp. 55–7.

Hamalainen, O. (1999). Thoracolumbar pain among fighter pilots. *Military Medicine*, 164, pp. 595–6.

Hamalainen, O. and Vanharanta, H. (1992). Effect of +Gz forces and head movements on cervical erector spinae muscle strain. *Aviation Space & Environmental Medicine*, 63, pp. 709–16.

Hamalainen, O., Vanharanta, H. and Bloigu, R. (1993a). Determinants of +Gz-related neck pain: a preliminary survey. *Aviation Space & Environmental Medicine*, 64, pp. 651–2.

Hamalainen, O., Vanharanta, H. and Bloigu, R. (1994a). +Gz-related neck pain: a follow-up study. *Aviation Space & Environmental Medicine*, 65, pp. 16–18.

Hamalainen, O., Vanharanta, H., Hupli, M., Karhu, M., Kuronen, P. and Kinnunen, H. (1996). Spinal shrinkage due to+ Gz forces. *Aviation Space & Environmental Medicine*, 67, pp. 659–61.

Hamalainen, O., Vanharanta, H. and Kuusela, T. (1993b). Degeneration of cervical intervertebral disks in fighter pilots frequently exposed to high +Gz forces. *Aviation Space & Environmental Medicine*, 64, pp. 692–6.

Hamalainen, O., Visuri, T., Kuronen, P. and Vanharanta, H. (1994b). Cervical disk bulges in fighter pilots. *Aviation Space & Environmental Medicine*, 65, pp. 144–6.

Hamalainen, O., Toivakka-Hamalainen, S.K. and Kuronen, P. (1999). + Gz associated stenosis of the cervical spinal canal in fighter pilots. *Aviation Space & Environmental Medicine*, 70, pp. 330–34.

Hamilton, W.F., Woodbury, R.A. and Harper, H.T. (1944). Arterial, cerebrospinal and venous pressures in man during cough and strain. *American Journal of Physiology*, 141, pp. 42–50.

Hanada, R., Hisada, T., Tsujimoto, T. and Ohashi, K. (2004). Arrhythmias observed during high-G training: proposed training safety criterion. *Aviation Space & Environmental Medicine*, 75, pp. 688–91.

Hanson, P., Slane, P.R., Rueckert, P.A. and Clark, S.V. (1995). Squatting revisited: comparison of haemodynamic responses in normal individuals and heart transplant recipients. *British Heart Journal*, 74, pp. 154–8.

Harding, R.M. and Bomar, J.B. Jr. (1990). Positive pressure breathing for acceleration protection and its role in prevention of inflight G-induced loss of consciousness. *Aviation Space & Environmental Medicine*, 61, pp. 845–9.

Harrison, M.H., Rittenhouse, D. and Greenleaf, J.E. (1986). Effect of posture on arterial baroreflex control of heart rate in humans. *European Journal of Applied Physiology*, 55, pp. 367–73.

Harsch, V. (2000). German acceleration research from the very beginning. *Aviation Space & Environmental Medicine*, 71, pp. 854–6.

Harsch, V. (2006). Centrifuge 'therapy' for psychiatric patients in Germany in the early 1800s. *Aviation Space & Environmental Medicine*, 77, pp. 157–60.

Haruna, Y., Bonde-Petersen, F., Takenaka, K., Suzuki, Y., Kawakubo, K. and Gunji, A. (1997). Effects of the rennin-angiotensin-aldosterone system on the cardiovascular system during 20-days bed rest. *Journal of Gravitational Physiology*, 4, pp. S62–68.

Hasser, E.M., Cunningham, J.T., Sullivan, M.J., Curtis, K.S., Blaine, E.H. and Hay, M. (2000). Area postrema and sympathetic nervous system effects of vasopressin and angiotensin II. *Clinical and Experimental Pharmacology and Physiology*, 27, pp. 432–6.

Haswell, M.S., Tacker Jr, W.A., Balldin, U.I. and Burton, R.R. (1986). Influence of inspired oxygen concentration on acceleration atelectasis. *Aviation Space & Environmental Medicine*, 57, pp. 432–7.

Hatton, P.D. and Harford, F.J. (1985). Calcified hematoma of the greater omentum in an F-15 fighter pilot. *Aviation Space & Environmental Medicine*, 56, pp. 1009–10.

Helleur, C.D., Gracovetsky, S.A. and Farfan, H.F. (1984). Tolerance of the human cervical spine to high acceleration: a modeling approach. *Aviation Space & Environmental Medicine*, 55, pp. 903–9.

Hendriksen, I.J. and Holewijn, M. (1999). Degenerative changes of the spine of fighter pilots of the Royal Netherlands Air Force (RNLAF). *Aviation Space & Environmental Medicine*, 70, pp. 1057–63.

Henry, J.P., Gauer, O.H., Kety, S.S. and Kramer, K. (1950). Factors maintaining cerebral circulation during gravitational stress. *Journal of Clinical Investigation*, 30, pp. 292–300.

Hermes, E.D.A., Webb, T.S. and Wells, T.S. (2010). Aircraft type and other risk factors for spinal disorders: data from 19,673 military cockpit aircrew. *Aviation Space & Environmental Medicine*, 81, pp. 850–56.

Hickman, J.R. (1991). Panel summary: from Zen riddle to the razor's edge. *Aviation Space & Environmental Medicine*, 62, pp. 632–7.

Hoek van Dijke, G.A., Snijders, E.R., Roosch, E.R., Burgers, P.I.C.J. (1993). Analysis of biomechanical and ergonomic aspects of the cervical spine in F-16 flight situations. *Journal of Biomechanics*, 26, pp. 1017–25.

Holland, D.A. and Freeman, J.E. (1995). A ten-year overview of USAF F-16 mishap attributes from 1980–89. *Proceedings of the Human Factors and Ergonomics Society 39th Annual Meeting*, HFES: San Diego.

Holmgren, A., Mossfeldt, F., Jostrand, T.S. and Strom, G. (1960). Effect of training on work capacity, total haemoglobin, blood volume, heart volume and pulse rate in recumbent and upright positions. *Acta Physiologica Scandinavica*, 50, pp. 72–83.

Houghton, J.D., McBride, D.K. and Hannah, K. (1985). Performance and physiological effects of acceleration-induced (+Gz) loss of consciousness. *Aviation Space & Environmental Medicine*, 56, pp. 956–65.

Howard, P. (1965). The physiology of positive acceleration. In: Gillies, J.A. (ed.), *A Textbook of Aviation Physiology*. New York: Pergamon Press.

Howard, P. and Garrow, J.S. (1958). Changes in the vascular resistance of the forearm and hand during radial acceleration. *Journal of Physiology*, 143, pp. P83–P84.

Hrebien, L. (1988). Current and emerging technology in G-LOC detection: pulse wave delay for +Gz tolerance assessment. *Aviation Space & Environmental Medicine*, 59, pp. 29–31.

Hrebien, L. and Hendler, E. (1985). Factors affecting human tolerance to sustained acceleration. *Aviation Space & Environmental Medicine*, 56, pp. 19–26.

Hyatt, K.H., Jacobson, L.B. and Schneider, V.S. (1975). Comparison of 70° tilt, LBNP, and passive standing as measures of orthostatic tolerance. *Aviation Space & Environmental Medicine*, 46, pp. 801–8.

Ille, H., Didier, A. and Allegrini, N. (1985). Selection et surveillance medicales des pilotes de Mirage 2000 apport de l'echocardiographie, *AGARD Conference Proceedings Medical Selection and Physiologic Training of Future Fighter Aircrew.* CP-396,1985. 32–1–32–13.

Jacobs, I., Bell, D.G., Pope, J. and Lee, W. (1987). Effects of hydraulic resistance circuit training on physical fitness components of potential relevance to +Gz tolerance. *Aviation Space & Environmental Medicine*, 58, pp. 754–60.

Jaeger, E.A., Severs, R.J., Weeks, S.D. and Duane, T.D. (1964). Visual field changes during positive acceleration. *Aviation Space & Environmental Medicine*, 35, pp. 969–72.

Jáuregui-Renaud, K., Reynolds, R., Bronstein, A.M. and Gresty, M.A. (2006). Cardio-respiratory responses evoked by transient linear acceleration. *Aviation Space & Environmental Medicine*, 77, pp. 114–20.

Jellema, W.T., Imholz, B.P.M., Van Goudoever, J., Wesseling, K.H. and Van Lieshout, J.J. (1996). Finger arterial versus intrabrachial pressure and continuous cardiac output during head-up tilt testing in healthy subjects. *Clinical Science*, 91, pp. 193–200.

Jennings, R.T., Stepanek, J.P., Scott, L.R. and Voronkov, Y.I. (2010). Frequent premature ventricular contractions in an orbital spaceflight participant. *Aviation Space & Environmental Medicine*, 81, pp. 597–601.

Jennings, T., Tripp, L.D. Jr, Howell, L., Seaworth, J., Ratino, D. and Goodyear, C. (1990). The effect of various straining maneuvers on cardiac volumes at 1G and during +Gz acceleration. *SAFE Journal*, 20, pp. 22–8.

Jia, H., Cui, G., Xie, S., Tian, D., Bi, H. and Guo, S. (2009). Vestibular function in military pilots before and after 10 s at +9 G_z on a centrifuge. *Aviation Space & Environmental Medicine*, 80, pp. 20–23.

Jian, B.J., Cotter, L.A., Emanuel, B.A., Cass, S.P. and Yates, B.J. (1999). Effects of bilateral vestibular lesions on orthostatic tolerance in awake cats. *Journal of Applied Physiology*, 86, pp. 1552–60.

Jing, X., Wu, P., Liu, F., Wu, B. and Miao, D. (2011). Guided imagery, anxiety, heart rate, and heart rate variability during centrifuge training. *Aviation Space & Environmental Medicine*, 82, pp. 92–6.

Johanson, D.C. and Pheeny, H.T. (1988). A new look at the loss of consciousness experience within the US Naval Forces. *Aviation Space & Environmental Medicine*, 59, pp. 6–8.

Jones, D.R. (1991). A review of central nervous system effects of G-induced loss of consciousness on volunteer subjects. *Aviation Space & Environmental Medicine*, 62, pp. 624–7.

Jones, J.A. (2000). Human and behavioral factors contributing to spine-based neurological cockpit injuries in pilots of high-performance aircraft: recommendations for management and prevention. *Military Medicine*, 165, pp. 6–12.

Jouanin, J.-C., Dussault, C., Tran, D. and Guézennec, C-Y. (2005). Aerobatic flight effects on baroreflex sensitivity and sympathovagal balance in experienced pilots. *Aviation Space & Environmental Medicine*, 76, pp. 1151–5.

Kalmus, H. (1966). *Regulation and Control in Living Systems*. London: John Wiley and Sons.

Kane, J.W. and Sternheim, M.M. (1984). *Physics*. 2nd edn. New York: John Wiley and Sons.

Kang, S., Hwang, S., Lee, E.T., Yang, S. and Park, J. (2011). Measuring the cumulative effect of G force on aviator neck pain. *Aviation Space & Environmental Medicine*, 82, pp. 1042–8.

Kasting, G.A., Eckberg, D.L., Fritsch, J.M. and Birkett, C.L. (1987). Continuous resetting of the human carotid baroreceptor-cardiac reflex. *American Journal of Physiology*, 252, pp. R732–6.

Kaufmann, H. (1996). Consensus statement on the definition of orthostatic hypotension, pure autonomic failure and multiple system atrophy. *Clinical Autonomic Research*, 6, pp. 125–6.

Kikukawa, A., Tachibana, S. and Yagura, S. (1994). G-related musculoskeletal spine symptoms in Japan Air Self Defence Force F-15 pilots. *Aviation Space and Environmental Medicine*, 65, pp. 269–72.

Kircheim, H.R. (1976). Systemic arterial baroreceptor reflexes. *Physiological Reviews*, 56, pp. 100–176.

Kirkham, W.R., Wicks, S.M. and Lowrey, D.L. (1982). *G Incapacitation in Aerobatic Pilots: A Flight Hazard* (No. FAA-AM-82-13). Federal Aviation Administration Washington, DC Office of Aviation Medicine.

Klein, K.E., Bruner, H., Jovy, D., Vogt, L. and Wegmann, H.M. (1969). Influence of stature and physical fitness on tilt-table and acceleration tolerance. *Aerospace Medicine*, 40, pp. 293–7.

Knapp, C.J. and Johnson, R. (1996). F-16 Class A mishaps in the U.S. Air Force, 1975–93. *Aviation Space & Environmental Medicine*, 67, pp. 777–83.

Knight, J.F. and Baber, C. (2004). Neck muscle activity and perceived pain and discomfort due to variations of head load and posture. *Aviation Space & Environmental Medicine*, 75, pp. 123–31.

Knudson, R., McMillan, D., Doucette, D. and Seidel, M. (1988). A comparative study of G-induced neck injury in pilots of the F/A-18, A-7 and A-4. *Aviation Space & Environmental Medicine*, 59, pp. 758–60.

Kobayashi, A., Kikukawa, A., Kimura, M., Inui, T. and Miyamoto, Y. (2012). Cerebral near-infrared spectroscopy to evaluate anti-G straining maneuvers in centrifuge training. *Aviation Space & Environmental Medicine*, 83, pp. 790–94.

Kobayashi, A., Tong, A. and Kikukawa, A. (2002). Pilot cerebral oxygen status during air-to-air combat maneuvering. *Aviation Space & Environmental Medicine*, 73, pp. 919–24.

Kotovskaya, A.R., Vil-Viliams, I.F. and Lukjanuk, V.Y. (2003). Human physiological responses to the G-load accompanying the orbiting and descent of Soyuz spacecraft. *Human Physiology*, 29, pp. 677–84.

Kovitaya, M., Tripp, L.D. and Chelette, T.L. (1997). Middle cerebral artery blood flow velocity after exposure to sustained +Gz. Dayton, OH: Armstrong Laboratory, 1997. AL/CF.-TR-1997–0159.

Krieger, E.M. (1970). Time course of baroreceptor resetting in acute hypertension. *American Journal of Physiology*, 218, p. 486.

Krock, L.P., Balldin, U.I., Harms-Ringdahl, K., Singstad, C.P., Linder, J. and Siegborn, J. (1997). Influence of a reduced G-suit pressure schedule on G-duration tolerance using enhanced G-protection ensembles. *Aviation Space & Environmental Medicine*, 68, pp. 403–9.

Krock, L.P., Russell, R.L., Siegborn, J. and Balldin, U.I. (1994). Reduced pressure in extended coverage anti-G-trousers with assisted pressure breathing. *Aviation Space & Environmental Medicine*, 65, pp. 287–92.

Krol, J.R. and Holewijn, M. (1995). The incidence of arrhythmias in F-16 pilots during combat flight. *Aviation Space & Environmental Medicine*, 66, p. 459.

Krutz, R.W., Rositano, S.A. and Mancini, R.E. (1975). Comparison of techniques for measuring +Gz tolerance in man. *Journal of Applied Physiology*, 38, pp. 1143–45.

Krutz, R.W. Jr., Sawin, C.F., Stegmann, B.J. and Burton, R.R. (1994). Preinflation before acceleration on tolerance to simulated Space Shuttle reentry G profiles in dehydrated subjects. *Journal of Clinical Pharmacology*, 34, pp. 480–83.

Kydd, G.H. (1972). Physiologic responses to short duration Gz. *Aviation Space & Environmental Medicine*, 43, pp. 1014–19.

Lalande, S. and Buick, F. (2009). Physiologic +G_z tolerance responses over successive +G_z exposures in simulated air combat maneuvers. *Aviation Space & Environmental Medicine*, 80, pp. 1032–8.

Lamb, L.E., Green, H.C., Combs, J.J., Cheeseman, S.A. and Hammond, J. (1960). Incidence of loss of consciousness in 1,980 Air Force personnel. *Aviation Space & Environmental Medicine*, 31, pp. 973–88.

Lambert, E.H. and Wood, E.H. (1946). The problem of blackout and unconsciousness in aviators. *Medical Clinics of North America*, 30, pp. 833–44.

Landau, D.-A., Chapnick, L., Yoffe, N., Azaria, B., Goldstein, L. and Atar, E. (2006). Cervical and lumbar MRI findings in aviators as a function of aircraft type. *Aviation Space & Environmental Medicine*, 77, pp. 1158–61.

Lange, B., Murray, M., Chreiteh, S.S., Toft, P., Jorgensen, M.B., Sogaard, K. and Sjogaard, G. (2014). Postural control and shoulder steadiness in F-16 pilots: a randomized controlled study. *Aviation Space & Environmental Medicine*, 85, pp. 420–25.

Lange, B., Nielsen, R.T., Skejo, P.B. and Toft, P. (2013a). Centrifuge-induced neck and back pain in F-16 pilots: a report of four cases. *Aviation Space & Environmental Medicine*, 84, pp. 734–8.

Lange, B., Toft, P., Myburgh, C. and Sjogaard, G. (2013b). Effect of targeted strength, endurance, and coordination exercise on neck and shoulder pain among fighter pilots: a randomized-controlled trial. *The Clinical Journal of Pain*, 29, pp. 50–59.

Lange, B., Torp-Svendsen, J. and Toft, P. (2011). Neck pain among fighter pilots after the introduction of the JHMCS helmet and NVG in their environment. *Aviation Space & Environmental Medicine*, 82, pp. 559–63.

Lau, D. and Steinleitner, J.M. (1994). Dynamic characteristics of centrifuges. *Aviation Space & Environmental Medicine*, 65, pp. 1134–9.

Laughlin, M.H. (1982). An analysis of the risk of human cardiac damage during +Gz stress: a review. *Aviation Space & Environmental Medicine*, 53, pp. 423–31.

Lauritzen, L.P. and Pfitzner, J. (2003). Pressure breathing in fighter aircraft for G accelerations and loss of cabin pressurization at altitude – a brief review. *Canadian Journal of Anesthesia*, 50, pp. 415–19.

Lecompte, J., Maisetti, O., Guillaume, A., Skalli, W. and Portero, P. (2008). Neck strength and EMG activity in fighter pilots with episodic neck pain. *Aviation Space & Environmental Medicine*, 79, pp. 947–52.

Lee, S.M.C., Guined, J.R., Brown, A.K., Stenger, M.B. and Platts, S.H. (2011). Metabolic consequences of garments worn to protect against post-spaceflight orthostatic intolerance. *Aviation Space & Environmental Medicine*, 82, pp. 648–53.

Levin, B., Andersson, J. and Karlsson, T. (2007). Memory performance during G exposure as assessed by a word recognition task. *Aviation Space & Environmental Medicine*, 78, pp. 587–92.

Lightfoot, J.T., Febles, S. and Fortney, S.M. (1989). Adaptation to repeated presyncopal lower body negative pressure exposures. *Aviation Space & Environmental Medicine*, 60, pp. 17–22.

Lim, D.J., Stith, J.A., Stockwell, C.W. and Oyama, J. (1974). Observations on saccules of rats exposed to long-term hypergravity. *Aerospace Medicine*, 45, pp. 705–10.

Linde, L. and Balldin, U. (1998). Arm pain among Swedish fighter pilots during +Gz flight and centrifuge exposures. *Aviation Space & Environmental Medicine*, 69, pp. 639–42.

Lipnicki, D.M., Gunga, H.C., Belavý, D.L. and Felsenberg, D. (2009). Bed rest and cognition: effects on executive functioning and reaction time. *Aviation Space & Environmental Medicine*, 80, pp. 1018–24.

Lipsitz, L.A., Mukai, S., Hamner, J., Gagnon, M. and Babikian, V. (2000). Dynamic regulation of middle cerebral artery blood flow velocity in aging and hypertension. *Stroke*, 31, pp. 1897–903.

Liu, Y., Zhang, L.-F., Lu, H.-B., Zhang, G.-P. and Pu, H.-S. (2009). Mathematical modeling of the push-pull effect for various acceleration profiles and countermeasures. *Aviation Space & Environmental Medicine*, 80, pp. 781–9.

Liu, Y., Zhang, L.-F., Zhang, K.-L. and Lu, H.-B. (2012). Role of carotid baroreflex and sympathetic responses in the push-pull effect: a simulation study. *Aviation Space & Environmental Medicine*, 83, pp. 841–9.

Livingston, P.C. (1939). The problem of 'black out' in aviation (amaurosis fugax). *British Journal of Surgery*, 26, pp. 749–56.

Logan, J.S., Veghte, J.H., Frey, M.A.B., Robillard, L.M.J., Mann, B.L. and Luciani, R.J. (1983). Cardiac function monitored by impedance cardiography during changing seatback angles and anti-G suit inflation. *Aviation Space & Environmental Medicine*, 54, pp. 328–33.

Lombard, C.F., Roth, H.P. and Drury, D.R. (1948). The influence of radial acceleration (centrifugal force) on respiration in human beings. *Journal of Aviation Medicine*, 19, pp. 355–64.

Low, R., Teoh, T., Loh, A. and Ooi, A. (2008). Vertebral fracture in a pilot during centrifuge training: finding of osteopenia. *Aviation Space & Environmental Medicine*,79, pp. 1067–70.

Lu, H., Liu, X., Zhang, L.F. and Bai, J. (2005). Combining protection of different anti-G techniques to +12 Gz: a computer simulation study. *Conference Proceedings IEEE Engineering in Medicine and Biology Society*, 5, pp. 4505–8.

Lu, H.-B., Zhang, L.-F., Bai, J., Liu, X. and Zhang, G. (2007). Mathematical modeling of high G protection afforded by various anti-G equipment and techniques. *Aviation Space & Environmental Medicine*, 78, pp. 100–109.

Lu, W.-H., Hsieh, K.-S., Li, M.-H., Ho, C.-W., Wu, Y.-C., Ger, L.-P., Wang, J.-S. and Chu, H. (2008). Heart status following high G exposure in rats and the effect of brief preconditioning. *Aviation Space & Environmental Medicine*, 79, pp. 1086–90.

Ludwig, D.A. and Convertino, V.A. (1994). Predicting orthostatic intolerance: physics or physiology? *Aviation Space & Environmental Medicine*, 65, pp. 404–11.

Ludwig, D.A. and Krock, L.P. (1991). Errors in measurement of +Gz acceleration tolerance. *Aviation Space & Environmental Medicine*, 62, pp. 261–5.

Lyons, T.J., Davenport, C., Copley, G.B., Binder, H., Grayson, K. and Kraft, N.O. (2004). Preventing G-induced loss of consciousness: 20 years of operational experience. *Aviation Space & Environmental Medicine*, 75, pp. 150–53.

Lyons, T.J., Harding, R., Freeman, J. and Oakley, C. (1992). G-induced loss of consciousness accidents: USAF experience 1982–1990. *Aviation Space & Environmental Medicine*, 63, pp. 60–66.

Lyons, T.J., Kraft, N.O., Copley, G.B., Davenport, C., Grayson, K. and Binder, H. (2004). Analysis of mission and aircraft factors in G-induced loss of consciousness in the USAF: 1982–2002. *Aviation Space & Environmental Medicine*, 75, pp. 479–82.

Lyons, T.J., Marlowe, B.L., Michaud, V.J. and McGowan, D.J. (1997). Assessment of the anti-G straining maneuver (AGSM) skill performance and reinforcement program. *Aviation Space & Environmental Medicine*, 68, pp. 322–4.

Mack, G.W., Quigley, B.M., Nishiyasu, T., Shi, X. and Nadel, E.R. (1991). Cardiopulmonary baroreflex control of forearm vascular resistance after acute blood volume expansion. *Aviation Space & Environmental Medicine*, 62, pp. 938–43.

Mack, G.W., Shi, X., Nose, H., Tripathi, A. and Nadel, E.R. (1987). Diminished baroreflex control of forearm vascular resistance in physically fit humans. *Journal of Applied Physiology*, 63, pp. 105–10.

Makela, M., Heliovaara, M., Sievers, K., Impivaara, O., Knekt, P. and Aromaa, A. (1991). Prevalence, determinants, and consequences of chronic neck pain in Finland. *American Journal of Epidemiology*, 134, pp. 1356–67.

Mancia, G. and Mark, A.L. (1983). Arterial baroreflexes in humans. In: *Handbook of Physiology. The Cardiovascular System*, Sect. 2, vol. III, Ch. 20. Bethesda: American Physiological Society.

Manen, O., Perrier, E. and Généro, M. (2011). Ground vasovagal presyncopes and fighter pilot fitness: aeromedical concerns. *Aviation Space & Environmental Medicine*, 82, pp. 917–20.

Maningas, P.A., DiJulio, M.A. and Dronen, S.C. (1983). Diaphragmatic rupture during G-maneuvers in a T33 jet trainer. *Aviation Space & Environmental Medicine*, 54, pp. 1037–38.

Manoogian, S.J., Kennedy, E.A., Wilson, K.A., Duma, S.M. and Alem, N.M. (2006). Predicting neck injuries due to head-supported mass. *Aviation Space & Environmental Medicine*, 77, pp. 509–14.

Marfella, R., Giugliano, D., di Maro, G., Acampora, R., Giunta, R. and D'Onofrio, F. (1994). The squatting test: a useful tool to assess both parasympathetic and sympathetic involvement of the cardiovascular autonomic neuropathy in diabetes. *Diabetes*, 43, pp. 607–12.

Martin, D.S., D'Aunno, D.S., Wood, M.L. and South, D.A. (1999). Repetitive high G exposure is associated with increased occurrence of cardiac valvular regurgitation. *Aviation Space & Environmental Medicine*, 70, pp. 1197–200.

Matzen, S., Perko, G., Groth, S., Friedman, D.B. and Secher, N.H. (1991). Blood volume distribution during head-up tilt induced central hypovolaemia in man. *Clinical Physiology*, 11, pp. 411–22.

McCloskey, K.A., Tripp, L.D., Chelette, T.L. and Popper, S.E. (1992). Test and evaluation metrics for use in sustained acceleration research. *Human Factors*, 34, pp. 409–28.

McGowan, D.G. (1997). 'A-LOC'– Almost loss of consciousness and its importance to fighter aviation [abstract]. *Aviation Space & Environmental Medicine*, 68, p. 632.

McKenzie, I. and Gillingham, K.K. (1993). Incidence of cardiac dysrhythmias occurring centrifuge training. *Aviation Space & Environmental Medicine*, 64, pp. 687–91.

McKinley, R.A. and Gallimore, J.J. (2013). Computational model of sustained acceleration effects on human cognitive performance. *Aviation Space & Environmental Medicine*, 84, pp. 780–88.

McKinley, R.A., Tripp, L.D. Jr, Bolia, S.D. and Roark, M.R. (2005). Computer modeling of acceleration effects on cerebral oxygen saturation. *Aviation Space & Environmental Medicine*, 76, pp. 733–8.

Michaud, V.J., Lyons, T.J. and Hansen, C.M. (1998). Frequency of the 'Push-Pull effect' in US Air Force fighter operations. *Aviation Space & Environmental Medicine*, 69, pp. 1083–6.

Mikuliszyn, R., Zebrowski, M. and Kowalczuk, K. (2005). Centrifuge training program with 'push-pull' elements. *Aviation Space & Environmental Medicine*, 76, pp. 493–5.

Milhorn, H.T. (1966). *The Application of Control Theory to Physiological Systems*. Philadelphia: Saunders.

Miller, H., Riley, M.B., Bondurant, S. and Hiatt, E.P. (1959). The duration of tolerance to positive acceleration. *Aviation Space & Environmental Medicine*, 30, pp. 360–66.

Miller, P.B., Johnson, R.L. and Lamb, L.E. (1964). The effects of four weeks of absolute bed rest on circulatory function in man. *Aerospace Medicine*, 35, pp. 1194–2000.

Montgomery, L.D. (1987). Body volume changes during simulated weightlessness: an overview. *Aviation Space & Environmental Medicine*, 58(9, Suppl.), pp. A80–85.

Montgomery, L.D. (1993). Body volume changes during simulated microgravity I: technique and comparison of men and women during horizontal bed rest. *Aviation Space & Environmental Medicine*, 64, pp. 893–8.

Montmerle, S. and Linnarsson, D. (2005). Cardiovascular effects of anti-G suit inflation at 1 and 2 G. *European Journal of Applied Physiology*, 94, pp. 235–41.

Moore, T. and Thornton, W.E. (1987). Space Shuttle inflight and postflight fluid shifts measured by leg volume changes. *Aviation Space & Environmental Medicine*, 58(9, Suppl.), pp. A91–6.

Morgan, T.R., Hill, R.C., Burns, J.W. and Vanderbeek, R.D. (1994). Effects of G-layoff on subsequent tolerance to +Gz [abstract]. *Aviation Space & Environmental Medicine*, 65, p. 448.

Morgan, T.R., Travis, T.W. and Hill, R.C. (1993). Air Force flight experience with the advanced technology anti-G suit (ATAGS) [abstract]. *Aviation Space & Environmental Medicine*, 64, p. 450.

Morrissette, K.L. and McGowan, D.G. (2000). Further support for the concept of a G-LOC syndrome: a survey of military high-performance aviators. *Aviation Space & Environmental Medicine*, 71, pp. 496–500.

Muller, T.U. (2002). G-induced vestibular dysfunction ('the wobblies') among aerobatic pilots: a case report and review. *Ear Nose & Throat Journal*, 81, pp. 269–72.

Mürbe, D., Lindner, P., Zöllner, S., Welsch, H., Kuhlisch, E., Hüttenbrink, K.-B. and Sundberg, J. (2004). Change of voice characteristics during +3 Gz acceleration. *Aviation Space & Environmental Medicine*, 75, pp. 1081–5.

Musgrave, F.S., Zechman, F.W. and Mains, R.C. (1969). Changes in total leg volume during lower body negative pressure. *Aerospace Medicine*, 40, pp. 602–6.

Musgrave, F.S., Zechman, F.W. and Mains, R.C. (1971). Comparison of the effects of 70o tilt and several levels of lower body negative pressure on heart rate and blood pressure in man. *Aerospace Medicine*, 42, pp. 1065–9.

Narlikar, J.V. (1996). *The Lighter Side of Gravity*. 2nd edn. Cambridge: Cambridge University Press.

Naumann, F.L., Bennell, K.L. and Wark, J.D. (2001). The effects of+ Gz force on the bone mineral density of fighter pilots. *Aviation Space & Environmental Medicine*, 72, pp. 177–81.

Naumann, F.L., Grant, M.C. and Dhaliwal, S.S. (2004). Changes in cervical spine bone mineral density in response to flight training. *Aviation Space & Environmental Medicine*, 75, pp. 255–9.

Nelson, J.G. (1987). Hydrostatic theory and G protection using tilting aircrew seats. *Aviation Space & Environmental Medicine*, 58, pp. 169–73.

Nelson, W.T., Bolia, R.S., McKinley, R.L., Chelette, T.L., Tripp, L.D. and Esken, R.L. (1998). Localization of virtual auditory cues in a high +Gz environment. In: *Proceedings of the Human Factors and Ergonomics Society Annual Meeting*, 42, pp. 97–101.

Netto, K.J. and Burnett, A.F. (2006). Neck muscle activation and head postures in common high performance aerial combat maneuvers. *Aviation Space & Environmental Medicine*, 77, pp. 1049–55.

Netto, K.J., Burnett, A.F. and Coleman, J.L. (2007). Neck exercises compared to muscle activation during aerial combat maneuvers. *Aviation Space & Environmental Medicine*, 78, pp. 478–84.

Newman, D.G. (1996). Cervical intervertebral disc protrusion in a RAAF F-111C pilot: a case report. *Aviation Space & Environmental Medicine*, 67, pp. 351–3.

Newman, D.G. (1997a). +Gz-induced neck injuries in Royal Australian Air Force fighter pilots. *Aviation Space & Environmental Medicine*, 68, pp. 520–24.

Newman, D.G. (1997b). Head positioning for high +Gz loads: an analysis of the techniques used by F/A-18 pilots. *Aviation Space & Environmental Medicine*, 68, pp. 732–5.

Newman, D.G. (1998). The biodynamic and physiological implications of supermanoeuvrable flight. *Australian Military Medicine*, 7, pp. 3–10.

Newman, D.G. (1999). Acquired left bundle branch block in an asymptomatic fighter pilot: a case report. *Aviation Space & Environmental Medicine*, 70, pp. 1219–22.

Newman, D.G. (2002). Helmet-mounted equipment in the high +Gz environment. *Aviation Space & Environmental Medicine*, 73, pp. 730–31.

Newman, D.G. (2006). Multi-sensor integration systems for the tactical combat pilot. *Aviation Space & Environmental Medicine*, 77, pp. 85, 88.

Newman, D.G. (2012). An analysis of accidents involving aerobatic aircraft in Australia, 1980–2011 [abstract]. *Aviation Space & Environmental Medicine*, 83, p. 349.

Newman, D.G. (2014). *Flying Fast Jets: Human Factors and Performance Limitations*. Farnham: Ashgate Publishing.

Newman, D.G. and Callister, R. (1999). Analysis of the Gz environment during air combat maneuvering in the F/A-18 fighter aircraft. *Aviation Space & Environmental Medicine*, 70, pp. 310–15.

Newman, D.G. and Callister, R. (2008). Cardiovascular training effects in fighter pilots induced by occupational high G exposure. *Aviation Space & Environmental Medicine*, 79, pp. 774–8.

Newman, D.G. and Callister, R. (2009). Flying experience and cardiovascular response to rapid head-up tilt in fighter pilots. *Aviation Space & Environmental Medicine*, 80, pp. 723–6.

Newman, D.G. and Ostler, D. (2011). The geometry of high angle of attack manoeuvres and the implications for Gy-induced neck injuries. *Aviation Space & Environmental Medicine*, 82, pp. 819–24.

Newman, D.G., White, S.W. and Callister, R. (1998). Evidence of baroreflex adaptation to repetitive +Gz in fighter pilots. *Aviation Space & Environmental Medicine*, 69, pp. 446–51.

Newman, D.G., White, S.W. and Callister, R. (1999). Patterns of physical conditioning in Royal Australian Air Force F/A-18 pilots and the implications for +Gz tolerance. *Aviation Space & Environmental Medicine*, 70, pp. 739–44.

Newman, D.G., White, S.W. and Callister, R. (2000). The effect of baroreflex adaptation on the dynamic cardiovascular response to head-up tilt. *Aviation Space & Environmental Medicine*, 71, pp. 255–9.

Nicogossian, A.E. (1989). Countermeasures to space deconditioning. In: Nicogossian, A.E., Huntoon, C.L. and Pool, S.L. (eds), *Space Physiology and Medicine*. Philadelphia: Lea and Febiger.

Nicogossian, A.E. and Nachtwey, D.S. (1989). Orbital flight. In: Nicogossian, A.E., Huntoon, C.L. and Pool, S.L. (eds), *Space Physiology and Medicine*. Philadelphia: Lea and Febiger.

Njemanze, P.C., Antol, P.J. and Lundgren, C.E. (1993). Perfusion of the visual cortex during pressure breathing at different high-G stress profiles. *Aviation Space & Environmental Medicine*, 64, pp. 396–400.

Noddeland, H., Myhre, K., Balldin, U.I. and Andersen, H.T. (1986). Proteinuria in fighter pilots after +Gz exposure. *Aviation Space & Environmental Medicine*, 57, pp. 122–5.

Nunneley, S.A., Dowd, P.J., Myhre, L.G. and Stribley, R.F. (1978). Physiological and psychological effects of heat stress simulating cockpit conditions. *Aviation Space & Environmental Medicine*, 49, pp. 763–7.

Nunneley, S.A., French, J., Vanderbeek, R.D. and Stranges, S.F. (1995). Thermal study of anti-G ensembles aboard F-16 aircraft in hot weather. *Aviation Space & Environmental Medicine*, 66, pp. 309–12.

Nunneley, S.A. and Myhre, L.G. (1976). Physiological effects of solar heat load in a fighter cockpit. *Aviation Space & Environmental Medicine*, 47, pp. 969–73.

Nunneley, S.A. and Stribley, R.F. (1979). Heat and dehydration effects on acceleration response in man. *Journal of Applied Physiology*, 47, pp. 197–200.

Nunneley, S.A., Stribley, R.F. and Allan, J.R. (1981). Heat stress in front and rear cockpits of F-4 aircraft. *Aviation Space & Environmental Medicine*, 54, pp. 287–90.

Obmiński, Z., Wojtkowiak, M., Stupnicki, R., Golec, L. and Hackney, A.C. (1997). Effect of acceleration stress on salivary cortisol and plasma cortisol and testosterone levels in cadet pilots. *Journal of Physiology and Pharmacology: An Official Journal of the Polish Physiological Society*, 48, pp. 193–200.

O'Hare, D., Chalmers, D. and Scuffham, P. (2003). Case-control study of risk factors for fatal and non-fatal injury in crashes of civil aircraft. *Aviation Space & Environmental Medicine*, 74, pp. 1061–6.

Ohashi, K. and Igarashi, M. (1985). Statoconia displacement in squirrel monkey ears. *ORL; Journal for Otorhinolaryngology and its Related Specialties*, 47, pp. 242–8.

Oksa, J., Hamalainen, O., Rissanen, S., Myllyniemi, J. and Kuronen, P. (1996). Muscle strain during aerial combat manoeuvring exercises. *Aviation Space & Environmental Medicine*, 67, pp. 1138–43.

Oksa, J., Hamalainen, O., Rissanen, S., Salminen, M. and Kuronen, P. (1999). Muscle fatigue caused by repeated aerial combat manoeuvring exercises. *Aviation Space & Environmental Medicine*, 70, pp. 556–60.

Oksa, J., Linja, T. and Rintala, H. (2003). The effect of lumbar support on the effectiveness of anti-G straining maneuvers. *Aviation Space & Environmental Medicine*, 74, pp. 886–90.

Olschewski, H. and Bruck, K. (1990). Cardiac responses to the Valsalva manoeuvre in different body positions. *European Journal of Applied Physiology*, 61, pp. 20–25.

Oscai, L.B., Williams, B.T. and Hertig, B.A. (1968). Effect of exercise on blood volume. *Journal of Applied Physiology*, 24, pp. 622–4.

Ossard, G., Clere, J.M., Kerguelen, M., Melchior, F. and Seylaz, J. (1994). Response of human cerebral blood flow to +Gz accelerations. *Journal of Applied Physiology*, 76, pp. 2114–18.

Ossard, G., Kerguelen, M. and Clere, J.M. (1995). +Gz tolerance with 70 and 100 hPa/G inflation schedules of the extended ARZ 830 anti-G suit [abstract]. *Aviation Space & Environmental Medicine*, 66, p. 469.

Ostrowski, V.B. and Bojrab, D.I. (2005). Otolith dysfunction and semicircular canal dysfunction. In: Jackler, R.K. and Brackmann, D.E. (eds), *Neurotology*, 2nd edn. Philadelphia: Mosby, Inc.

Parker, D.E., Covell, W.P. and von Gierke, H.E. (1968). Exploration of vestibular damage in guinea pigs following mechanical stimulation. *Acta Otolaryngolica*, Suppl. 239, p. 7.

Parkhurst, M.J., Leverett, S.D. and Shubrooks, S.J. (1972). Human tolerance to high, sustained +Gz acceleration. *Aerospace Medicine*, 43, pp. 708–12.

Paul, M.A. (1996). Extended-coverage-bladder G-suits can provide improved G-tolerance and high Gz foot pain. *Aviation Space & Environmental Medicine*, 67, pp. 253–5.

Paul, M.A. and Ackles, K.N. (1993). Improved G-tolerance with an extended-coverage-bladder G-suit [abstract]. *Aviation Space & Environmental Medicine*, 64, p. 450.

Pecaric, M. and Buick, F. (1992). Determination of a pressure breathing schedule for improving +Gz tolerance. *Aviation Space & Environmental Medicine*, 63, pp. 572–8.

Pendergast, D.R., Olszowka, A. and Farhi, L.E. (2012). Cardiovascular and pulmonary responses to increased acceleration forces during rest and exercise. *Aviation Space & Environmental Medicine*, 83, pp. 488–95.

Perez, S.A., Charles, J.B., Fortner, G.W., Hurst, V. IV, and Meck, J.V. (2003). Cardiovascular effects of anti-G suit and cooling garment during space shuttle re-entry and landing. *Aviation Space & Environmental Medicine*, 74, pp. 753–7.

Peterson, D.F., Bishop, V.S. and Erickson, H.H. (1975). Cardiovascular changes during and following 1-min exposure to +Gz stress. *Aviation Space & Environmental Medicine*, 46, pp. 775–9.

Peterson, D.F., Bishop, V.S. and Erickson, H.H. (1977). Anti-G suit effect on cardiovascular dynamic changes due to +Gz stress. *Journal of Applied Physiology*, 43, pp. 765–9.

Petren-Mallmin, M. and Linder, J. (1999). MRI cervical spine findings in asymptomatic fighter pilots. *Aviation Space & Environmental Medicine*, 70, pp. 1183–8.

Petren-Mallmin, M. and Linder, J. (2001). Cervical spine degeneration in fighter pilots and controls: a 5-yr follow-up study. *Aviation Space & Environmental Medicine*, 72, pp. 443–6.

Phillips, C.A. and Petrofsky, J.S. (1983). Neck muscle loading and fatigue: systematic variation of headgear weight and center-of-gravity. *Aviation Space & Environmental Medicine*, 54, pp. 901–5.

Pickering, T.G., Gribbin, B., Petersen, E.S., Cunningham, D.J.C. and Sleight, P. (1971). Comparison of the effects of exercise and posture on the baroreflex in man. *Cardiovascular Research*, 5, pp. 582–6.

Platts, S.H., Tuxhorn, J.A., Ribeiro, L.C., Stenger, M.B., Lee, S.M.C. and Meck, J.V. (2009). Compression garments as countermeasures to orthostatic intolerance. *Aviation Space & Environmental Medicine*, 80, pp. 437–42.

Pluta, J.C. (1984). LOC survey. *Flying Safety*, pp. 25–8.

Powell, T.J., Carey, T.M., Brent, H.P. and Taylor, W.J.R. (1957). Episodes of unconsciousness in pilots during flight in 1956. *Journal of Aviation Medicine*, 28, pp. 374–86.

Rahn, H., Otis, A.B., Chadwick, L.E. and Fenn, W.O. (1946). The pressure-volume diagram of the thorax and lung. *American Journal of Physiology*, 146, pp. 161–78.

Ramsey, C.S., Werchan, P.M., Isdahl, W.M., Fischer, J. and Gibbons, J.A. (2008). Acceleration tolerance at night with acute fatigue and stimulants. *Aviation Space & Environmental Medicine*, 79, pp. 769–73.

Ray, C.A., Hume, K.M. and Shortt, T.L. (1997). Skin sympathetic outflow during head-down neck flexion in humans. *American Journal of Physiology, (Regulatory Integrative Comp Physiol 42)*, 273, pp. R1142–46.

Rayman, R.B. (1973a). In-flight loss of consciousness. *Aerospace Medicine*, 44, pp. 679–81.

Rayman, R.B. (1973b). Sudden incapacitation in flight 1 Jan 1966–30 Nov 1971. *Aerospace Medicine*, 44, pp. 953–5.

Rayman, R.B., Antuñano, M.J., Garber, M.A., Hastings, J.D., Illig, P.A., Jordan, J.L., Landry, R.F., McMeekin, R.R., Northrup, S.E., Ruehle, C., Saenger, A. and Schneider, V.S. (2002). Medical guidelines for space passengers--II. *Aviation Space & Environmental Medicine*, 73, pp. 1132–4.

Rayman, R.B. and McNaughton, G.B. (1983). Sudden incapacitation: USAF experience, 1970–80. *Aviation Space & Environmental Medicine*, 54, pp. 161–4.

Rickards, C.A. and Newman, D.G. (2002). The effect of low-level normobaric hypoxia on orthostatic responses. *Aviation Space & Environmental Medicine*, 73, pp. 460–65.

Rickards, C.A. and Newman, D.G. (2003). A comparative assessment of two techniques for investigating initial cardiovascular reflexes under acute orthostatic stress. *European Journal of Applied Physiology*, 90, pp. 449–57.

Rickards, C.A. and Newman, D.G. (2005). G-induced visual and cognitive disturbances in a survey of 65 operational fighter pilots. *Aviation Space & Environmental Medicine*, 76, pp. 496–500.

Rook, A.F. (1938). Hypotension and flying. *Lancet*, 2, pp. 1503–10.

Ross, J.A. (1990). A case of G-LOC in a propeller aircraft. *Aviation Space & Environmental Medicine*, 61, pp. 567–8.

Rossberg, R. and Penaz, J. (1988). Initial cardiovascular response on change of posture from squatting to standing. *European Journal of Applied Physiology*, 57, pp. 93–7.

Rossen, R., Kabat, H., and Anderson, J.P. (1943). Acute arrest of cerebral circulation in man. *Archives of Neurology and Psychiatry*, 50, pp. 510–28.

Rowell, L.B. (1986). *Human Circulation: Regulation during Physical Stress*. New York: Oxford University Press.

Rowell, L.B. (1993). *Human Cardiovascular Control*. New York: Oxford University Press.

Rushmer, R.F. (1947). A roentgenographic study of the effect of a pneumatic anti-blackout suit on the hydrostatic columns in man exposed to positive radial acceleration. *American Journal of Physiology*, 151, pp. 459–68.

Rushmer, R.F., Beckman, E.L. and Lee, D. (1947). Protection of the cerebral circulation by the cerebrospinal fluid under the influence of radial acceleration. *American Journal of Physiology*, 151, pp. 355–65.

Sagawa, K. (1983). Baroreflex control of systemic arterial pressure and vascular bed. In: *Handbook of Physiology. The Cardiovascular System*, Sect. 2, vol. III, Ch. 14. Bethesda: American Physiological Society.

Sand, D.P., Girgenrath, M., Bock, O. and Pongratz, H. (2003). Production of isometric forces during sustained acceleration. *Aviation Space & Environmental Medicine*, 74, pp. 688–7.

Sandor, P.M.B., McAnally, K.I., Pellieux, L. and Martin, R.L. (2005). Localization of virtual sound at 4 Gz. *Aviation Space & Environmental Medicine*, 76, pp. 103–7.

Sandor, P.M.B., Pellieux, L., Godfroy, M., Ossard, G. and Dancer, A. (2004). Hearing thresholds during Gz acceleration with masking noise. *Aviation Space & Environmental Medicine*, 75, pp. 952–5.

Sasaki, S. and Dampney, R.A. (1990). Tonic cardiovascular effects of angiotensin II in the ventrolateral medulla. *Hypertension*, 15, pp. 274–83.

Sather, T.M., Goldwater, D.J., Montgomery, L.D. and Convertino, V.A. (1986). Cardiovascular dynamics associated with tolerance to lower body negative pressure. *Aviation Space & Environmental Medicine*, 57, pp. 413–19.

Schall, D.G. (1989). Non-ejection cervical spine injuries due to +Gz in high performance aircraft. *Aviation Space & Environmental Medicine*, 60, pp. 445–56.

Schlegel, T.T., Benavides, E.W., Barker, D.C., Brown, T.E., Harm, D.L., DeSilva, S.J. and Low, P.A. (1998). Cardiovascular and valsalva responses during parabolic flight. *Journal of Applied Physiology*, 85, pp. 1957–65.

Schlegel, T.T., Wood, S.J., Brown, T.E., Harm, D.L. and Rupert, A.H. (2003). Effect of 30-min +3 Gz centrifugation on vestibular and autonomic cardiovascular function. *Aviation Space & Environmental Medicine*, 74, pp. 717–24.

Schmidt-Neilsen, K. (1991). *Animal Physiology: Adaptation and Environment.* 4th edn. Cambridge: Cambridge University Press.

Schneider, S., Guardiera, S., Kleinert, J., Steinbacher, A., Abel, T., Carnahan, H. and Strüder, H.K. (2008). Centrifugal acceleration to 3Gz is related to increased release of stress hormones and decreased mood in men and women: Research Report. *Stress: The International Journal on the Biology of Stress,* 11, pp. 339–47.

Scott, J.M., Esch, B.T., Goodman, L.S., Bredin, S.S., Haykowsky, M.J. and Warburton, D.E. (2007). Cardiovascular consequences of high-performance aircraft maneuvers: implications for effective countermeasures and laboratory-based simulations. *Applied Physiology, Nutrition & Metabolism,* 32, pp. 332–9.

Scott, J.P.R., Jungius, J., Connolly, D. and Stevenson, A.T. (2013). Subjective and objective measures of relaxed +G_z tolerance following repeated +G_z exposure. *Aviation Space & Environmental Medicine,* 84, pp. 684–91.

Seagard, J.L., Dean, C. and Hopp, F.A. (2000). Neurochemical transmission of baroreceptor input in the nucleus tractus solitaries. *Brain Research Bulletin,* 51, pp. 111–18.

Seidel, H., Herzel, H. and Eckberg, D.L. (1997). Phase dependencies of the human baroreceptor reflex. *American Journal of Physiology,* 272, pp. H2040–53.

Sekiguchi, C., Iwane, M. and Oshibuchi, M. (1986). Anti-G training of Japanese Air Self Defense Force fighter pilots. *Aviation Space & Environmental Medicine,* 57, pp. 1029–34.

Self, B.P., Balldin, U.I., Shaffstall, R.M. and Morgan, T.R. (2000). Pressurized sleeves and gloves for protection against acceleration-induced arm pain. *Aviation Space & Environmental Medicine,* 71, pp. 501–5.

Self, D.A., White, C.D., Shaffstall, R.M., Mtinangi, B.L., Croft, J.S. and Hainsworth, R. (1996). Differences between syncope resulting from rapid onset acceleration and orthostatic stress. *Aviation Space & Environmental Medicine,* 67, pp. 547–54.

Seng, K.-Y., Lam, P.-M. and Lee, V.-S. (2003). Acceleration effects on neck muscle strength: pilots vs. non-pilots. *Aviation Space & Environmental Medicine,* 74, pp. 164–8.

Sevilla, N.L. and Gardner, J.W. (2005). G-induced loss of consciousness: case-control study of 78 G-LOCs in the F-15, F-16, and A-10. *Aviation Space & Environmental Medicine,* 76, pp. 370–74.

Shaffstall, R.M. and Burton, R.R. (1979). Evaluation of assisted positive pressure breathing on +Gz tolerance. *Aviation Space & Environmental Medicine,* 50, pp. 820–24.

Shender, B.S. (2001). Human tolerance to acceleration loads generated in high-performance helicopters. *Aviation Space & Environmental Medicine,* 72, pp. 693–703.

Shender, B.S., Forster, E.M., Hrebien, L., Ryoo, H.C. and Cammarota, J.P. Jr. (2003). Acceleration-induced near-loss of consciousness: the 'A-LOC' syndrome. *Aviation Space & Environmental Medicine,* 74, pp. 1021–8.

Shender, B.S. and Heffner, P.L. (2001). Dynamic strength capabilities of small-stature females to perform high-performance flight tasks. *Aviation Space & Environmental Medicine*, 72, pp. 89–99.

Shinners, S.M. (1998). *Modern Control System Theory and Design*. 2nd edn. New York: John Wiley and Sons.

Shortt, T.L. and Ray, C.A. (1997). Sympathetic and vascular responses to head-down neck flexion in humans. *American Journal of Physiology (Heart Circ Physiol 41)*, 272, pp. H1780–1784.

Shubrooks, S.J., Jr. (1973). Positive-pressure breathing as a protective technique during +Gz acceleration. *Journal of Applied Physiology*, 25, pp. 294–8.

Shubrooks, S.J., Jr. and Leverett S.D., Jr. (1973). Effects of the Valsalva manoeuvre on tolerance to +Gz acceleration. *Journal of Applied Physiology*, 34, pp. 460–66.

Shvartz, E. and Meyerstein, N. (1970). Tilt tolerance of young men and young women. *Aerospace Medicine*, 41, pp. 253–5.

Shvartz, E. and Meyerstein, N. (1972). Relation of tilt tolerance to aerobic capacity and physical characteristics. *Aerospace Medicine*, 43, pp. 278–80.

Shy, G. and Drager, G.A. (1960). A neurological syndrome associated with orthostatic hypotension: a clinical-pathologic study. *AMA Archives of Neurology*, 2, pp. 511–27.

Siitonen, S.L., Kauppinen, T., Leino, T.K., Vanninen, E., Kuronen, P. and Länsimies, E. (2003). Cerebral blood flow during acceleration in flight measured with SPECT. *Aviation Space & Environmental Medicine*, 74, pp. 201–6.

Sjostrand, T. (1952). The regulation of the blood distribution in man. *Acta Physiologica Scandinavica*, 26, pp. 312–27.

Skyttä, J., Karjalainen, J., Aho, J. and Laitinen, L.A. (1994). Heart rate and cardiac arrhythmia during high-Gz flight. *Military Medicine*, 159, pp. 490–93.

Smith, J.J., Bonin, M.L., Weidmeier, V.T., Kalbfleisch, J.H. and McDermott, D.J. (1974). Cardiovascular response of young men to diverse stresses. *Aerospace Medicine*, 45, pp. 583–90.

Smith, M.L., Fritsch, J.M. and Eckberg, D.L. (1994). Rapid adaptation of vagal baroreflexes in humans. *Journal of the Autonomic Nervous System*, 47, pp. 75–82.

Snyder, Q.C. and Kearney, P.J. (2002). High +Gz induced acute inguinal herniation in an F-16 aircrew member: case report and review. *Aviation Space & Environmental Medicine*, 73, pp. 68–72.

Sondag, H.N.P.M., Jong, H.A.A.D. and Oosterveld, W.J. (1996). Altered behavior of hamsters by prolonged hypergravity: adaptation to 2.5 G and re-adaptation to 1 G. *Acta Otolaryngolica*, 116, pp. 192–7.

Sovelius, R., Oksa, J., Rintala, H., Huhtala, H. and Siitonen, S. (2007). Ambient temperature and neck EMG with +Gz loading on a trampoline. *Aviation Space & Environmental Medicine*, 78, pp. 574–8.

Sovelius, R., Oksa, J., Rintala, H., Huhtala, H. and Siitonen, S. (2008a). Neck muscle strain when wearing helmet and NVG during acceleration on a trampoline. *Aviation Space & Environmental Medicine*, 79, pp. 112–16.

Sovelius, R., Oksa, J., Rintala, H., Huhtala, H., Ylinen, J. and Siitonen, S. (2006). Trampoline exercise vs. strength training to reduce neck strain in fighter pilots. *Aviation Space & Environmental Medicine*, 77, pp. 20–25.

Sovelius, R., Oksa, J., Rintala, H. and Siitonen, S. (2008b). Neck and back muscle loading in pilots flying high G_z sorties with and without lumbar support. *Aviation Space & Environmental Medicine*, 79, pp. 616–19.

Sovelius, R., Salonen, O., Lamminen, A., Huhtala, H. and Hamalainen, O. (2008c). Spinal MRI in fighter pilots and controls: a 13-year longitudinal study. *Aviation Space & Environmental Medicine*, 79, pp. 685–8.

Sowood, P.J. and O'Connor, E.M. (1994). Thermal strain and G protection associated with wearing an enhanced anti-G protection system in a warm climate. *Aviation Space & Environmental Medicine*, 65, pp. 992–8.

Spodick, D.H. and Lance, V.Q. (1977). Comparative orthostatic responses: standing versus head-up tilt. *Aviation Space & Environmental Medicine*, 48, pp. 432–3.

Sprangers, R.L.H., Wesseling, K.H., Imholz, A.L.T., Imholz, B.P.M. and Wieling, W. (1991). Initial blood pressure fall on stand up and exercise explained in total peripheral resistance. *Journal of Applied Physiology*, 70, pp. 523–30.

Stanford, W. (1961). Use of an air force antigravity suit in a case of severe postural hypotension. *Annals of Internal Medicine*, 55, pp. 843–5.

Stegemann, J., Busert, A. and Brock, D. (1974). Influence of fitness on the blood pressure control system in man. *Aerospace Medicine*, 45, pp. 45–8.

Stevenson, A.T. and Scott, J.P. (2014). +Gz tolerance, with and without muscle tensing, following loss of anti-G trouser pressure. *Aviation Space & Environmental Medicine*, 85, pp. 426–32.

Stevenson, A.T., Scott, J.P.R., Chiesa, S., Sin, D., Coates, G., Bagshaw, M. and Harridge, S. (2014). Blood pressure, vascular resistance, and +Gz tolerance during repeated +Gz exposures. *Aviation Space & Environmental Medicine*, 85, pp. 536–42.

Stevenson, A.T., Lythgoe, D.T., Darby, C.L.J., Devlin, J.M., Connolly, D.M. and Scott, J.P.R. (2013). Garment fit and protection from sustained +G_z acceleration with 'full-coverage' anti-G trousers. *Aviation Space & Environmental Medicine*, 84, pp. 600–607.

Stewart, W.K. (1945). Some observations on the effect of centrifugal force in man. *Journal of Neurology and Psychiatry*, 8, pp. 24–33.

Stoll, A.M. (1956). Human tolerance to positive G as determined by the physiological end points. *Journal of Aviation Medicine*, 27, pp. 356–67.

Stromme, S.B., Ingjer, F. and Meen, H.D. (1977). Assessment of maximal aerobic power in specifically trained athletes. *Journal of Applied Physiology*, 42, pp. 833–7.

Tachibana, S., Akamatus, T., Nakamura, A. and Yagura, S. (1994). Serious arrhythmias coinciding with alteration of consciousness in aircrew during +Gz stress. *Aviation Space & Environmental Medicine*, 65, pp. 60–66.

Tacker Jr, W.A., Balldin, U.I., Burton, R.R., Glaister, D.H., Gillingham, K.K. and Mercer, J.R. (1987). Induction and prevention of acceleration atelectasis. *Aviation Space & Environmental Medicine*, 58, pp. 69–75.

Takahata, T., Shouji, I., Maruyama, S., Sato, Y., Nishida, Y. and Ueno, T. (2011). Teeth clenching and positive acceleration-induced cerebral arterial hypotension in rats. *Aviation Space & Environmental Medicine*, 82, pp. 442–7.

Tanaka, H., Sjoberg, B.J. and Thulesius, O. (1996). Cardiac output and blood pressure during active and passive standing. *Clinical Physiology*, 16, pp. 157–70.

Tarui, H. and Nakamura, A. (1987). Saliva cortisol: a good indicator for acceleration stress. *Aviation Space & Environmental Medicine*, 58, pp. 573–5.

Taylor, M.K., Hodgdon, J.A., Griswold, L., Miller, A., Roberts, D.E. and Escamilla, R.F. (2006). Cervical resistance training: effects on isometric and dynamic strength. *Aviation Space & Environmental Medicine*, 77, pp. 1131–5.

Ten Harkel, A.D.J., Baisch, F. and Karemaker, J.M. (1992). Increased orthostatic blood pressure variability after prolonged head-down tilt. *Acta Physiologica Scandinavica*, 144, pp. S604:89–99.

Tesch, P.A., Hjort, H. and Balldin, U.I. (1983). Effects of strength training on G tolerance. *Aviation Space & Environmental Medicine*, 54, pp. 691–5.

Thompson, C.A., Tatro, D.L., Ludwig, D.A. and Convertino, V.A. (1990). Baroreflex responses to acute changes in blood volume in man. *American Journal of Physiology*, 259, pp. R792–8.

Thornton, W.E., Hedge, V., Coleman, E., Uri, J.J. and Moore, T.P. (1992). Changes in leg volume during microgravity simulation. *Aviation Space & Environmental Medicine*, 63, pp. 789–94.

Thornton, W.E., Moore, T.P. and Pool, S.L. (1987). Fluid shifts in weightlessness. *Aviation Space & Environmental Medicine*, 58(9, Suppl.), pp. A86–90.

Thrasher, T.N. (1994). Baroreceptor regulation of vasopressin and renin secretion: low-pressure versus high-pressure receptors. *Frontiers in Neuroendocrinology*, 15, pp. 157–96.

Tolga Aydog, S., Türbedar, E., Akin, A. and Doral, M.N. (2004). Cervical and lumbar spinal changes diagnosed in four-view radiographs of 732 military pilots. *Aviation Space & Environmental Medicine*, 75, pp. 154–7.

Tomaselli, C.M., Frey, M.A.B., Kenny, R.A. and Hoffler, G.W. (1990). Effect of a central redistribution of fluid volume on response to lower body negative pressure. *Aviation Space & Environmental Medicine*, 61, pp. 38–42.

Tong, A., Balldin, U.I., Dooley, J.W. and Hill, R.C. (1998a). Tactical vs other simulated aerial combat maneuvers. *Aviation Space & Environmental Medicine*, 69, pp. 525–7.

Tong, A., Balldin, U.I., Hill, R.C. and Dooley, J.W. (1998b). Improved anti-G protection boosts sortie generation ability. *Aviation Space & Environmental Medicine*, 69, pp. 117–20.

Tong, A., Hill, R.C., Tripp, L. and Webb, J.T. (1994). The effect of head and body position on +Gz acceleration tolerance. *Aviation Space & Environmental Medicine*, 65(5 Suppl), pp. A90–94.

Toth, D.N., Repperger, D.W. and Frazier, J.W. (1980). The effects of test and training intervals on performance evaluations in acceleration stress [abstract]. *Aviation Space & Environmental Medicine*, 51, pp. 98–9.

Travis, T.W. and Morgan, T.R. (1994). U.S. Air Force positive-pressure breathing anti-G system (PBG): subjective health effects and acceptance by pilots. *Aviation Space & Environmental Medicine*, 65(5 Suppl), pp. A75–9.

Tripp, L.D. Jr, Jennings, T.J., Seaworth, J.F., Howell, L.L. and Goodyear, C. (1994). Long-duration $+G_z$ acceleration on cardiac volumes determined by two-dimensional echocardiography. *Journal of Clinical Pharmacology*, 34, pp. 484–8.

Trippe, S. (2013). A simplified treatment of gravitational interaction on galactic scales. *Journal of The Korean Astronomical Society*, 46, pp. 41–7.

Truszczynski, O., Wojtkowiak, M., Lewkowicz, R., Biernacki, M.P. and Kowalczuk, K. (2013). Reaction time in pilots at sustained acceleration of +4.5 G_z. *Aviation Space & Environmental Medicine*, 84, pp. 845–9.

Tuckman, J. and Shillingford, J. (1966). Effect of different degrees of tilt on cardiac output, heart rate, and blood pressure in normal man. *British Heart Journal*, 28, pp. 32–9.

Vallejo Desviat, P., Esteban Benavides, B., López, J.A., Rios-Tejada, F., Bárcena, A., Álvarez–Sala, F. and Alonso Rodríguez, C. (2007). Surgical correction of disc pathology in fighter pilots: a review of 14 cases. *Aviation Space & Environmental Medicine*, 78, pp. 784–8.

Van Lieshout, J.J., Ten Harkel, A.D.J. and Wieling, W. (1992). Physical manoeuvres for combating orthostatic dizziness in autonomic failure. *Lancet*, 11, pp. 897–8.

Van Patten, R.E. (1988). Advances in anti-G valve technology: what's in the future? *Aviation Space & Environmental Medicine*, 59, pp. 32–5.

Vanderbeek, R.D. (1988). Period prevalence of acute neck injury in U.S. Air Force pilots exposed to high G forces. *Aviation Space & Environmental Medicine*, 59, pp. 1176–80.

Vartbaronov, R.A., Glod, G.D., Uglova, N.N., Rolik, I.S. and Krasnykh, I.G. (1986). [Adaptive and cumulative effects in the dog exposed to routine+ Gz acceleration]. *Kosmicheskaia biologiia i aviakosmicheskaia meditsina*, 21, pp. 37–40.

Vayenas, C.G. and Souentie, S.N.A. (2012). *Gravity, Special Relativity, and the Strong Force: A Bohr-Einstein-de Broglie Model for the Formation of Hadrons*. Berlin: Springer.

Vil-Viliams, I.F., Kotovskaya, A.R., Gavrilova, L.N., Lukjanuk, V.Y. and Yarov, A.S. (1998). Human +Gx tolerance with the use of anti-G suits during descent from orbit of the Soyuz space vehicles. *Journal of Gravitational Physiology*, 5, pp. 129–30.

Vinake, W.E. (1948). Aviator's vertigo. *Journal of Aviation Medicine*, 19, pp. 158–70.

Vogt, F.B. (1966). An objective approach to the analysis of tilt table data. *Aerospace Medicine*, 37, pp. 1195–204.

Von Beckh, H.J. (1981). The beginnings of aeromedical research. Warminster, PA: Naval Air Development Centre. NADC-81281–60:1–34.

Wagstaff, A.S., Jahr, K.I. and Rodskier, S. (2012). +Gz-induced spinal symptoms in fighter pilots: operational and individual associated factors. *Aviation Space & Environmental Medicine*, 83, pp. 1092–6.

Wald, R.M. (1984). *General Relativity*. Boston: University of Chicago Press.

Walker, T.B., Balldin, U., Fischer, J., Storm, W. and Warren, G.L. (2010). Acceleration tolerance after ingestion of a commercial energy drink. *Aviation Space & Environmental Medicine*, 81, pp. 1100–106.

Wanstall, B. (1990). Helping combat pilots survive. *Interavia Aerospace Review*, 45, pp. 231–4.

Ward, R.J., Danziger, F., Bonica, J.J., Allen, G.D. and Tolas, A.G. (1966). Cardiovascular effects of change of posture. *Aerospace Medicine*, 33, pp. 257–9.

Warren, J.V. (1974). The physiology of the giraffe. *Scientific American*, 231, pp. 96–105.

Watkins, S.M., Welch, L., Whitley, P. and Forster, E. (1998). The design of arm pressure covers to alleviate pain in high G maneuvers. *Aviation Space & Environmental Medicine*, 69, pp. 461–7.

Webb, J.T., Oakley, C.J. and Meeker, L.J. (1991). Unpredictability of fighter pilot G tolerance using anthropometric and physiologic variables. *Aviation Space & Environmental Medicine*, 62, pp. 128–35.

Weeks, S.D., Jaeger, E.A. and Duane, T.D. (1964). Plethysmographic goggles: a new type of ophthalmodynamometer. *Neurology*, 14, pp. 240–43.

Weigman, J.F., Burton, R.R. and Forster, E.M. (1995). The role of anaerobic power in human tolerance to simulated aerial combat maneuvers. *Aviation Space & Environmental Medicine*, 66, pp. 938–42.

Weiss, S. and Baker, J.P. (1933). The carotid sinus reflex in health and disease. *Medicine*, 12, pp. 297–354.

Wenning, G.K., Colosimo, C., Geser, F. and Poewe, W. (2004). Multiple system atrophy. *The Lancet Neurology*, 3, pp. 93–103.

Werchan, P.M. (1991). Physiologic bases of G-induced loss of consciousness (G-LOC). *Aviation Space & Environmental Medicine*, 62, pp. 612–14.

Werchan, P.M. and Shahed, A.R. (1992). Brain biochemical factors related to G-LOC. *The Physiologist*, 35(1, Suppl.), pp. S143–6.

Westfall, R. (1993). *The Life of Isaac Newton*. Cambridge: Cambridge University Press.

Whinnery, J.E. (1979). +Gz tolerance: correlation with clinical parameters. *Aviation Space & Environmental Medicine*, 50, pp. 736–41.

Whinnery, J.E. (1982a). G-tolerance enhancement: straining ability comparison of aircrewmen, non-aircrewmen, and trained centrifuge subjects. *Aviation Space & Environmental Medicine*, 53, pp. 232–4.

Whinnery, J.E. (1982b). Acceleration-induced atrioventricular dissociation: hemodynamic consequences. *Aviation Space & Environmental Medicine*, 53, pp. 432–4.

Whinnery, J.E. (1986). +Gz-induced loss of consciousness in undergraduate pilot training. *Aviation Space & Environmental Medicine*, 57, pp. 997–9.

Whinnery, J.E. (1987). Comparative distribution of petechial haemorrhages as a function of aircraft cockpit geometry. *Journal of Biomedical Engineering*, 9, pp. 201–5.

Whinnery, J.E. (1988). Converging research on +Gz-induced loss of consciousness. *Aviation Space & Environmental Medicine*, 59, pp. 9–11.

Whinnery, J.E. (1989). Observations on the neurophysiologic theory of acceleration (+Gz) induced loss of consciousness. *Aviation Space & Environmental Medicine*, 60, pp. 589–93.

Whinnery, J.E. (1990). Electrocardiographic response to high +Gz centrifuge training. *Aviation Space & Environmental Medicine*, 61, pp. 716–21.

Whinnery, J.E. and Burton, R.R. (1987). +Gz-induced loss of consciousness: a case for training exposure to unconsciousness. *Aviation Space & Environmental Medicine*, 58, pp. 468–72.

Whinnery, J.E., Burton, R.R., Boll, P.A. and Eddy, D.R. (1987). Characterization of the resulting incapacitation following unexpected +Gz-induced loss of consciousness. *Aviation Space & Environmental Medicine*, 58, pp. 631–6.

Whinnery, J.E., Fischer, J.R. and Shapiro, N.L. (1989). Recovery to +1 Gz and +2 Gz following +Gz-induced loss of consciousness: operational considerations. *Aviation Space & Environmental Medicine*, 60, pp. 1090–95.

Whinnery, J.E. and Jones, D.R. (1987). Recurrent +Gz-induced loss of consciousness. *Aviation Space & Environmental Medicine*, 58, pp. 943–7.

Whinnery, J.E., Laughlin, M.H. and Hickman, Jr J.R. (1979). Concurrent loss of consciousness and sino-atrial block during +Gz stress. *Aviation Space & Environmental Medicine*, 50, pp. 635–8.

Whinnery, J.E., Laughlin, M.H. and Uhl, G.S. (1980). Coincident loss of conscious and ventricular tachycardia during +Gz stress. *Aviation Space & Environmental Medicine*, 51, pp. 827–31.

Whinnery, J.E. and Murray, D.C. (1990). Enhancing tolerance to acceleration (+Gz) stress: the 'hook' manoeuvre. Report No. NADC-90088–60, Air Development Center, Warminster, PA.

Whinnery, J.E. and Parnell, M.J. (1987). The effects of long-term aerobic conditioning on +Gz tolerance. *Aviation Space & Environmental Medicine*, 58, pp. 199–204.

Whinnery, J.E. and Shaffstall, R.M. (1979). Incapacitation time for +Gz-induced loss of consciousness. *Aviation Space & Environmental Medicine*, 50, pp. 83–5.

Whinnery, J.E. and Whinnery, A.M. (1990). Acceleration-induced loss of consciousness: a review of 500 episodes. *Archives of Neurology*, 47, pp. 764–76.

Whinnery, A.M., Whinnery, J.E. and Hickman, J.R. (1990). High +Gz centrifuge training: the electrocardiographic response to +Gz-induced loss of consciousness. *Aviation Space & Environmental Medicine*, 61, pp. 609–14.

White, M. (1997). *Isaac Newton: The Last Sorcerer*. London: Fourth Estate Ltd.

Whitley, P.E. (1997). Pilot performance of the anti-G straining maneuver: respiratory demands and breathing system effects. *Aviation Space & Environmental Medicine*, 68, pp. 312–16.

Whitton, R.C. (ed.) (1992). *Flight Surgeon's Guide*. San Antonio: USAF School of Aerospace Medicine.

Wickes, S.J. and Greeves, J.P. (2005). Prevalance and associated factors of neck related flight pain. Qinetiq report 0601069. Farnborough, UK: Qinetiq.

Will, C.M. (1974). Gravitational theory. *Scientific American*, 231, pp. 24–33.

Will, C.M. (1998). Bounding the mass of the graviton using gravitational-wave observations of inspiralling compact binaries. *Physical Review D*, 57, pp. 2061–8.

Williams, C.A., Lind, A.R., Wiley, R.L., Douglas, J.E. and Miller, G. (1988). Effect of different body postures on the pressures generated during an L-1 maneuver. *Aviation Space & Environmental Medicine*, 59, pp. 920–27.

Williams, R.S., Werchan, P.M., Fischer, J.R. and Bauer, D.H. (1998). Adverse effects of Gz in civilian aerobatic pilots [abstract]. *Aviation Space & Environmental Medicine*, 69, p. 201.

Wilmore, J.H. and Costill, D.L. (1994). *Physiology of Sport and Exercise*. Champaign: Human Kinetics.

Wilson, G.F., Reis, G.A. and Tripp, L.D. (2005). EEG correlates of G-induced loss of consciousness. *Aviation Space & Environmental Medicine*, 76, pp. 19–27.

Winfield, D.A. (1999). Aircrew lumbar supports: an update. *Aviation Space & Environmental Medicine*, 70, pp. 321–4.

Wood, E.H. (1947). Do permanent effects result from repeated blackouts caused by positive acceleration? *Aerospace Medicine*, 18, pp. 471–82.

Wood, E.H. (1990). Hydrostatic homeostatic effects during changing force environments. *Aviation Space & Environmental Medicine*, 61, pp. 366–73.

Wood, E.H. (1992). Potential hazards of high anti-Gz suit protection. *Aviation Space & Environmental Medicine*, 63, pp. 1024–6.

Wood, E.H., Lambert, E.H., Baldes, E.J. and Code, C.F. (1946). Effects of acceleration in relation to aviation. *Federation Proceedings*, 5, pp. 327–44.

Wood, E.H. and Sturm, R.E. (1989). Human centrifuge non-invasive measurements of arterial pressure at eye level during Gz acceleration. *Aviation Space & Environmental Medicine*, 60, pp. 1005–10.

Woodring, S.F., Rossiter, C.D. and Yates, B.J. (1997). Pressor response elicited by nose-up vestibular stimulation in cats. *Experimental Brain Research*, 113, pp. 165–8.

Wu, B., Xue, Y., Wu, P., Gu, Z., Wang, Y. and Jing, X. (2012). Physiological responses of astronaut candidates to simulated +G$_x$ orbital emergency re-entry. *Aviation Space & Environmental Medicine*, 83, pp. 758–63.

Yacavone, D.W. and Bason, R. (1992). Cervical injuries during high G maneuvers: a review of Naval Safety Center data, 1980–1990. *Aviation Space & Environmental Medicine*, 63, pp. 602–5.

Yamazaki, F., Kawahara, C., Soga, I., Yamada, S. and Hamasaki, K. (2003). Baroreflex control of heart rate during heating in subjects with low orthostatic tolerance. *Aviation Space & Environmental Medicine*, 74, pp. 1237–42.

Yang, P., Frier, B.C., Goodman, L. and Duffin, J. (2007). Respiratory muscle training and the performance of a simulated anti-G straining maneuver. *Aviation Space & Environmental Medicine*, 78, pp. 1035–41.

Yates, B.J. (1992). Vestibular influences on the sympathetic nervous system. *Brain Research Reviews*, 17, pp. 51–9.

Yates, B.J. (1996). Vestibular influences on cardiovascular control. In: Yates, B.J. and Miller, A.D. (eds), *Vestibular Autonomic Regulation*. Boca Raton: CRC Press.

Yates, B.J. and Miller, A.D. (1994). Properties of sympathetic reflexes elicited by natural vestibular stimulation: implications for cardiovascular control. *Journal of Neurophysiology*, 71, pp. 2087–92.

Yates, B.J. and Miller, A.D. (1998). Physiological evidence that the vestibular system participates in autonomic and respiratory control. *Journal of Vestibular Research*, 8, pp. 17–25.

Yilmaz, U., Cetinguc, M. and Akin, A. (1999). Visual symptoms and G-LOC in the operational environment and during centrifuge training of Turkish jet pilots. *Aviation Space & Environmental Medicine*, 70, pp. 709–12.

Zawadzka-Bartczak, E.K. and Kopka, L.H. (2004). Centrifuge braking effects on cardiac arrhythmias occurring at high +Gz acceleration. *Aviation Space & Environmental Medicine*, 75, pp. 458–60.

Zawadzka-Bartczak, E.K. and Kopka, L.H. (2011). Cardiac arrhythmias during aerobatic flight and its simulation on a centrifuge. *Aviation Space & Environmental Medicine*, 82, pp. 599–603.

Zhang, L. (1999). Cognitive performance and physiological changes in females at high G while protected with COMBAT EDGE and ATAGS. *Aviation Space & Environmental Medicine*, 70, pp. 857–62.

Zhang, R., Claassen, J.A., Shibata, S., Kilic, S., Martin-Cook, K., Diaz-Arrastia, R. and Levine, B.D. (2009). Arterial-cardiac baroreflex function: insights from repeated squat-stand maneuvers. *American Journal of Physiology-Regulatory, Integrative and Comparative Physiology*, 297, pp. R116–23.

Zhang, S.X., Guo, H.Z., Jing, B.S. and Liu, S.F. (1992). The characteristics and significance of intrathoracic and abdominal pressures during Qigong (QG) maneuvering. *Aviation Space & Environmental Medicine*, 63, pp. 795–801.

Zhang, S.X., Guo, H.Z., Jing, B.S., Wang, X. and Zhang, L.M. (1991). Experimental verification of effectiveness and harmlessness of the Qigong maneuver. *Aviation Space & Environmental Medicine*, 62, pp. 46–52.

Zhang, S.X., Guo, H.Z., Zhu, J. and Jing, B.S. (1994). Qigong and L-1 straining maneuver oxygen system requirements with and without positive pressure breathing. *Aviation Space & Environmental Medicine*, 65, pp. 986–91.

Zhang, W.X., Zhan, C.L., Geng, X.C., Mu, D.W., Lu, X.I.A., Yan, G.D. and Chu, X. (2001). Decreased $+G_z$ tolerance following lower body positive pressure: simulated push–pull effect. *Aviation Space & Environmental Medicine*, 72, pp. 1045–7.

Zoller, R.P., Mark, A.L., Abboud, F.M., Schmid, P.G. and Heistad, D.D. (1972). The role of low pressure baroreceptors in reflex vasoconstrictor responses in man. *Journal of Clinical Investigation*, 51, pp. 2967–72.

Zuidema, G.D., Cohen, S.I., Silverman, A.J. and Riley, M.B. (1956). Human tolerance to prolonged acceleration. *Journal of Aviation Medicine*, 27, pp. 469–81.

Index

Abdomen, 78, 163, 164, 165, 166, 176
Abdominal
    belt, 163, 164, 186
    bladder, 78, 159, 165, 166, 167, 168,
        169, 170, 176, 177, 179, 186
    contents, 24, 77, 78, 80
    pressure, *see* Pressure, abdominal
    wall, 153
Acceleration
    angular, 8, 11, 12, 17, 19, 22
    applied, 8, 17, 19, 20, 40, 42, 57, 58,
        59, 63, 64, 65, 72, 141
    centrifugal, 12, 20, 22
    centripetal, 9, 12, 13, 20, 22
    linear, 22, 24, 79
    radial, 22
Accidents, 32, 33, 65, 68
    fatal, 32, 68
ACM, 21, 26, 27, 28, 29, 70, 83, 84, 85,
        86, 90, 93, 94, 107, 114, 115, 123,
        124, 126, 127, 147, 161, 169, 183
ACTH, 105
Adams
    John Couch, 6, 7
ADH, 25, 105, 140, 147
Adventitia, 48
Aerobatic
    aircraft, 17, 23, 30, 31, 32, 33, 35, 57,
        68, 70, 83, 96, 102, 117, 126, 127,
        133, 153, 161, 185
    flight, 21, 23, 25, 26, 30, 32, 34, 90,
        101, 102, 106, 127, 147
    pilot, 33, 70, 102, 106, 124
    box, 32
Aerobatics, 26, 30, 31, 32, 94
Aerobic, 120, 121, 122, 124, 140, 141
Aerofoil, 30
Aeromedical disposition, 89
Age, 89, 94, 95, 106, 118, 122, 126

AGSM, 73, 79, 107, 114, 120, 122, 123,
        129, 143, 153, 154, 155, 156, 157,
        158, 159, 160, 161, 167, 169, 170,
        171, 173, 174, 176, 177, 178, 180,
        183, 186
AGV, 165, 166, 168, 169, 172
Air
    combat manoeuvring, 28, 86, 98, 113,
        114, 115, 180
    leak, 184
Air spaces, 73, 74, 76, 78, 186
    apical, 75
    basilar, 78
Aircraft
    aerobatic, *see* Aerobatic, aircraft
    fast jet, 25, 26, 29, 31, 95, 113, 126,
        129, 163, 169, 185
    handling, 26
    transport, 95, 99
Air-to-air, 26, 84
Air-to-ground, 26
Airway
    collapse, 76, 78
    resistance, 75
Akinesia, 56
Alcohol, 101, 119
Aldosterone, 140, 146, 147
A-LOC, 61, 62, 63, 100, 159
Altimeter, 66
Altitudes, 30, 66
Aluminium, 4
Alveoli, 75, 76, 78
Amnesia, 62, 64, 67
Anaerobic, 120, 121, 122, 123, 124
Angiotensin, 146, 147
Angle of attack, *see* AOA
Anthropometric, 118
Anti-diuretic hormone, *see* ADH
Anti-G straining manoeuvre, *see* AGSM

Anti-G valve, *see* AGV
Anxiety, 67
AOA, 29, 87, 88
Aorta, 48
Aortic
    morphology, 99
    valve, 99
Apical bulla, 174
Apices, 74, 75, 76, 78
Apollo, 14, 33
Aresti, 31, 32
Aristotle, 6, 7
Arm, 24, 88
    pain, 184, 185, 186, 187
Arousal, 100
Arrested landing, 24
Arrhythmias, 25, 57, 97, 98, 99, 120, 121
Arterial pressure, *see* Pressure, arterial
Arteries, 47, 48, 65, 185, 201
Arterioles, 154
Artery
    carotid, 47, 48, 64, 106
    femoral, 40, 41, 48
    pulmonary, 48, 74
Astronauts, 14, 21, 33, 34, 119, 133, 134,
        137, 139, 140, 163, 168
Asystole, 72
ATAGS, 170, 173
Atelectasis, 77, 78
    acceleration, 78, 79, 80, 159, 177, 186
    basal, 76
Atmosphere, 14
Atria, 48
Atrioventricular, 141
Atrio-ventricular node, 49, 50, 52
Atrium, 45
ATSB, 32
Attention, 100, 169
Auditory
    cues, 103
    function, 103
    warnings, 103
Australia, 4, 32, 164
Autonomic
    failure, 56
    imbalance, 98
    insufficiency, 56
Autoregulation, 43, 59, 185

Avulsion, 108
Axial alignment, 85, 90

Baboon, 99
Balance, 49, 54, 62, 98, 101, 178
Baroreceptor, 45, 49, 50, 51, 52, 53, 117,
        138, 139, 140, 147
    sensitivity, 139
Baroreceptors, 48, 50, 54, 117, 131, 133,
        137, 138, 139, 140, 147
Baroreflex, 53, 55, 56, 116, 117, 120, 127,
        131, 132, 135, 139, 140, 142, 143,
        144, 145, 147, 148, 159, 166, 168
    activity, 53, 127, 131, 139
    adaptation, 139, 147
    sensitivity, 52, 143, 145, 148
Baroreflexes, 47, 49, 50, 51, 52, 53, 55, 71,
        72, 116, 117, 127, 131, 132, 135,
        138, 139, 140, 141, 147, 148, 149,
        159, 176
BFM, 21, 125
Birds, 141
Black holes, 4
Black-out, 60, 61, 70, 72, 104, 114, 115,
        117, 124, 125
Bladder, 78, 159, 165, 166, 167, 168, 169,
        170, 172, 176, 177, 178, 179, 184,
        186
Bladders, 164, 165, 166, 167, 171, 179
Blepharospasm, 184
Blood
    cell, 147
    density, 41
    flow, 39, 40, 43, 46, 58, 59, 60, 62,
        64, 65, 66, 67, 69, 70, 71, 74, 105,
        136, 144, 154, 167, 171, 174, 176,
        185, 186
    plasma, 140
    pooling, 168, 176
    pressure, *see* BP
    vena caval, 46
    vessels, 40, 43, 47, 48, 71, 106, 108,
        166, 174
    volume, 42, 43, 45, 46, 54, 80, 119,
        133, 134, 135, 139, 140, 145, 146,
        147, 148, 149, 166, 176, 177
Bone
    mineral density, 95, 99

Bones, 83, 86
BP, 39, 41, 47, 49, 50, 51, 52, 53, 54, 58,
    60, 64, 71, 72, 74, 102, 103, 116,
    117, 118, 119, 120, 121, 122, 124,
    125, 127, 132, 133, 134, 135, 138,
    139, 140, 144, 145, 146, 153, 155,
    156, 158, 163, 168, 171, 182
Brain, 40, 44, 57, 58, 59, 62, 64, 66, 67,
    118, 119, 124, 125, 154, 174, 176,
    181, 182
Brainstem, 47
Breathing, 24, 46, 73, 75, 77, 78, 79, 80,
    81, 155, 156, 158, 168, 173, 174,
    178, 180, 181, 183, 184, 186
    positive pressure, 158, 167, 170, 173,
        175, 177, 179, 181, 182, 183, 184,
        185, 186, 187
    work of, 75, 77, 78, 81, 156, 174, 178,
        180
Brightness, 104

Caffeine, 119, 120
Caloric stimulation, 54
Canada, 64
Canadian Forces, 123
Canard foreplanes, 29
Canines, 142
Canopy, 92
Capacitance, 43, 44, 45, 46, 134, 166
    vessels, 43, 44, 134, 166
Capillaries, 108, 109
Capillary, 45, 109
Capstan suits, 164
Cardiac
    chambers, 47
    contractility, 43, 49, 50, 52, 117, 127,
        140
    damage, 99
    morphology, 98
    output, *see* CO
    valve, 99
Cardiopulmonary, 47, 48, 54, 133, 138,
    139, 140, 147, 148, 149
Cardiovascular
    adaptation, 126, 131, 132, 133, 134,
        135, 137, 138, 140, 141, 142, 143,
        144, 148, 149, 159, 160
    compromise, 60, 70, 118

control, 53, 54, 55, 139, 148
deconditioning, 134
efficiency, 120, 121
function, 131, 132, 144, 147
index of deconditioning, 134
performance, 141, 142, 159, 167
reflex, 138
responses, 127, 134, 136, 138, 142,
    143, 144, 145, 146
system, 57, 60, 63, 64, 65, 70, 71, 72,
    73, 117, 120, 127, 131, 133, 135,
    136, 139, 141, 142, 143, 144, 148,
    149, 166, 167, 168, 176
Carotid sinus, 48, 51
Carrier, 21, 22, 24, 34
Catecholamine, 25, 97, 124, 185
Cats, 54
Cavendish
    experiment, 6
    Henry, 6
CCPG, 79, 173, 178, 179, 180, 181, 182,
    183, 186, 187
Central
    light loss, 114
    nervous system, 68, 69, 119
Centre of gravity, 41, 85, 86, 136
Centrifuge, 98, 100, 101, 103, 104, 105,
    107, 109, 114, 115, 120, 121, 122,
    125, 128, 129, 137, 142, 143, 145,
    148, 154, 156, 158, 159, 160, 164,
    170, 171, 172, 177, 180, 183, 185,
    187
Cerebral
    circulation, 44, 69, 71
    cortex, 67, 69, 154
    function, 62
    ischaemia, 100
    shut-down, 67
Cerebrospinal fluid, 58, 71
Cerebrovascular, 144
Cervical
    occlusion cuff, 69
    vertebrae, 88
Check 6, 85, 86, 92, 102
Chest, 20, 24, 79, 153, 154, 176, 178, 179,
    181, 186
    counterpressure, 178, 186
    counterpressure garment, *see* CCPG

wall, 24, 77, 79, 81, 154, 155, 156, 174, 176, 177, 178, 179
Chickens, 141
Circadian desynchronosis, 120
Circle, 8, 10, 11, 15, 16, 19, 22, 23
Circulatory
  compromise, 44, 45
  system, 40, 42, 44, 48, 49, 56, 134, 166, 168
Circumference, 10, 11, 16
CO, 39, 43, 46, 117, 133, 136, 144, 155, 174, 176, 181
Cognition, 62
Cognitive
  abnormalities, 63
  functions, 61
  impairment, 63
  impairments, 100
Collagen, 48
Collisions
  mid-air, 21
Colour, 104, 105
Combat Edge, 170, 173, 187
Communications, 160, 184
Compensatory
  mechanisms, 44, 45, 46, 135, 136
Competition
  aerobatic, 23, 30, 31, 32, 35, 70, 102, 117, 123, 153, 163, 171, 185
Compliance, 40, 42, 45, 75, 78, 80, 140, 154, 155
Confusion, 3, 19, 20, 61, 66, 67, 71, 106, 113
Conjunctival suffusion, 184
Contractility, 43, 49, 50, 52, 117, 127, 140
Contrast sensitivity, 104
Control
  authority, 29, 87
  column, 25, 70, 127, 128
  laws, 87
  theory, 47
Copernicus, Nicholas, 6, 15
Cortisol, 25, 105
Cosmonauts, 168
Cutaneous circulation, 53

Danish Air Force, 88

Deceleration, 29, 34
Degenerative changes, 89, 94, 95
Dehydration, 30, 113, 119, 134, 187
Density, 6, 14, 40, 41, 95, 125
Denver, 13
Diabetes mellitus, 56
Diaphragm, 41, 46, 75, 76, 77, 78, 107, 124, 154, 158, 166
Diaphragmatic rupture, 107
Diastolic, 39, 57, 74, 99, 133, 134, 142
  pressure, *see* DP
Disc degeneration, 95
Disorientation, 66
Display and sighting systems, 94
Dissection, 106, 107
Distraction, 184
Dizziness, 103
Dogs, 47, 53, 54, 142
Doppler, 144, 167
Dorsal motor nucleus, 48
DP, 39, 43, 44, 134, 136, 145
Dream, 67, 69
Dynamic Flight Simulation, 128
Dysrhythmias, 141

Ear, 101, 108, 158, 184
  pain, 184
Earth, 5, 6, 8, 9, 12, 13, 14, 15, 17, 20, 21, 22, 30, 33, 34, 119, 133, 134, 135, 140, 163, 168
ECG, 99
ECGS, 169, 170, 171, 172
Echocardiographic, 99
Einstein, Albert, 4
Ejection, 94
  fraction, 43, 140
  seat, 92, 95, 126
  spinal injuries, 94, 126
Elastic, 42, 44, 48, 75, 76, 166, 168, 176, 177
  recoil, 75, 177
Elastin, 48
Elbow, 108
Electromyography, 160
Ellipse, 15, 16
Emphysema, 79
Encoding, 101

Endocrine, 25, 105
Endurance, 92, 115, 120, 121, 122, 140, 147, 187
Epinephrine, 105
Error, 103, 115
    signal, 47
Errors, 62, 104
Erythropoiesis, 133
ERV, 74
Eurofighter, 27, 170, 173, 187
Eustachian tube, 184
Executive
    functions, 100
Exercise, 31, 73, 74, 75, 91, 92, 107, 118, 121, 122, 123, 140, 141, 145, 147, 155
Exhalation, 73, 79, 158, 179
Expiration, 46, 75, 155, 178
Expiratory, 73, 74, 77, 79, 153, 154, 155, 156, 157, 158, 159, 174, 177, 178, 180
Expiratory reserve volume, *see* ERV
Extended coverage G-suit, *see* ECGS
Extension, 85
Extra 300, 31, 106
Extravascular, 45, 46, 61
Eye, 25, 60, 71, 104, 184
Eyelid, 72

F/A-18, 22, 26, 28, 29, 68, 84, 85, 92, 93, 170
F-111C, 88
F-15, 27, 29, 65, 83, 87, 167, 170
F-16, 23, 27, 29, 30, 65, 68, 84, 87, 90, 92, 94, 95, 98, 102, 107, 108, 125, 128, 167, 170, 187
Face, 24, 85, 180, 184
Facial puffiness, 25, 71, 133
FAI, 31
Fast jet, 23, 25, 26, 27, 29, 30, 31, 70, 83, 84, 85, 87, 88, 89, 90, 92, 94, 95, 96, 102, 103, 105, 108, 113, 119, 124, 126, 129, 153, 157, 163, 166, 169, 172, 173, 182, 185, 186
    aircrew, 83, 84, 90, 92, 94, 96, 157, 186
    cockpit, 103, 186

pilot, 27, 84, 85, 87, 95, 124, 169, 173, 182
pilots, 70, 85, 89, 92, 94, 95, 96, 163, 166
Fast jets, 87, 161
Fatigue, 30, 90, 96, 115, 120, 122, 124, 142, 160, 161, 177, 183, 185, 187
    penalty, 24, 159, 160, 161, 173, 182
FCAGT, 170, 173
Feet, 26, 45, 70
Fighter
    aircraft, 22, 23, 29, 30, 35, 57, 65, 70, 79, 87, 88, 102, 123, 125, 128, 132, 144, 149, 169, 170, 173, 187
    basic manoeuvres, *see* BFM
    pilot, 26, 27, 70, 84, 107, 132, 133, 144, 148, 149, 172, 187
    pilots, 60, 61, 63, 65, 83, 84, 89, 90, 91, 92, 94, 99, 121, 123, 131, 142, 144, 145, 148, 149, 159, 160, 166
    sixth generation, 29
Filtration, 44, 45, 46, 133
Finger, 25
Finland, 83, 89
Finnish Air Force, 170, 171
Flexion, 54, 85, 87, 107
Flight
    aerobatic, *see* Aerobatic, flight
    control systems, 29, 87
    envelope, 29, 87, 128, 132
    helmet, *see* Helmet
    model, 128
    safety, 67, 100, 101, 103, 104
    simulation, 128
    training, 26
Flight Operations
    military, 23, 26
Fluid
    redistribution, 135, 137
    shift, 133
    shifts, 57, 137, 146
Flying experience, 84, 95, 118, 126, 143
Foot, 22, 39, 40, 41, 104, 168, 170
Force
    centrifugal, 8, 9, 12, 13, 22, 70
    centripetal, 8, 9, 10, 12, 22
    inertial, 22, 24, 80, 117

isometric, 101
multiplier, 183
tangential, 8
Forearm
venous pressure, *see* FVP
venous resistance, *see* FVR
Fracture
compression, 88, 95
Fractures
vertebral, 85
Frank-Starling, 43
FRC, 74, 76, 78, 80
Friction, 7
Functional
buffer period, 67, 69, 115, 119
residual capacity, *see* FRC
FVP, 185
FVR, 185

G adaptation, 127, 131, 144, 147, 159
G duration, 113, 161, 173
G intensity, 113, 114, 161, 171
G tolerance, 30, 61, 69, 98, 99, 104, 105,
109, 113, 114, 115, 116, 117, 118,
119, 120, 123, 124, 125, 126, 127,
129, 131, 160, 170, 179, 185
Gain, 55, 140
Gait, 101, 102
Galileo, 6, 7
Gas
compression, 156
exchange, 155
Gender, 94, 118
Giraffe, 43, 44, 59, 166
GIVD, 101, 102, 103
G-LOC, 25, 27, 30, 32, 58, 62, 63, 64, 65,
66, 67, 68, 69, 70, 72, 95, 100, 101,
115, 116, 117, 118, 121, 124, 126,
127, 129, 131, 132, 141, 149, 155,
159, 161, 163, 167, 169, 180, 183
Glossopharyngeal nerve, 47, 48
Glottis, 153, 157, 160, 184
Gloves, 186
Gondola, 114
GOR, 113, 128, 187
Gravitational
attraction, 4, 6, 8, 13
constant, 6

field, 17, 20, 22, 43, 56, 133, 135, 141
force, 5, 6, 9, 12, 13, 14, 17, 20, 21,
22, 59
spectrum, 133
waves, 4, 5
Gravity, 3, 4, 5, 7, 9, 11, 12, 13, 14, 15, 17,
19, 20, 21, 22, 33, 40, 41, 44, 46,
75, 85, 86, 125, 133, 136, 137, 168
Grey-out, 60, 61, 70, 72, 104, 115, 117,
159
Gripen, *see* JAS-39
Grounding, 89
G-suit, 73, 76, 78, 79, 80, 99, 108, 109,
156, 159, 163, 164, 165, 166, 167,
168, 167, 168, 169, 170, 171, 172,
173, 176, 177, 179, 181, 182, 183,
186
G-time tolerance curve, 115, 116, 117, 132

Haematoma, 108
Haemorrhage, 42, 45, 108
subconjunctival, 71
Hawk 127, 68
Hawk T1, 90
HDNF, 54
Head, 22, 23, 25, 39, 40, 41, 44, 54, 58, 60,
66, 70, 71, 72, 83, 85, 86, 88, 90,
92, 93, 96, 102, 103, 126, 127, 136,
145, 146, 153, 155, 182, 184
down neck flexion, *see* HDNF
up tilt, *see* HUT
Headache, 71
Hearing, 62, 103
Heart, 39, 40, 41, 42, 43, 44, 45, 46, 47,
48, 49, 50, 51, 52, 55, 57, 58, 59,
60, 65, 74, 81, 97, 98, 100, 107,
118, 124, 125, 137, 144, 145, 146,
154, 155, 164, 166, 167, 168, 174,
176, 177, 181, 186
rate, *see* HR
volume, 43
Heat, 89, 187
stress, 42, 119, 134
Helicopter, 30
operations, 30
pilots, 94
Helmet, 25, 83, 85, 86, 93, 94, 108, 173,
184

Helmet-mounted displays, *see* HMD
Hepatic, 46
  venous outflow, 46
Hering, 47
Hernia
  inguinal, 107
HIP, 41, 42, 53, 134
HMD, 85
Hook, 157, 158, 160
Horizon, 102
Hormones, 105
HOTAS, 25
HP, 40, 41, 42, 43, 44, 45, 57, 60, 74, 117,
    125, 135, 154, 166, 176, 181
HR, 39, 40, 43, 47, 49, 52, 54, 55, 72, 97,
    117, 119, 121, 124, 127, 133, 134,
    136, 137, 140, 142, 143, 144, 145,
    146, 148, 159
Hue, 104
HUT, 54, 121, 135, 136, 137, 138, 143,
    144, 145, 146, 147, 148, 166
Hydration, 41
Hydrostatic
  barrier, 44
  column, 41, 45
  differential, 124, 125, 186
  force, 55, 56, 57, 58, 60, 65, 71, 77,
    133, 136, 144, 171
  forces, 44, 57, 58, 64, 105
  indifference Point, *see* HIP
  penalties, 148
  pressure, *see* HP
  theory, 64
Hyperaemia, 138
Hyperextension, 85
Hypertension, 139
Hypertensive, 134, 139
Hyperventilating, 155
Hypoglycaemia, 124
Hypotension, 54, 56, 139, 168
Hypotensive, 139
Hypovolaemia, 143
Hypovolaemic, 168
Hypoxia, 119

IC, 74

Impact
  forces, 21
  ground, 21, 30, 32, 66, 72
Incapacitation period
  absolute, 66, 67
  relative, 66, 68
  total, 66
Incontinence, 161
Individual variation, 69, 88, 93, 118, 144,
    167, 175
Inertia, 8, 52
Inertial vectors, 20, 21
Infections, 124
Inflation, 24, 73, 75, 156, 159, 164, 165,
    166, 167, 168, 171, 172, 181
Information processing, 29
Inhalation, 155
Injury
  patterns, 22
Inspiration, 24, 46, 73, 75, 78, 79, 80, 155,
    157, 160, 182
Inspiratory, 74, 75, 77, 79, 156, 158, 180
Inspiratory
  capacity, *see* IC
  reserve volume, *see* IRV
Interferometers, 4
Internal jugular vein, 174
International
  Acceleration Research Workshop, 61
  Space Station, 13, 21
Intervertebral
  disc, 88
Intravenous, 163
Inverse-Square Law, 13, 15
IRV, 74
Isometric, 101, 122, 153, 154

JAS-39, 23, 27, 125, 170
JHMCS, 85
Judgement, 67
Jugular
  bulb, 59
  siphon, 59
Jupiter, 14

Kentavr, 168

Kepler, Johannes, 6, 15, 16, 17
Kidney, 43, 106
Koch, 47

L-1, 155, 157, 158, 160
Laplace, Pierre Simon, 6
Lateral G, 73, 81, 88
Launch, 17, 22, 24, 33, 57, 73, 79, 108
    catapult, 21, 24
Laws
    of motion, 3, 5, 6, 7, 8, 15, 17, 19, 22
    of planetary motion, 6, 15
Lay-off, 132, 143, 148, 149
LBNP, 135, 137, 143
Le Verrier, Urbain Jean Joseph, 6
Leg, 133, 137, 154, 165, 176
Length–tension relationship, 43
Lift, 22, 80
    vector, 22
Ligaments, 83, 85, 88
Lipoprotein, 75
Locomotion, 46
Lomcovak, 31
Loop, 22, 31, 32, 39, 47, 70, 71, 73, 128,
    136, 176
Loss
    of consciousness, 45, 47, 57, 61, 62,
        63, 69, 70, 71, 72, 98, 118
    of vision, 60, 61, 72
Lumbar supports, 96, 161
Luminance, 104, 105
Lung, 73, 74, 75, 76, 78, 80, 81, 107, 176,
    177, 178, 186
    function, 73
    volume, 74, 76, 77, 78, 80, 156, 157,
        186
Lungs, 24, 73, 74, 75, 76, 77, 80, 81, 156,
    174, 176, 177, 178, 180, 184

M-1, 157, 158, 160
Mach, 9, 26, 29
Macrogravity, 146
Magnetic resonance imaging, *see* MRI
Manoeuvrability, 29, 84, 87
MAP, 39, 40, 43, 44, 58, 119, 120, 127,
    134, 136, 144, 145, 146, 148
Mass, 5, 6, 7, 8, 12, 13, 14, 16, 17, 20, 22,
    76, 86, 122, 133, 140, 179

Matter, 8, 13, 14
Mayo Clinic, 65, 157
Mean arterial pressure, *see* MAP
Mechanoreceptors, 47, 48
Mediastinum, 24, 79, 81
Medical guidelines, 34, 79
Medulla oblongata, 47, 48, 50, 51
Medullary, 49, 139
Memory, 62, 100
Mercury, 33
Metabolic energy reserve, 115, 117, 131
MFD, 104, 105
Microcirculatory, 45
Microgravity, 14, 17, 21, 33, 131, 133,
    134, 135, 137, 139, 140, 141, 145,
    146, 147
Microvascular, 45
Mirage 2000, 99
Mission performance, 104
Mobility, 24, 171
Monkeys, 139
Mood, 100
Moon, 5, 14
Motion sickness, 121
Motivation, 67
MRI, 87, 95
MSDRS, 29
Multi-axial, 31, 87, 102
Multi-function displays, *see* MFD
Multiple system atrophy, 56
Muscle
    conditioning, 90, 91, 92, 93, 96
    pump, 45, 46
    skeletal, 43, 53, 153, 154, 155
    tensing, 154, 158, 159, 161
Muscles, 25, 46, 75, 79, 83, 85, 86, 87, 88,
    90, 91, 92, 93, 96, 123, 137, 154,
    158, 160, 171, 177, 178
    cervical, 85, 87, 88, 91
    inspiratory, 79
    intercostal, 75
Musculoskeletal
    system, 72, 83, 96
Myocardial ischaemia, 99
Myoclonic convulsions, 66, 67, 69

Nap-of-the-earth, 30
NASA, 168

Naso-lacrimal ducts, 184
NATO, 99
Natriuretic, 147
Nausea, 102, 107
Naval Air Development Centre, 61
Neck
    chamber, 51, 52
    injuries, 25, 83, 84, 85, 86, 87, 88, 89,
        90, 91, 92, 93, 94, 96
    muscles, 83, 85, 86, 90, 92, 93, 123
    pain, 83, 84, 87, 89, 91, 92
Negative feedback, 47
Neptune, 7
Neurologic impairment, 106
Newton, Isaac, 5, 17
Niacin, 125
Night vision goggles, *see* NVG
Niobium, 4
Nitrogen, 78, 186
Nomex, 165, 178
Norepinephrine, 105
NTS, 48
Nucleus Tractus Solitarius, *see* NTS
NVG, 85

Oedema, 45, 46
Omentum, 108
Operations
    fast jet, 25, 26, 30, 119
Orbit, 5, 7, 8, 9, 13, 15, 16, 17, 21, 33, 119,
        133, 134
    low-Earth, 9, 17
Orthostasis, 45, 134
Orthostatic
    challenge, 35, 42, 44, 45, 120, 134,
        135, 136, 138, 141, 144, 145, 147,
        148, 166
    intolerance, 117, 119, 133, 134, 135,
        137, 139, 140, 141, 148, 163, 168
    tolerance, 121, 134, 168
Osteopenia, 95
Osteoporosis, 95
Othematoma, 108
Otoconia, 103
Otolith, 55, 103, 104
Overdistension, 178, 185

Oxygen, 60, 61, 62, 64, 66, 67, 74, 77, 78,
        80, 83, 85, 86, 104, 119, 120, 143,
        154, 155, 158, 159, 173, 176, 180,
        182, 186
    mask, 83, 85, 86, 173, 182
Oxygenation, 81, 82, 154, 160
Oxyhaemoglobin, 77, 80

Pain
    abdominal, 24, 31, 106
    chest, 80, 186
    epigastric, 107
    inguinal, 107
    low back, 94
    neck, *see* Neck, pain
Parachute, 33
Paralysis, 106
Parasympathetic, 48, 49, 50, 55, 98, 104,
        121, 140
Parenchymal
    disruption, 174
PBG, 73, 79, 170, 171, 173, 174, 175, 176,
        177, 178, 180, 181, 182, 183, 185,
        186, 187
Peptide, 147
Perception, 63, 104, 105
    colour, 104, 105
Perfusion, 25, 53, 56, 59, 68, 74, 75, 76,
        77, 78, 80, 81, 154, 176
    cerebral, 25, 43, 44, 45, 47, 59, 63, 68,
        71, 72, 82, 117, 132, 141, 154, 155,
        161, 174, 176
    deficit, 68
Periorbital, 133
Peripheral
    light loss, 114
    pooling, 43, 44, 45, 55, 154, 166
    sequestration, 46
Petechiae, 108, 109
PFD, 104
Physical
    conditioning, 113, 120, 124, 140
    fitness, 84, 121, 124
Physiotherapy, 89
Pitch, 29, 31, 55, 184
Planetary motion, 5, 6, 7, 15

Planets, 6, 15, 16
Plasma, 57, 140, 146, 147
   volume, 57, 140, 147
Pleural cavity, 76
Pneumatic, 163, 164, 165, 168, 171
Pneumomediastinum, 107
Pneumothorax, 76, 174
Pons, 48
Positioning strategies, 90, 92, 93, 96
Posture, 40, 41, 42, 43, 44, 45, 46, 53, 55,
     56, 57, 58, 73, 74, 76, 87, 117, 135,
     136, 137, 176
PPE, 34, 127, 128
Pressure
   abdominal, 24
   aortic, 44
   arterial, 39, 40, 45, 47, 49, 50, 51, 52,
     53, 54, 55, 58, 60, 61, 71, 137, 138,
     139, 145, 146, 148, 154, 155, 156,
     168
   arterial perfusing, 53
   arteriovenous, 58, 71
   central venous, 46, 53
   differential, 44, 58, 59, 60, 71, 75, 125
   distending, 47, 52
   dynamic, 39, 43
   extravascular, 46
   filling, 42, 43, 46
   gradient, 40, 58, 76, 78, 137, 154, 158,
     164, 167, 174, 176, 181
   internal ocular, 60
   intra-abdominal, 46, 107, 137, 138
   intrapleural, 75
   intrathoracic, 46, 79, 154, 155, 156,
     157, 159, 160, 167, 174, 176, 177
   intravascular, 42, 45
   oscillations, 181
   perfusion, 53, 56
   pleural, 76, 78
   pulmonary artery, 74
   schedule, 166, 173, 175, 181
   syncope, 167, 176, 181
   transmission, 174, 176, 177, 178, 179
   transmural, 44, 45, 46, 51, 71, 109, 185
   venous, 71
Primary flight displays, *see* PFD

Prolactin, 105
Propanolol, 124
Proprioceptive, 47
Proteins, 147
Proteinuria, 25, 105, 106
Psychiatric illness, 100
Psychomotor, 101
Ptolemy, 6
Pulitzer Air Race, 63
Pulmonary
   sequestration, 107
   valve, 99
Push–pull effect, *see* PPE

Q10, 125
Q-G, 158
Qigong, *see* Q-G
Quantum Field Theory, 5

RAAF, 26, 60, 61, 63, 68, 84, 88, 89, 90,
     92, 93, 123
Rabbits, 139, 142
Radius, 10, 11, 12, 15, 19, 23, 29, 71
RAF, 68, 83, 90, 170, 187
Rafale, 172
Rapid onset, 62, 68, 69, 95, 120, 137, 169
Ratio
   power-to-weight, 30
   ventilation-perfusion, 75, 77, 80, 81
   V/Q, *see* V/Q
Rats, 139, 142, 154
Red cell, 133, 140
Red-out, 72
Re-entry, 17, 33, 34, 73, 79, 108, 119, 168
Reflex arcs, 47, 148
Regulator, 173, 180, 181
Relativity Theory
   General, 4, 15
   Special, 14, 15
REM, 67
Renal, 105, 106, 133, 136, 139, 147
Renin, 146, 147
Republic of Korea Air Force, 98
Republic of Singapore Air Force, 95, 107
Resetting, 135, 139
Residual volume, *see* RV

Resistance
  peripheral, 40, 42, 44, 55, 136, 142,
    145, 168
  training, 122, 123
  vascular, 51, 52, 53, 55, 136, 154, 166,
    168, 185
Respiration, 52, 158
Respiratory
  demand, 75
  demands, 156
  effects, 24, 73, 75, 76, 77, 78, 79, 81,
    107
  function, 24, 76
  illnesses, 79
  movements, 46
  muscle, 75, 158, 160
  pump, 45
  rate, 75, 76, 77
  system, 24, 25, 33, 72, 73, 81, 107
  trauma, 107
  volume, 75
  work, 78
  workload, 160
Reticular formation, 67, 69
Retina, 60, 61
Retinal
  ischaemia, 60
Rib cage, 75, 171
Rocket, 13, 24, 33
Roll, 30, 31, 32, 55, 70, 88, 127
ROR, 69, 113, 128, 129, 158
Royal Australian Air Force, *see* RAAF
Royal Air Force, *see* RAF
Royal Norwegian Air Force, 84
Rudder, 31, 154
RV, 73, 74

SA, 62, 63, 85, 100, 103
SACM, 114, 115, 120, 122, 123, 126, 143,
    160, 171, 180, 183
Saline, 119, 139
  loading, 119
Satellite, 8, 13
Saturation, 77, 80, 104
Scalar, 3
Scissors
  rolling, 27
Seat, 33, 64, 72, 87, 88, 126

  back angle, 87, 125, 126, 174
  ejection, *see* Ejection, seat
Sensitivity, 52, 73, 104, 139, 143, 145,
    148, 149
Set point, 139
Shortness of breath, 78, 186
Shoulders, 93
Shunt, 77, 80, 81
Shy–Drager syndrome, 56, 168
Sighting and display systems, 85, 86, 96,
    184
Sino-atrial
  block, 98, 141
  node, 49, 50
Sinus, 48, 51, 98, 133
Situational awareness, *see* SA
Skin, 43, 53, 55, 108, 166
Sleep, 67
Sleeves, 186
Socks, 170
Sodium, 147
Soldiers, 46
Sound
  localisation, 103
Soyuz, 13, 33
Space Shuttle, 9, 13, 14, 21, 33, 34, 119,
    134
Spacecraft, 8, 9, 13, 22, 35
Spaceflight, 17, 21, 23, 24, 26, 33, 34, 57,
    73, 79, 81, 99, 100, 108, 128, 133,
    134, 137, 139, 141, 163, 168
  commercial, 26, 33, 34, 79, 128
  suborbital, 34
Space–time, 4
  continuum, 4, 15
Spatial
  disorientation, 62, 101
  orientation, 54
Spectroscopy, 154
Speed, 3, 5, 7, 8, 9, 12, 13, 14, 22, 26, 29,
    30, 31, 87
  of light, 14
  of sound, 9
  supersonic, 26
Spin, 31
Spinal
  column, 98, 99
  injuries, 94, 96, 106

injury, 95
Spine, 83, 85, 86, 87, 88, 89, 90, 92, 94,
        95, 96, 108, 123, 126
    cervical, 85, 86, 87, 88, 89, 90, 92, 94,
        96, 123
    lumbar, 94, 95, 108
    thoracic, 95
    thoracolumbar, 94, 96
Spitfire, 164
Splanchnic, 42, 43, 53, 136, 138, 166
Squatting, 138, 144
SST, 135, 138, 144
Stability criteria, 29, 87
Stall, 29, 31, 32
Standard operating procedure, 77, 168
Standing, 12, 42, 44, 46, 47, 134, 135, 137,
        138, 144
Starling-Landis principle, 46
Stimulus, 52, 67, 131, 136, 142, 147, 166
Stoll, 115, 116, 131
Stomach, 124
Strain, 93, 107, 122, 153, 154, 155, 156,
        157, 158, 159, 174, 175, 178
Straining, 114, 122, 155, 157, 174, 178
    manoeuvre, *see* AGSM
Stress, 25, 42, 46, 54, 57, 58, 64, 69, 98,
        105, 117, 119, 127, 134, 141, 142,
        143, 148, 171, 187
Stressor, 142
Stroke, 106
    volume, *see* SV
Su-31, 31, 106
Sun, 6, 15
Super-agile, 29, 30, 79, 87, 88, 172
Supraventricular premature beats, 98
Surface tension, 75
Surfactant, 75
Surgery, 89
Survival, 133, 141, 161, 187
SV, 39, 40, 43, 46, 99, 117, 133, 136, 140,
        144, 145, 167, 176
Swedish Air Force, 170
Swine, 99
Sympathetic, 48, 49, 50, 51, 52, 53, 54, 55,
        97, 98, 117, 185
    activity, 54, 98
    drive, 97, 98, 117, 185
Syncopal episode, 121

Syncope, 44, 46, 56, 61, 67, 121, 134, 137,
        167, 176, 181
Systolic, 57, 74, 134, 140
    pressure, 39, 43, 134, 136, 145
    pressures, 39, 44
    volumes, 140

T-33, 107
TACM, 115
Teeth, 154
Tendon, 108
Terrain, 32, 128
Terrestrial, 14, 20, 133, 147
Test pilot, 108
Testosterone, 105
Thermal burden, 169, 187
Thoracic
    cage, 154, 177, 178
    cavity, 24, 80, 174
    volume, 156
Thoracolumbar, 94, 96
Thorax, 46, 78, 80, 107, 108, 164, 167,
        168, 177
Throttle, 25
Thrust vectoring, 29
Tidal volume, *see* TV
Tilt, 54, 133, 136, 137, 144, 145, 146
    testing, 133
Tissue resistance, 75
TLC, 73, 76, 78
Tolerance
    human, 19, 24, 30, 58, 64
    time, 119, 122, 123, 160, 183
Torsion balance, 6
Total
    lung capacity, *see* TLC
    peripheral resistance, *see* TPR
Tourniquet, 138
TPR, 40, 43, 53, 144, 145, 166
Tracking, 101, 143
Training effect, 91, 146, 148
Trampoline, 90
Translocation, 44, 133
Triceps, 108
Tricuspid valve, 99
Tubes, 42
Turkish Air Force, 132
TV, 73, 74, 75, 76, 77, 80, 180

Unconsciousness, 59, 63, 65, 66, 67, 69, 70, 155
United Kingdom, 64, 166
United States, 33, 64, 164, 166, 170, 172
    Air Force, *see* USAF
Universal law of gravitation, 5, 6, 12, 13, 15, 17
Unusual attitudes, 26
Uranus, 7
Urine, 105, 106
US Navy, *see* USN
USAF, 27, 68, 84, 127, 129, 157, 159, 164, 170, 172, 173
USN, 61, 123, 163

V/Q, 75, 77, 80
Vagal
    centre, 48, 49
    excitation, 50
    impulses, 50
    tone, 121, 122, 140, 141
Vagus
    nerve, 48, 50, 51
Valsalva, 154, 155, 156, 159, 161
Valve, 99, 172
Valves, 44, 45, 46, 172, 176
Vascular
    bed, 42, 45
    container, 42, 146
    pressure, 40, 185
    system, 41, 42, 154, 174, 176
    tone, 40
Vasoactive, 145, 148
Vasoconstriction, 40, 49, 53, 117, 145, 185
Vasoconstrictor, 48
Vasodilatation, 50, 127, 138, 185
Vasodilate, 47
Vasodilation, 125
Vasomotor, 50
    centre, 47, 48, 49, 50, 51
Vasopressin, 147
VC, 73, 74, 76, 78, 80
Vector, 3, 19, 20, 22, 41, 70, 80, 81, 88
Veins, 42, 44, 45, 46, 59, 133, 154, 176, 185
Velocity, 3, 7, 8, 10, 11, 12, 16, 19, 23, 88, 144, 167
    angular, 8, 11, 12

tangential, 10, 11
vector, 88
Venoatrial junctions, 48
Venoconstriction, 53
Venous
    capacitance, 46
    compliance, 140
    distension, 185
    return, *see* VR
    system, 42, 43, 44, 58
Ventilation, 74, 77, 81
Ventilation–perfusion, 75, 77, 80, 81
Ventricular
    contractions, 98
    diameter, 99
    fibrillation, 98
    filling, 43
    filling pressure, 43, 46
    sump, 46
    tachycardia, 98
Vertebral
    bodies, 85
    body, 88, 95
Vertigo, 64, 101, 102, 103
Vestibular
    afferents, 54
    dysfunction, 101, 102
    impairment, 101, 103
    inputs, 54, 149
    nerves, 54
    nuclei, 54
    problems, 64
    signals, 55
    stimulation, 54, 55
    system, 54, 55, 101, 103, 104, 148
Vestibulo-ocular, 55
Vestibulosympathetic
    reflex, *see* VSR
    responses, 55
Vibration, 4, 95
Virgin Galactic, 33, 34
Viscoelastic, 46
Viscosity, 75
Visual
    contact, 83
    field, 60, 72
    impairment, 57, 104, 184
    input, 61

phenomena, 60
pursuit, 104
scanning, 126
symptoms, 61, 70, 72, 113, 115, 116,
126, 132
system, 55, 60
threshold, 117
warning, 61, 70, 115, 126
Vital capacity, *see* VC
Vocal cords, 160
Voice, 103
Volume
intravascular, 42, 43, 44
Vomiting, 107
VR, 42, 43, 44, 45, 46, 55, 99, 117, 137,
154, 155, 158, 167, 168, 170, 171,
172, 176, 181

VSR, 55, 148

Water immersion, 171
Weber
bar, 4
Joseph, 4
Weight, 5, 12, 13, 14, 22, 24, 30, 33, 75,
76, 78, 79, 81, 83, 85, 97, 99, 118,
119, 120, 122, 123, 124, 126, 148,
156, 164, 174, 179, 185
Weight-bearing, 83
Weightless, 9, 137
Weightlessness, 133
White Knight Two, 34
Workload, 93, 124, 143, 160, 181, 182,
183, 187
Wright brothers, 163